NEW CONCEPTS IN ASTHMA

Pierre Fabre Monograph Series

Series Editors:

D. BIGG, M. BRILEY, F. COLPAERT, R. KISS, P. LENOBLE,
J. TISNE-VERSAILLES
Centre de Recherche Pierre Fabre
Avenue Jean Moulin 17
81106 Castres cédex
France

Created in 1961, the Pierre Fabre Group is one of Europe's youngest research-based ethical pharmaceutical and beauty-care groups. From its base in Castres in south-west France, the group has expanded to become one of the major privately owned French companies in its field.

The Pierre Fabre Research Centre has adopted a strategy of encouraging communication between its own research centre in Castres and academic research scientists throughout the world. The creation of the Pierre Fabre Monograph Series is a further development of this strategy. Certain monographs in this series will be based on international symposia organized or sponsored by the Pierre Fabre Research Centre. Others will group together chapters from acknowledged international experts and dynamic young scientists destined to become tomorrow's experts. In all cases, the subjects of these monographs will be those presenting a major challenge to therapeutic medicine.

PIERRE FABRE MONOGRAPH SERIES

NEW CONCEPTS IN ASTHMA

Edited by

J. P. TARAYRE
Centre de Recherche Pierre Fabre
17 avenue Jean Moulin
81100 Castres
France

B. VARGAFTIG
Institut Pasteur
25 rue du Dr Roux
75015 Paris
France

and

E. CARILLA
Centre de Recherche Pierre Fabre
17 avenue Jean Moulin
81100 Castres
France

150th YEAR
M
MACMILLAN

First published 1993 by
THE MACMILLAN PRESS LTD
Houndmills, Basingstoke, Hampshire RG21 2XS
and London
Companies and representatives
throughout the world

ISBN 0–333–56430–8

A catalogue record for this book is available
from the British Library

Printed and bound in Great Britain

Contents

v

Contents (Posters)

Preface

During recent years the role of inflammation in physiopathology of asthma has been well demonstrated, but its underlying mechanisms and relationships with bronchopulmonary hyperresponsiveness are still largely unknown. The cellular mechanisms of bronchopulmonary inflammation in asthma were the topic of the International Symposium organized in September 1991, at Castres, in southwest France, by the Centre de Recherche Pierre Fabre.

The participation of eosinophils, but also of T lymphocytes, macrophages, endothelial cells and mast cells was evoked. The increasingly recognized role of some mediators in cell interactions was discussed. In particular, interleukine-5 of course, but also interleukines-1, -3 and -6, TNF and GM-CSF; leukotrienes; and PAF-acether. A topic was devoted to receptors of IgE and the growing interest on adhesion proteins was noted. A special session of the meeting was devoted to animal models of asthma in guinea-pigs, rats and mice.

This fifth volume of the Pierre Fabre Monograph series, which contains all the conferences and the abstracts of the posters of this symposium, is in fact an up-to-date review on this important subject which opens new ventures for therapeutics.

We would like to thank many active members of the Centre de Recherche Pierre Fabre for their help and most particularly Helene Duflos, secretary of the Congress.

Castres and Paris, 1991   J. P. T.
                                                            B. V.
                                                            E. C.

The Contributors

Arch, J. R. S.
  Smithkline Beecham Pharmaceuticals
  Yew Tree Bottom Road
  Epsom Surrey KT18 5XQ
  UK

Arm, J. P.
  Department of Allergy and Allied
    Respiratory Disorders
  4th Floor, Hunt's House
  Guy's Hospital
  London SE1 9RT
  UK

Bronner, C.
  Neuroimmunopharmacologie
    Pulmonaire
  INSERM CJF-9105
  Université Louis Pasteur–Strasbourg 1
  BP 24
  67401 Illkirch Cédex
  France

Bruijnzeel, P. L. B.
  Department of Pharmacology
  MBL/TNO
  Lange Kleiweg 139
  NL 2288 GJ Rijswijk
  Netherlands

Buijs, J.
  National Institute of Public Health and
    Environmental Protection
  P.O. Box 1
  3720 BA Bilthoven
  Netherlands

Cadieux, A.
  Department of Pharmacology
  Faculty of Medicine
  University of Sherbrooke
  Sherbrooke (Quebec) J1H 5N4
  Canada

Capron, A.
  Centre d'Immunologie et de Biologie
    Parasitaire
  INSERM U167–CNRS 624
  Institut Pasteur
  1 rue du Pr A. Calmette
  59019 Lille Cédex
  France

Capron, M.
  Centre d' Immunologie et de Biologie
    Parasitaire
  INSERM U167–CNRS 624
  Institut Pasteur
  1 rue du Pr A. Calmette
  59019 Lille Cédex
  France

Cavaillon, J.-M.
  Unité d'Immuno-Allergie
  Institut Pasteur
  28 rue du Dr Roux
  75015 Paris
  France

Coëffier, E.
  Unité de Pharmacologie Cellulaire
  Unité Associés Institut Pasteur–
    INSERM N°285
  25 rue du Dr Roux
  75015 Paris
  France

Corrigan, C. J.
  Department of Allergy and Immunology
  National Heart and Lung Institute
  Dovehouse Street
  London SW3 6LY
  UK

Desquand, S.
  Unité de Pharmacologie Cellulaire
  Unité Associés Institut Pasteur–
    INSERM N°285
  25 rue du Dr Roux
  75015 Paris
  France

Eisenburger, R.
  Klinge Pharma GmbH
  28 Weihenstephaner Strasse
  8000 Munich 80
  Germany

Englert, H. C.
  Hoechst AG
  SBU Cardiovascular Bldg G 838
  P.O. Box 80 03 20
  6230 Frankfurt am Main 80
  Germany

Fattah, D.
  Glaxo Group Research Ltd
  Biochemistry Department
  Greenford Road Middx UB6 0HE
  UK

Fischer, M. J. E.
  University of Utrecht
  Faculty of Pharmacy
  Department of Biomedical Pharmacy
  16 Sorbonnelaan
  3584 CA Utrecht
  Netherlands

Folkerts, G.
  Faculty of Pharmacy
  Department of Pharmacology
  University of Utrecht
  P.O. Box 80.082 Utrecht
  Netherlands

Fournier, M.
  Service Pneumologie et Réanimation
  Hôpital Beaujon
  100 bld du Général Leclerc
  92110 Clichy
  France

Gorenne, I.
  C. C. M. Lannelongue
  133 avenue de la Résistance
  92350 Plessis Robinson
  France

Hammond, M.
  Bayer UK Limited
  Strawberry Hill
  Newbury RG13 1JA
  UK

Hropot, M.
  Cardiovascular Agents, H 821
  Hoechst AG
  Postfach 80 01 20
  6230 Frankfurt am Main 80
  Germany

Jones, T. R.
  Merck Frosst Centre for Therapeutic
    Research
  16711 Trans Canada Highway
  Kirkland H9R 3L1
  Canada

Landry, Y.
  Neuroimmunopharmacologie
    Pulmonaire
  INSERM CJF-9105
  Université Louis Pasteur–Strasbourg 1
  BP 24
  67401 Illkirch Cédex
  France

Lapa e Silva, J. R.
  Unité de Pharmacologie Cellulaire
  Unité Associés Institut Pasteur–
    INSERM N°285
  25 rue du Dr Roux
  75015 Paris
  France

Lassalle, P.
Institut Pasteur
BP 245
59019 Lille
France

Lavezzo, A.
Dompe' Farmaceutici S.p.A.
12 Via San Martino
20122 Milano
Italy

Lawrence, C. E.
Rhône Poulenc Rorer Ltd
Rainham Road South
Dagenham Essex RM10 7XS
UK

Nijkamp, F. P.
Faculty of Pharmacy
Department of Pharmacology
University of Utrecht
P.O. Box 80.082 Utrecht
Netherlands

Paciorek, P.
Bronchopulmonary Department
Roche Products Ltd
P.O. Box 8 Welwyn Garden City
Hertfordshire AL73 3AY
UK

Pauwels, R.
Department of Respiratory Diseases
University Hospital
185 De Pintelaan
B 9000 Ghent
Belgium

Payard, M.
Faculté de Pharmacie
31 allée Jules Guesde
31000 Toulouse
France

Payne, A. N.
Department of Pharmacology
The Wellcome Research Laboratories
Langley Court
South Eden Park Road
Beckenham Kent BR3 3BS
UK

Pearce, F. L.
Department of Chemistry
University College of London
20 Gordon Street
London WC1H 0AJ
UK

Pipy, B.
Laboratoire de la Signalisation et de la
    Différenciation des Macrophages
Université Paul Sabatier – CHU
    Rangueil
1 avenue Jean Poulhes
31054 Toulouse Cédex
France

Pretolani, M.
Unité de Pharmacologie Cellulaire
Unité Associés Institut Pasteur–
    INSERM N°285
25 rue du Dr Roux
75015 Paris
France

Sanderson, C. J.
Department of Biochemistry
Searle Research Group
South Park Road
Oxford OX1 3QU
UK

Schellenberg, R. R.
Pulmonary Research Laboratory
University of British Columbia
1081 Burrard Street
Vancouver B.C. V6Z 1Y6
Canada

Tarayre, J. P.
Department de Pharmacologie Générale
Centre de Recherche Pierre Fabre
17 avenue Jean Moulin
81106 Castres Cédex
France

Tonnel, A.-B.
  Institut Pasteur
  1 rue du Pr Calmette
  59019 Lille
  France

Vachier, I.
  INSERM U 58
  60 rue de Navacelles
  34000 Montpellier
  France

Vardey, C. J.
  Glaxo Group Research Ltd
  Park Road
  Ware SG12 0DP
  UK

Varley, J. G.
  Immunopharmacology Group
  University of Southhampton
  Centre Block
  Southhampton General Hospital
  Tremona Road
  Southhampton SO9 4XY
  UK

Venge, P.
  Laboratory for Inflammation Research
  Department of Clinical Chemistry
  University Hospital
  751 85 Uppsala
  Sweden

Vignola, A. M.
  Hôpital de l'Aiguelongue
  avenue du Major Flandre
  34059 Montpellier
  France

Wegner, C. D.
  Department of Pharmacology
  Boehringer Ingelheim Pharmaceuticals
    Inc.
  90 East Ridge P.O. Box 368
  Ridgefield, CT 06877
  USA

Wei, E. T.
  School of Public Health
  University of California
  Berkeley, California 94720
  USA

Wilhelms, O. H.
  Boehringer Mannheim GmbH
  116 Sandhofer strasse
  6800 Mannheim
  Germany

Wood, L. J.
  Dagenham Research Centre
  Rhône Poulenc Rorer Ltd
  Dagenham Essex RM10 7XS
  UK

1

Allergy and Immune Defence: Common IgE-dependent Mechanisms or Divergent Pathways

A. Capron, J. P. Dessaint and M. Capron

1.1 Introduction

When considered at a global level, exposure to environmental allergens and to parasitic organisms certainly represents the main sources of discomfort or morbidity in children and young adults. It is striking that, since the early days of the basic studies on immediate-type hypersensitivity and of parasitic diseases, emphasis was given to the existence, in both pathological situations, of so-called reaginic antibodies, which was exemplified by the description of anaphylaxis by Richet and Portier (1902) on the one hand and Casoni's reaction on the other. It is also striking that, many years later, the description of passive cutaneous anaphylaxis by Ovary was accompanied by the pioneering observation made by Ogilvie *et al.* (1966) regarding the production of reaginic antibodies during experimental schistosome infection, raising the question of the participation of such antibodies in immune defence. Likewise, entering its molecular phase, the discovery of immunoglobulin E (IgE) and of its association with allergy was rapidly followed by the demonstration of elevated IgE production in helminthic infections (Johansson *et al.*, 1971) reflecting the massive IgE antibody response to parasites (Dessaint *et al.*, 1975; Jarrett and Miller, 1982; Dessaint, 1982).

For many years, we have lived with the concept of a proverbial association of most helminthic infections with an elevated IgE antibody response and hypereosinophilia, both of which are also observed in allergic diseases

1

(although often at lower levels), but without knowing their biological significance and the reasons for their appearance late in phylogeny. Contrasting with this elevated IgE production and the reasonable expectation of a high incidence of allergic manifestations during parasitic diseases, a number of epidemiologic reports indicated the paucity of symptoms related to immediate-type reactions to parasitic antigens, and even the lack of positive association between allergy and parasitism in endemic areas (Dessaint, 1982). This is all the more remarkable since contemporary experimental studies pointed to the existence of the potentiation of IgE antibody production by parasite infection such as described by Orr and Blair (1969) and extensively investigated by Jarrett and Miller (1982) in the *Nippostrongylus brasiliensis* model. It is noteworthy that these early studies of IgE potentiation constituted the experimental system for the description of the regulation of IgE production, leading to the discovery of a complex feed-back control by soluble IgE-binding factors (Ishizaka, 1984). It is also of interest that the demonstration of the role of interleukins, mainly IL-4 and IFN-γ, in the regulation of IgE response *in vivo* is also derived from the utilization of experimental helminthic infections (Finkelman *et al.*, 1988).

In parallel, at the level of effector cell populations, mast cell degranulation and mast-cell-derived mediators were considered as the single component of IgE-dependent reactions in allergy (Holgate *et al.*, 1986) as well as an essential cellular factor of the 'self-cure' phenomenon in immunity to intestinal nematodes or cestodes (Lee and Wakelin, 1986). Mast cells may play an exclusive role in worm expulsion from the gut mucosa. However, the direct helminthotoxicity of mast-cell-derived vasoactive amines and leakage of other immune effectors does not seem to be relevant to systemic helminthic infections such as schistosomiasis. In fact, a series of observations initiated in experimental and human schistosomiasis and confirmed in allergic diseases clearly points to the diversity of the cellular targets of IgE, and has led to the description of a second type of IgE Fc receptor, now called $Fc_\epsilon R_{II}$, on a wide variety of bone-marrow-derived cells (A. Capron *et al.*, 1986).

One can see through this brief historical introduction that the most significant biological observations leading to our present basic knowledge of the molecular and cellular mechanisms of allergy have in fact been provided by the extensive study of parasitic models in which allergic symptoms are not a predominant feature. This naturally led to the concept of a dual function of IgE in immunopathology and immune defence against helminths which may also apply to some protozoan parasites (A. Capron *et al.*, 1987; Ridel *et al.*, 1988).

The purpose of this review is to analyse common mechanisms or divergent pathways in the effector or regulatory phases of both allergic manifestations and parasitic infections.

1.2 IgE Antibody-dependent Cell Activation

Immunoglobulin E (IgE), a class of antibody of short half-life in the circulation, but of long persistence in tissues, exerts its biological function only through its interaction with cell surface receptors that are specific for its Fc_ε region. The dramatic result of the discharge of an array of potent proinflammatory mediators triggered by the aggregation of Fc_ε receptors has long been recognized in anaphylaxis and allergic diseases. Most mediators responsible for increase in vascular permeability, bronchoconstriction, bronchial hyperreactivity, and infiltration with inflammatory cells were initially considered as derived from mast cells or basophils. However, their cellular sources *in vivo* now appear to be more diverse, since most of these mediators of anaphylaxis, including chemotactic peptides, leukotrienes, and platelet-activating factor (PAF), are in fact produced and released by many of the inflammatory cells that accumulate at the site of allergic reactions (Holgate *et al.*, 1986).

The Second Class of Receptor for IgE

In vitro studies of correlates of immunity to schistosomes led to the demonstration of IgE antibody-dependent cytotoxicity (ADCC) mediated by monocytes–macrophages, eosinophils, and platelets both in experimental rat infection and in human schistosomiasis (A. Capron *et al.*, 1975; Joseph *et al.*, 1978, 1983a; M. Capron *et al.*, 1981, 1984a). Rosetting with IgE-coated erythrocytes, labelled IgE binding, and the use of polyclonal and monoclonal (BB10) anti-Fc_ε receptor antibodies allowed the demonstration of specific receptors for IgE on subsets of monocytes, macrophages, eosinophils, and platelets in man and rodents. These receptors differ from the classical mast cell or basophil receptor ($Fc_\varepsilon R_I$) by exhibiting a hundredfold lower affinity for IgE. The absence of antigenic cross-reactivity with the $Fc_\varepsilon R_I$ α chain of mast cells and basophils, when polyclonal and monoclonal (BB10) antibodies to inflammatory cell receptors bind similarly to macrophages, eosinophils, and platelets (A. Capron *et al.*, 1986) justifies the characterization of subsets of inflammatory cells. The essential role of IgE antibody in ADCC against helminth parasites was also indicated by the use of an anti-schistosome monoclonal antibody of the rat IgE class, which triggered rat macrophages, eosinophils or platelets to kill schistosome targets. These particular ADCC mechanisms are all the more remarkable since most classical killing processes do not appear to damage schistosome larvae *in vitro*.

Although the $Fc_\varepsilon R_{II}$ is of lower affinity than the mast cell or basophil receptor, the increased extrinsic affinity of $Fc_\varepsilon R_{II}$ for IgE dimers or complexes (Dessaint *et al.*, 1979; Finbloom and Metzger, 1982) gives this class of receptors a particular significance in all situations where IgE complexes are produced. This is the case not only of parasitic infections (Dessaint, 1982) but also of various allergic diseases (Brostoff *et al.*, 1977; Stevens and Bridts, 1984; Swainson *et al.*, 1985). In addition, the number of $Fc_\varepsilon R_{II}$-bearing cells increases in all pathological or experimental situations associated with elevated IgE levels. Furthermore, *ex vivo* studies of cell populations from parasitized or allergic individuals indicated the existence of surface-bound (cytophilic) IgE on a large proportion of monocytes, alveolar macrophages, peripheral blood or tissue eosinophils, and platelets (Joseph *et al.*, 1983a, b; Capron *et al.*, 1985; Joseph *et al.*, 1986).

One can accept therefore the general view that, both *in vitro* and *in vivo*, subsets of monocytes, macrophages, eosinophils, and platelets can, like mast cells or basophils, selectively bind IgE molecules. The important question is thus the possible participation, through mediators released after their activation, of these cells in IgE-dependent reactions.

As in the case of mast cells or basophils, the initial step in the stimulation of cells through IgE bound to $Fc_\varepsilon R_{II}$ receptors is the aggregation of the receptors. It has been shown, particularly for macrophages (Dessaint *et al.*, 1980), that dimers of IgE constitute the 'unit signal' for cell stimulation which can be detected 10–30 min after IgE-dependent $Fc_\varepsilon R_{II}$ aggregation (Dessaint *et al.*, 1990).

Monocytes–macrophages respond to IgE by releasing lysosomal enzymes, neutral proteases, interleukin-1, reactive oxygen metabolites, and also such potent mediators of anaphylaxis as sulphidopeptide leukotrienes (LTC4, LTD4), (LTB4), prostaglandins, and PAF. These observations initially made with purified monoclonal IgE were confirmed after the passive sensitization of normal alveolar macrophages with serum from allergic patients, by adding either anti-human IgE or the specific allergen. The release was dependent on IgE antibody in patients' sera, as shown by its disappearance after the depletion of IgE of the sensitizing serum. Moreover, alveolar macrophages collected from patients allergic to house mite or to grass pollen release lysosomal enzymes and PAF in similar amounts after addition of specific allergen, anti-IgE, or the F(ab')2 fragments of anti-IgE.

Likewise, platelets can produce reactive oxygen metabolites, a property unravelled by studies on IgE-dependent activation, and cytotoxic mediators that kill schistosomula *in vitro*; they also release a granule-stored mediator (histamine) but no serotonin and do not aggregate on triggering via their $Fc_\varepsilon R_{II}$. Platelets from allergic asthmatics, with mite- or grass-pollen-positive skin tests and high levels of specific IgE, generate such responses in the presence of the appropriate purified allergen or anti-human IgE, whereas anti-IgG has no such effect.

In the case of eosinophils, IgE triggers the release of proinflammatory granule components (basic proteins), mainly eosinophil peroxidase (EPO) and the major basic protein (MBP), but the eosinophil cationic protein

(ECP) is not liberated. When human eosinophils from patients with hypereosinophilia and increased IgE levels were incubated with either anti-IgE antibodies or the specific allergen, significant levels of PAF-acether were likewise produced (M. Capron *et al.*, 1989).

Comparison of IgE-dependent release of mediators by mast cells and basophils through $Fc_\varepsilon R_I$ on the one hand and through $Fc_\varepsilon R_{II}$ on mononuclear phagocytes and eosinophils reveals that both degranulation and exocytosis of preformed, stored mediators and new synthesis and secretion of lipidic mediators such as eicosanoids and PAF can be stimulated by IgE on its aggregation by the corresponding multivalent antigen. These observations open the question of the selectivity of the secretory response that is triggered by aggregation of the $Fc_\varepsilon R_{II}$ molecules on inflammatory cells. In the case of monocytes–macrophages, induction of leukotriene production, although faster by IgE-dependent reaction, is equivalent in quantity for both classes of immunoglobulins (Rankin *et al.*, 1984; Ferreri *et al.*, 1986), but, in the case of eosinophils, preferential release of EPO and PAF depends on IgE, when IgG triggers the secretion of ECP but not of EPO. Likewise, platelets release serotonin and tend to aggregate when stimulated by IgG, but they produce oxygen metabolites and cytotoxic factors after cross-linking of surface-bound IgE, but both IgG and IgE can stimulate platelets to liberate histamine as mentioned previously (Dessaint *et al.*, 1990).

In fact, this apparent selectivity in mediator release may be related in the case of eosinophils to the heterogeneity of this population. A particular subset of human eosinophils, sometimes found in blood in hypereosinophilic patients, but prominent in tissues, is characterized by its low density of metrizamide gradients, high expression of IgE receptors, and binding of the BB10 monoclonal antibody, and this 'hypodense' subset has also the selective capacity of releasing EPO and MBP by IgE antibody challenge (M. Capron *et al.*, 1989). In contrast, eosinophils with normal density are activated by IgG antibodies to release mainly cationic proteins (MBP, ECP) but no EPO (M. Capron *et al.*, 1989). It should be stressed that it is the human hypodense eosinophil subset that is the most efficient at killing schistosome targets in cooperation with human IgE antibodies (M. Capron *et al.*, 1984b) despite the fact that eosinophils can participate in ADCC reactions against helminth parasites *in vitro* in the presence of either IgG or IgE antibodies and the granule proteins released can cause parasite attrition.

Role of IgE in Defence Against Helminth Parasites

In contrast with these experimental demonstrations of *in vitro* activation by IgE of $Fc_\varepsilon R_{II}$-bearing cells to kill parasite targets, we have only circumstantial evidence for the involvement of this cooperation *in vivo*. A close chronological relationship has been observed between the development of protective immunity in rats infected by schistosomes and the evolution both of their levels of anaphylactic antibodies and of the ability of their cells and serum to kill parasites in *in vitro* cytotoxicity assays. Moreover, transfer of macrophages, eosinophils, or platelets collected from immune rats and shown to bear surface IgE each induced high levels of protein in recipient rats (Joseph *et al.*, 1983a; M. Capron *et al.*, 1984b), whereas administration of anti-schistosome monoclonal IgE antibody conferred on naive rats significant protection to a challenge schistosome infection (Verwaerde *et al.*, 1987).

In fact, a clear demonstration of the role of IgE antibodies in immune defence against helminth parasites *in vivo* has only recently been gained through a series of convergent epidemiological studies of humans in endemic schistosomiasis areas. In the Gambia, P. Hagan and coworkers convincingly demonstrated by multiple logistic regression that resistance to re-infection by *Schistosoma haematobium* was positively correlated with the presence of serum anti-parasite IgE antibody, individuals with low IgE being ten times more susceptible to the re-infection (Hagan *et al.*, 1991). Similarly, in Kenyan teenagers exposed to *S. mansoni*, acquired resistance was found to be correlated with levels of anti-schistosome antibody of the IgE class (Dunne *et al.*, 1992). Similar correlation was observed in Brazil (A. Dessein *et al.*, personal communication).

Macrophages, Eosinophils, and Platelets in Allergy

The heterogeneity of the receptors for IgE, $Fc_\varepsilon R_I$ being expressed only by basophils, mast cells, and their progenitors whereas $Fc_\varepsilon R_{II}$ is borne by subsets of most leukocytes and platelets, together with the range of cellular responses, from degranulation to synthesis and secretion of pro-inflammatory or cytotoxic mediators, may be considered to account for the differences in the consequences of IgE antibody-dependent reactions, from immune defence against helminth parasites to allergy.

Apart from the *ex vivo* studies demonstrating the occupation of $Fc_\varepsilon R_{II}$ by IgE on alveolar macrophages, eosinophils, and platelets of allergic patients, and the role of this cytophilic antibody in triggering mediator release on addition of the specific allergen, supportive evidence for the participation of alveolar macrophages in allergic reactions has been afforded by the demonstration of a decrease in the concentration of lysosomal enzymes in alveolar macrophages after a local provocation test, while the enzyme levels in bronchoalveolar lavage fluids were significantly higher than in the control lung (Tonnel *et al.*, 1983). The selectivity of the mediators released after IgE- or IgG-dependent stimulation of human eosinophils is also consistent with *in vivo* observations showing that release of MBP is linked to hypersensitivity states, including allergic asthma, whereas ECP levels are lower in asthmatic patients than in other hypereosinophilic individuals without bronchospasm (Gleich and Adolphson, 1986). Accordingly, lung eosinophils collected by bronchoalveolar lavage in patients with the hypereosinophilic syndrome or with drug hypersensitivity show important alterations with a loss of the granule core, reflecting a loss of MBP. Although no clear-cut demonstration of the nature of the antibodies involved and of the direct involvement of $Fc_\varepsilon R_{II}$ in triggering eosinophil degranulation in tissues has been provided, one may wonder whether locally activated hypodense eosinophils could participate in the pathogenesis of such diseases as pulmonary interstitial eosinophilia (PIE), lung interstitial fibrosis or eosinophilic gastroenteritis, in which ultrastructural alterations similar to those triggered through $Fc_\varepsilon R_{II}$ can be detected (Gleich and Adolphson, 1986; Torpier et al., 1988).

Other indirect evidence for the in vivo participation of $Fc_\varepsilon R_{II}$-positive cells in allergy may be drawn from the study of changes in cell reactivity induced by antiallergic treatment. Some antiallergic drugs such as disodium cromoglycate (DSCG) exert an inhibitory activity on IgE-dependent activation on cell populations expressing $Fc_\varepsilon R_{II}$. Alveolar macrophages, eosinophils, and platelets have been tested in allergic diseases, and a significant inhibition of their response to IgE-dependent stimulation has been observed with a dose of DSCG and similar to that found in vivo (Tsicopoulos et al., 1988a). It may therefore be considered that the action of antiallergic drugs such as DSCG and nedocromil is not restricted solely to their controversial direct effects on mast cells and basophils, but that they also interfere with $Fc_\varepsilon R_{II}$-positive cells, leading to a reduction of the inflammatory response in allergic diseases, which gives new insights into the mechanisms of action of these drugs in allergy.

Other suggestive evidence is provided by platelets from individuals sensitized to Hymenoptera stings, in whom platelets exposed in vitro to purified allergen (yellow-jacket or honey-bee venom) produce cytocidal factors and oxygen metabolites, previously shown to be a characteristic feature of activation by IgE. After rush desensitization to the corresponding venom, the ex vivo reactivity of platelets to the allergen was shown to be significantly decreased, indicating a close correlation between IgE-dependent activation of platelets and the clinical response of the patients to allergen therapy (Tsicopoulos et al., 1988b).

1.3 T Cell Control of IgE-dependent Reactions

Studies of the cellular mechanisms of allergy have been enriched during the last 10 years by extensive investigation of the control of IgE production by

T and B cell populations. In this respect, the discovery of IgE Fc receptors on B and some T cells and the functional and molecular characterization of soluble binding factors for IgE have represented important steps in our understanding of the regulation of IgE responses. At the same time, the successive identification and molecular cloning of various members of the interleukin cascade has allowed the demonstration of their crucial intervention both at the level of the induction of IgE responses and of the differentiation of potential target cells for IgE-dependent activation. We therefore have a broad but incomplete picture of the various cellular events and of the chemical signals which influence them that underlie the initiation, regulation, and expression of IgE-dependent reactions. Here again, it is striking that most of the knowledge acquired has been based on experimental studies involving a parasite infection in rodents, and although the general concepts derived from such studies are widely accepted as applicable to the field of allergy, the only evidence we have of their *in vivo* relevance is still limited to parasitic infections. Even the appealing concept of helper T cell subsets and the now classical (Th1 vs Th2) dichotomy, derived from the study of rodent T cell clones, finds more direct applicability and biological significance in murine parasitic infection such as leishmaniasis and schistosomiasis (Mosmann and Coffman, 1989; Pearce *et al.*, 1991). In brief, it seems clear, at least in mice, that two inducer cell subsets with distinct secretion profiles play a key role in the switch of antibody isotypes and inflammatory responses. Th1 cells essentially secrete IL-2 and IFN-γ and are responsible for delayed-type hypersensitivity reactions whereas Th2 cells are specifically implicated in the production of IL-4 and IL-5. A most important observation is the demonstration that Th1-derived IFN-γ acts as an essential factor of negative regulation of the IL-4 induced IgE production, whereas Th2 cells inhibit IL-2 dependent proliferation of Th1 cells. More broadly, it can be admitted that the privileged orientation of the immune response towards IgE-dependent reactions or T-cell-mediated hypersensitivity is closely related to the signals provided by specific interleukins, their production being controlled by the balance between activation of Th1 and Th2 cells.

In addition to their essential role in the induction and maintenance of IgE antibody responses, several interleukins are key factors for the functional differentiation of effector cells. The prominent roles of IL-3 and IL-4 in the recruitment and differentiation of T-dependent mast cells (Stevens and Austen, 1989), of IL-5 in eosinophil maturation (Silberstein and David, 1987) and of IFN-γ in platelet activation are now well established (Pancré *et al.*, 1988a; Boltz-Nitulescu *et al.*, 1988). If these interleukins can exert multiple functions on their target cells, one of these is certainly the induction or up-regulation of membrane receptors for IgE: this is the case of IFN-γ for macrophages and platelets (Boltz-Nitulescu *et al.*, 1988; Pancré *et al.*, 1988b) of IL-4 for monocyte–macrophage Fc$_\varepsilon$R$_{II}$ (Vercelli *et al.*, 1988) and of IL-3, GM-CSF and IL-5 on eosinophils (Dessaint *et al.*, 1990).

The relative contributions of interleukins and IgE binding factors (soluble $Fc_\varepsilon R_{II}$) to IgE responses is difficult to assess. Recent observations indicate that isotypic switching leading to IgE production is related to the action of IL-4 on B cells with membrane bound IgM (Bμ cells) whereas IgE binding factors amplify ongoing IgE responses by interacting with B cells with membrane-bound IgE (BE cells) (Delespesse *et al.*, 1989). The negative regulation of IgE seems to depend on isotypic switching induced by IFN-γ whereas BE lymphocytes are the sole target of putative IgE suppressive factors.

Since other interleukins, such as IL-5 and IL-6, play a role alone or in conjunction with IL-4 in the maturation of antibody producing cells and can also act as growth factors for T helper and B lymphocytes, we are confronted with a complex machinery of cells, lymphokines and soluble $Fc_\varepsilon R_{II}$ controlling IgE antibody production and IgE-dependent cell activation. Are these pathways common to both allergy and to the immune defence against helminth parasites and is there evidence of their *in vivo* relevance?

The concepts outlined above are derived from *in vivo* observations of murine models. The extension of these ideas to man is at this time based on the fragmentary evidence that IFN-γ and IL-4 can exert similar effects on CD23–$Fc_\varepsilon R_{II}$ expression and IgE production *in vitro* to those observed with murine cells (Delespesse *et al.*, 1989; Pene *et al.*, 1988a,b). Although the interleukin secretory patterns of CD4⁺ T cell clones from atopic and non-atopic donors (Wierenga *et al.*, 1990) appeared to be compartmentalized, the patterns were not consistent with the Th1–Th2 dichotomy of lymphokine secretion observed during parasitic infections in murine models. The combined use of recombinant massive IgE antibody response and the hypereosinophilia which accompanies helminth infections can be regulated by T cell products (Finkelman *et al.*, 1988; Mosmann and Coffman, 1989; Pearce *et al.*, 1991). The results obtained with such studies shed more light on the effects of interleukins in cell differentiation than on their role in the initiation of humoral and cellular events. It seems likely that such mechanisms are significant in the response to helminth infection and allergens given the similarities in their humoral and cellular components. However, as IgE-dependent reactions do not appear to be an essential component of immunity to schistosomes in mice, their participation in essential protective pathways against helminths remains open to debate. At present there is good evidence that Th1 (cell-mediated) responses can be protective in murine schistosomiasis (Pearce *et al.*, 1991) but there is no evidence to show that T-cell-mediated reactions are related to immunity to re-infection in human populations.

At the level of the effector cells, there is now evidence that $Fc_\varepsilon R_{II}$, on monocytes and on an eosinophil cell line, shares a strong homology with the IL-4 inducible B cell CD23b–Fc$_\varepsilon$R$_{II}$ (Yokota *et al.*, 1988). Although it cannot be excluded that some inflammatory cell populations such as alveolar macrophages, eosinophils and platelets express an IgE receptor with a different extracellular domain, their expression of Fc$_\varepsilon$R$_{II}$, or related structures, appears to be essential *in vivo* and *in vitro* for their activation as cytotoxic effectors against helminths and participation in allergic reactions (Dessaint *et al.*, 1990).

The apparent discrepancies between human and murine reactivities may be partly reconciled by the evidence that IgE binding is only one of the many functions of the CD23 family of molecules.

At the B cell level CD23b–Blast 2–Fc$_\varepsilon$R$_{II}$ has been shown to be an early activation market, a B cell growth factor (BCGF), a receptor for low molecular weight BCGF and a putative animal lectin (Delespesse *et al.*, 1989). In addition, the existence of the arginin–glycine–aspartic acid (DGR) adhesion sequence in CD23 (Gordon *et al.*, 1989), the inhibitory effect of the synthetic tetrapeptides arginine–glycine–aspartic acid–serine (RGDS) and serine–aspartic acid–glycine–arginine (SDGR) on IgE antibody-dependent cytotoxicity by eosinophils and on the recognition by the BB10 monoclonal antibodies (Grangette *et al.*, 1989) as well as the interaction of Fc$_\varepsilon$R$_{II}$ with platelet integrins (gpIIbIIIa) (Ameisen *et al.*, 1986) point to a more general role for IgE receptors in cellular interactions. This may be extended to Fc$_\varepsilon$R$_I$ since IgE-dependent activation of mast cells causes the release of immunomodulatory molecules including interleukins (Gordon *et al.*, 1990).

1.4 Biological Significance of the Diversity of the Cellular Targets of IgE

The demonstration that the expression of Fc$_\varepsilon$R$_{II}$ is increased in allergic patients and may be up-regulated by IgE indicates that immediate-type hypersensitivity involves multiple changes in many reactive cells. The elaboration of many inflammatory mediators from mononuclear phagocytes, eosinophils, and platelets in response to IgE immune complexes points to the primary effector function of cells until now considered only to be involved in non-specific inflammatory responses. In addition, these cells, along with Fc$_\varepsilon$R$_I$-bearing mast cells or basophils, may also be direct cellular partners of IgE. In allergy, increased production of IgE and the formation of circulating IgE complexes or, alternatively, local formation of IgE immune complexes capable of high affinity binding with Fc$_\varepsilon$R$_{II}$ can lead to activation of proinflammatory cells. Although monomeric IgE rapidly dissociates from the cell surface, preformed or newly formed IgE immune complexes will persist and confer on Fc$_\varepsilon$R$_{II}$-positive cells a direct role in the pathophysiology of allergic disorders. The selective activation of inflammatory cell subpopulations through their $Fc_\varepsilon R_{II}$ does not exclude their cooperation with cells bearing the $Fc_\varepsilon R_I$ at the effector phase. An array of lymphokines may be involved in the control of the effector cells themselves but the role of these lymphokines in the control of IgE antibody production has also to be considered.

One may consider that in both allergy and immune defence to helminths there is an integrated system for the regulation of IgE production and its functional expression through the maturation of its $Fc_\varepsilon R_{II}$ positive target cells. It would seem unreasonable to claim that all allergic manifestations are related only to IgE-dependent reactions, and it would seem equally unreasonable to postulate that immune defence to helminth parasites relies exclusively on IgE. The fact that two major mechanisms, i.e. lymphokine-dependent macrophage activation and IgE antibody dependent cell-mediated cytotoxicity, appear as alternative pathways of protective immunity to helminths depending on the animal model used (as exemplified by the rat–mouse schistosomiasis controversy) naturally raises the question of the phylogenic emergence of IgE as a basic mechanism of defence. The dichotomy in the function of IgE and its cellular partners in allergy and parasitic diseases raises the fundamental question of the evolutionary significance of an immunoglobulin molecule which is produced and active at hormone-like levels.

The late appearance of IgE in phylogeny as well as the high rate of evolution of the E chain in comparison with other immunoglobulin heavy chains (Ishida et al., 1982) suggest selection for the continuous existence of this fifth class of immunoglobulins. If a major biologic function of IgE is in the immune response to parasitic infection, then a number of clinically significant allergic responses to environmental antigens may reflect the inappropriate activation of immunologic circuits or effector pathways ordinarily initiated by helminths.

IgE, contrary to other classes of antibody that may interact with complement components, exerts its biological function only through interaction with cell surface receptors. Available evidence on the molecular structure of various Fc receptors indicates that, in general, their extracellular domains are homologous to each other and to other members of the immunoglobulin superfamily. A remarkable exception is afforded by IgE receptors: even though the α chain which binds IgE with high affinity on mast cells or basophils is homologous to other Fc receptors, $Fc_\varepsilon R_I$ is only expressed when the α chain is associated with non-immunoglobulin-related β and γ chains (Miller et al., 1989). The study of $Fc_\varepsilon R_{II}$ mutants has revealed that the binding site for IgE is confined to the domain homologous to animal lectins, although $Fc_\varepsilon R_{II}$ can bind recombinant IgE molecules lacking carbohydrate (Bettler et al., 1989). The unusual structure of the various Fc_ε receptors might thus reflect a specialized function of IgE in triggering the discharge of potent proinflammatory or cytotoxic mediators.

Although the heterotypic interactions among certain pairs of immuno-globulin superfamily members can be attributed to parallel or tandem evolution from a common ancestral molecule, the demonstration that IgE and CD23/$Fc_\varepsilon R_{II}$ have distinct ancestral origins and that IgE appeared late in the phylogeny suggests a remarkable covergence conferring on mammals benefits not provided by other molecules.

The homology, but also the diversity, of $Fc_\varepsilon R_{II}$s may reflect differences in biological function of the corresponding cells. A first series of $Fc_\varepsilon R_{II}$ molecules appears to be related to immunoregulation: this is the case of the receptors borne by B and T cells (Delespesse et al., 1989), and by Langerhans cells which have recently been shown to bind IgE (Bruijnzeel-Koomen et al., 1988). These $Fc_\varepsilon R_{II}$ found either on the cell surface or as soluble IgE-binding factors can participate in control of lymphocyte growth and differentiation, especially in the isotypic regulation of IgE production. Interestingly, at least in B cells, the CD23–$Fc_\varepsilon R_{II}$ molecules may interact with class II major histocompatibility complex products (Bonnefoy et al., 1988) and/or with membrane IgM or IgD. This may indicate their parti-cipation in the general processes of antigen-driven B cell activation or cognate interaction with helper T cells.

A second series of receptors appears to trigger IgE-dependent cytotoxic-ity and the release of many potent proinflammatory mediators by mono-nuclear phagocytes, eosinophils and platelets, which may indicate that this receptor is capable of transducing a signal either by itself or through its interaction with integrins such as gpllbllla on platelets (Ameisen et al., 1986) or iC3b receptor (CD11b) on eosinophils (M. Capron et al., 1987), suggesting a remarkable intersection between members of three major superfamilies (i.e. IgE, animal lectins, and integrins) exploited to eliminate parasites that resist destruction by conventional lymphoid-cell-mediated cytotoxicity, but also involved in the triggering of potent bioactive mediators implied in adverse allergic reactions.

Through its interaction with one or the other of its receptors, IgE can thus trigger multiple cell populations and play a key role in many biological reactions, either in immune defence against helminth parasites or as direct effector cells in allergic disorders. In both cases, the network of cells responsive to IgE appears to be highly complex and interconnected through IgE itself, cytokines, and so-called factors of anaphylaxis. It is thus perhaps not surprising that common IgE-dependent mechanisms might appear to diverge in their functional consequences in parasitized and parasite-free individuals.

The recent demonstration in human populations of a close correlation between IgE antibodies and acquired resistance to schistosomiasis (Hagan et al., 1991), while confirming our original working hypothesis and our experimental approach, gives additional support to the views expressed in this report.

References

Ameisen, J. C., Joseph, M., Caen, J. P., Kusnierz, J. P., Capron, M., Boizard, B., Wautier, J. L., Levy-Toledano, S., Vorng, H. and Capron, A. (1986). A role for glycoprotein IIb–IIIa complex in the binding of IgE to human platelets and in platelet IgE-dependent cytotoxic functions. *Br. J. Haematol.*, **64**, 21–32.

Bettler, B., Maier, R., Ruegg, D. and Hofstetter, H. (1989). Binding site for IgE of the human Fc$_\varepsilon$ receptor II (Fc$_\varepsilon$R$_{II}$/CD23) is confined to the domain homologous with animal lectins. *Proc. Natl. Acad. Sci. USA*, **86**, 7118–23.

Boltz-Nitulescu, G., Wiltsche, C., Langer, K., Nemet, H., Holzinger, C., Gessl, A., Forster, O. and Penner, E. (1988). Augmentation of IgE receptor expression and IgE receptor-mediated phagocytosis of rat bone-marrow derived macrophages by murine interferons. *Immunology*, **63**, 529–35.

Bonnefoy, J. Y., Guillot, O., Spits, H., Blanchard, D., Ishizaka, K. and Banchereau, J. (1988). The low affinity receptor for IgE (CD23) spatially associated with HLA-DR antigens. *J. Exp. Med.*, **167**, 57–70.

Brostoff, J., Johns, P. and Stanworth, D. R. (1977). Immune complexed IgE in atopy. *Lancet*, **ii**, 741.

Bruijnzeel-Koomen, C. A. F. M., van der Donk, E. M. M., Mudde, G. C., Capron, M., Brujnzeel, P. L. B. and de Gost G. C. (1988). Associated expression of T6 antigen and Fc receptor for IgE on epidermal Langerhans cells from patients with atopic dermatitis. *Clin. Exp. Immunol.*, **74**, 137–42.

Capron, A., Dessaint, J. P., Capron, M. and Bazin, H. (1975). Specific IgE antibodies in immune adherence of normal macrophages to *Schistosoma mansoni* schistosomules. *Nature (London)*, **253**, 474–5.

Capron, A., Dessaint, J. P., Capron, M., Joseph, M., Ameisen, J. C. and Tonnel, A. B. (1986). From parasites to allergy: the second receptor for IgE (Fc$_\varepsilon$R$_{II}$). *Immunol. Today*, **7**, 15–18.

Capron, A., Dessaint, J. P., Capron, M., Ouma, A. and Butterworth, A. E. (1987). Immunity to schistosomes: progress toward vaccine. *Science*, **238**, 1065–72.

Capron, M., Bazin, H., Joseph, M. and Capron A. (1981). Evidence for IgE-dependent cytotoxicity by rat eosinophils. *J. Immunol.*, **126**, 1764–8.

Capron, M., Nogueira-Queiroz, J. A., Papin, J. P. and Capron, A. (1984a). Interactions between eosinophils and antibodies: *in vivo* protective role against rat schistosomiasis. *Cell. Immunol.*, **83**, 60–72.

Capron, M., Spiegelberg, H. L., Prin, L., Bennich, H., Butterworth, A. E., Pierce, R. J., Ouaissi, M. A. and Capron, A. (1984b). Role of IgE receptors in effector function of human eosinophils. *J. Immunol.*, **232**, 462–8.

Capron, M., Kusnierz, J. P., Prin, L., Spiegelberg, H. L., Ovlaque, G., Gosset, P., Tonnel, A. B. and Capron, A. (1985). Cytophilic IgE on human blood and tissue eosinophils: detection by flow microfluorometry. *J. Immunol.*, **134**, 3013–18.

Capron, M., Jouault, T., Prin, L., Ameisen, J. C., Butterworth, A. E., Papin, J. P., Kusnierz, J. P. and Capron, A. (1986). Functional study of a monoclonal antibody to IgE Fc receptor (Fc$_\varepsilon$R$_{II}$) of eosinophils, platelets, and macrophages. *J. Exp. Med.*, **164**, 72–89.

Capron, M., Kazatchkine, M. D., Fischer, E., Joseph, M., Butterworth, A. E., Kusnierz, J. P., Prin, L., Papin, J. P. and Capron, A. (1987). Functional role of the α chain of complement receptor type 3 in human eosinophil-dependent antibody-mediated cytotoxicity against schistosomes. *J. Immunol.*, **139**, 2059–65.

Capron, M., Grangette, C., Torpier, G. and Capron A. (1989). The second receptor for IgE in eosinophil effector function. *Chem. Immunol.*, **47**, 128–78.

Delespesse, G., Sarfati, M. and Hofstetter, H. (1989). Human IgE-binding factors. *Immunol. Today*, **10**, 159–64.

Dessaint, J. P. (1982). Anaphylactic antibodies and their significance. *Clin. Immunol. Allergy*, **2**, 621–37.

Dessaint, J. P., Capron, M., Bout, D. and Capron, A. (1975). Quantitative determination of specific IgE antibodies to schistosome antigens and serum IgE levels in patients with schistosomiasis (*S. mansoni* or *S. haematobium*). *Clin. Exp. Immunol.*, **20**, 427–436.

Dessaint, J. P. Torpier, G., Capron, M. and Bazin, H. (1979). Cytophilic binding of IgE to the macrophage. I. Binding characteristics of IgE on the surface of macrophages in the rat. *Cell. Immunol.*, **46**, 12–23.

Dessaint, J. P., Waksman, B. H., Metzger, H. and Capron, A. (1980). Cytophilic binding of IgE to the macrophage. III. Involvement of cyclic GMP and calcium in macrophage activation by dimeric or aggregated rat myeloma IgE. *Cell. Immunol.*, **51**, 280–92.

Dessaint, J. P., Capron, M. and Capron, A. (1990). Immunoglobulin E-stimulated release of mediators from mononuclear phagocytes, eosinophils, and platelets. In Metzger, H. (ed.), *Fc Receptors and the Action of Antibodies*, *American Society for Microbiology*, Washington, DC, 260–87.

Dunne, W. D., Butterworth, A. E., Fulford, A. J. C., Kariuki, H. C., Langley, J. G., Ouma, J. H., Capron, A., Pierce, R. J. and Sturrock, F. (1992). Immunity after treatment of human *Schistosomiasis mansoni* association between IgE antibodies to adult worm antigens and resistance to reinfection. *Eur. J. Immunol.*, in press.

Ferreri, N. R., Howland, W. C. and Spiegelberg, H. L. (1986). Release of leukotrienes C4 and B4 and prostaglandin E2 from human monocytes stimulated with aggregated IgG, IgA, and IgE. *J. Immunol.*, **136**, 4188–93.

Finbloom, D. S. and Metzger, H. (1982). Binding of immunoglobulin E to the receptor on rat peritoneal macrophages. *J. Immunol.*, **129**, 2004–8.

Finkelman, F. D., Katona, I. M., Urban, J. F., Jr, Holmes, J., Ohara, J., Tung, A. S., Sample, J. V. G. and Paul, W. E. (1988). IL-4 is required to generate and sustain *in vivo* IgE responses. *J. Immunol.*, **141**, 2335–41.

Gleich, G. J. and Adolphson, C. R. (1986). The eosinophil leukocyte. *Adv. Immunol.*, **39**, 177–253.

Gordon, J. R., Flores-Romo, L., Cairns, J. A., Millsum, M. J., Lane, P. J., Johnson, G. D. and MacLennan, I. C. M. (1989). CD23: a multi-functional receptor/lymphokine? *Immunol. Today*, **10**, 153–7.

Gordon, J. R., Burd, P. R. and Galli, S. J. (1990). Mast cells as a source of multifunctional cytokines. *Immunol. Today*, **11**, 458–64.

Grangette, C., Gruart, V., Ouaissi, M. A., Rizvi, F., Delespesse, G., Capron, A. and Capron, M. (1989). IgE receptor on human eosinophils (Fc$_\varepsilon$R$_{II}$): comparison with B cell CD23 and association with an adhesion molecule. *J. Immunol.*, **143**, 3580–8.

Hagan, P., Blumenthal, U. J., Dunn, D., Simpson, A. J. G. and Wilkins, H. A. (1991). Human IgE, IgG4 and resistance to reinfection with *Schistosoma haematobium*. *Nature (London)*, **349**, 243–5.

Holgate, S. T., Hardy, C., Robinson, C., Agius, R. M. and Howarth, P. R. (1986). The mast cell as a primary effector cell in the pathogenesis of asthma. *J. Allergy Clin. Immunol.*, **77**, 274–82.

Ishida, N., Ueda, S., Hayashida, T. and Honjo, T. (1982). The nucleotide sequence of the mouse immunoglobulin epsilon gene: comparison with the human epsilon gene sequence. *EMBO J.*, **1**, 1117–22.

Ishizaka, K. (1984). Regulation of IgE synthesis. *Annu. Rev. Immunol.*, **2**, 159–62.

Jarrett, E. E. E. and Miller, H. R. P. (1982). Production and activities of IgE in helminth infection. *Prog. Allergy*, **31**, 178–233.

Johansson, S. G. O., Bennich, H. H. and Berg, T. (1971). The clinical significance of IgE. *Prog. Allergy*, **1**, 157–8.

Joseph, M., Capron, A., Butterworth, A. E., Sturrock, R. F. and Houba, V. (1978). Cytotoxicity of human and baboon mononuclear phagocytes against schistosomula *in vitro*: induction by immune complexes containing IgE and *Schistosoma mansoni* antigens. *Clin. Exp. Immunol.*, **33**, 45–56.

Joseph, M., Auriault, C., Capron, A., Vorng, H. and Viens, P. (1983a). A role for platelets in IgE-dependent killing of schistosomes. *Nature (London)*, **303**, 810–11.

Joseph, M., Tonnel, A. B., Torpier, G., Capron, A., Arnoux, A. and Benveniste, J. (1983b). Involvement of immunoglobulin E in the secretory processes of alveolar macrophages from asthmatic patients. *J. Clin. Invest.*, **71**, 221–30.

Joseph, M., Capron, A., Ameisen, J. C., Capron, M., Vorng, H., Pancre, V., Kusnierz, J. P. and Auriault C. (1986). The receptor for IgE on blood platelets. *Eur. J. Immunol.*, **16**, 306–12.

Lee, T. D. G. and Wakelin, D. (1986). Mast cell responses to helminth infection. *Parasitol. Today*, **2**, 186–90.

Miller, L., Blanck, U., Metzger, H. and Kinet, J. P. (1989). Expression of high-affinity binding of human immunoglobulin E by transfected cells. *Science*, **244**, 334–6.

Mosmann, T. R. and Coffman, R. L. (1989). Heterogeneity of cytokine secretion patterns and functions of helper T cells. *Adv. Immunol.*, **46**, 111–47.

Ogilvie, B. M., Smithers, S. R. and Terry, R. J. (1966). Reagin-like antibodies in experimental infection of *Schistosoma mansoni* and the passive transfer of resistance. *Nature (London)*, **209**, 1221.

Orr, T. S. C. and Blair, A. M. J. N. (1969). Potentiated reagin response to egg albumin and conalbumin in *Nippostrongylus brasiliensis* infected rats. *Life Sci.*, **8**, 1073–82.

Pancre, V., Joseph, M., Mazingue, C., Wietzerbin, J., Kusnierz, J. P., Vorng, H. and Auriault, C. (1988a). Induction of platelet cytotoxic functions by lymphokines: role of interferon-γ. *J. Immunol.*, **138**, 4490–5.

Pancre, V., Joseph, M., Capron, A., Wietzerbin, J., Kusnierz, J. P., Vorng, H. and Auriault, C. (1988b). Recombinant human interferon-gamma induces increased IgE receptor expression on human platelets. *Eur. J. Immunol.*, **18**, 829–32.

Pearce, E. J., Caspar, P., Grzych, J. M., Lewis, F. A. and Sher, A. (1991). Downregulation of Th1 cytokine production accompanies induction of Th2 responses by a parasitic helminth, *Schistosoma mansoni*. *J. Exp. Med.*, **173**, 159–66.

Pene, S., Rousset, F., Briere, F., Chretien, I., Bonnefoy, J. Y., Spits, H., Yokota, T., Arai, N., Arai, K., Banchereau, J. and de Vries, J. E. (1988a). IgE production by normal human lymphocytes is induced by interleukin-4 and suppressed by interferons γ and α and prostaglandin E_2. *Proc. Natl. Acad. Sci. USA*, **85**, 6880–4.

Pene, J., Rousset, F., Briere, F., Chretien, I., Wideman, J., Bonnefoy, J. Y. and de Vries, J. E. (1988b). Interleukin-5 enhances interleukin 4-induced IgE production by normal human B cells. The role of soluble CD23 antigen. *Eur. J. Immunol.*, **18**, 929–35.

Rankin, J. A., Hitchcock, M., Merrill, W. W., Huang, S. S., Brashler, J. R., Bach,

M. K. and Askenase, P. W. (1984). IgE immune complexes induce immediate and prolonged release of leukotriene C4 (LTC4) from rat alveolar macrophages. *J. Immunol.*, **132**, 1993–9.

Richet, C. and Portier, P. (1902). De l'action anaphilactic de certains vaccins. *C.R. Soc. Biol. (Paris)*, **54**, 170–2.

Ridel, P. R., Auriault, C., Darcy, F., Pierce, R. J., Leite, P., Neyrinck, J. L., Kusnierz, J. P. and Capron, A. (1988). Protective role of IgE in immunocompromized rat toxoplasmosis. *J. Immunol.*, **141**, 978–83.

Silberstein, D. S. and David, J. R. (1987). The regulation of human eosinophil function by cytokines. *Immunol. Today*, **8**, 380–5.

Stevens, R. L. and Austen, K. F. (1989). Recent advances in the cellular and molecular biology of mast cells. *Immunol. Today*, **10**, 381–6.

Stevens, W. J. and Bridts, C. H. (1984). IgG-containing and IgE-containing circulating immune complexes in patients with asthma and rhinitis. *J. Allergy Clin. Immunol.*, **73**, 276–82.

Swainson, J. A., Wilson, P. B., Dore, P. and Pumphrey, R. S. H. (1985). Evidence for circulating complexes containing IgE in patients with atopic dermatitis. *Int. Arch. Allergy Appl. Immunol.*, **76**, 237–41.

Tonnel, A. B., Joseph, M., Gosset, P. and Fournier, E. (1983). Stimulation of alveolar macrophages in asthmatic patients after local provocation test. *Lancet*, **8339**, 1406–8.

Torpier, G., Colombel, J. F., Mathieu-Chandelier, C., Capron, M., Dessaint, J. P., Cortot, A., Paris, J. C. and Capron, A. (1988). Eosinophilic gastroenteritis: ultrastructural evidence for a selective release of eosinophilic major basic protein. *Clin. Exp. Immunol.*, **74**, 404–8.

Tsicopoulos, A., Lassalle, P., Joseph, M., Tonnel, A. B., Thorel, T., Dessaint, J. P. and Capron, A. (1988a). Effect of disodium cromoglycate on inflammatory cells bearing the Fc epsilon receptor type II (Fc$_\varepsilon$R$_{II}$). *Int. J. Immunopharmacol.*, **10**, 227–36.

Tsicopoulos, A., Tonnel, A. B., Wallaert, B., Joseph, M., Ameisen, J. C. and Ramon, P. H. (1988b). Decrease of IgE-dependent platelet activation in Hymenoptera hypersensitivity after specific rush desensitization. *Clin. Exp. Immunol.*, **71**, 433–8.

Vercelli, D., Jabara, H. H., Lee, B. W., Woodland, N., Geha, R. S. and Leung, D. Y. M. (1988). Human recombinant IL-4 induces Fc$_\varepsilon$R$_{II}$/CD23 on normal human monocytes. *J. Exp. Med.*, **167**, 1406–16.

Verwaerde, C., Joseph, M., Capron, M., Pierce, R. J., Damonneville, M., Velge, F., Auriault, C. and Capron, A. (1987). Functional properties of a rat monoclonal IgE antibody specific for *Schistosoma mansoni*. *J. Immunol.*, **138**, 4441–6.

Wierenga, E. A., Snoek, M., De Groot, C., Chretien, I., Bos, J. D., Jansen, H. M. and Kapsenberg, M. L. (1990). Evidence for compartmentalization of functional subsets of CD4$^+$ T lymphocytes in atopic patients. *J. Immunol.*, **144**, 4651–6.

Yokota, A., Kikutani, H., Tanaka, T., Sato, R., Barsumian, E. L., Suemura, M. and Kishimoto, T. (1988). Two species of human Fc$_\varepsilon$R$_{II}$ (Fc epsilon R$_{II}$/CD23): tissue-specific and IL-4 specific regulation of gene expression. *Cell*, **55**, 611–18.

2

Animal Models of Asthma

A. N. Payne

2.1 Introduction

Asthma is now recognized to be a multifactorial syndrome involving bronchial smooth muscle spasm, airway inflammation and non-specific bronchial hyperreactivity (BHR). As shown in Fig. 2.1, these pathophysiological components interact to produce intermittent episodes of airway narrowing in response to either intrinsic (e.g. emotion) or extrinsic (e.g. allergen) provocation factors. Such episodes usually remit either spontaneously or following drug treatment, but in the worst prognoses can prove irreversible and fatal. Even between acute asthma attacks, baseline airway calibre is often reduced, sometimes imperceptibly to the patient.

Despite the current availability of a range of different classes of established anti-asthmatic drugs (Payne, 1989), the prevalence, severity and mortality of asthma appears to be on the increase (Friday and Fireman, 1988).

Hence there exists a need for the identification and rapid progression into clinical evaluation of new and more efficacious drugs for asthma. Considered to be of particular importance in this respect is the need for new drugs to be 'disease modifying' rather than simply providing relatively short-term symptomatic relief.

It has yet to be proven whether recently developed potential anti-asthmatic drugs such as platelet-activating factor (PAF) antagonists (Gundel et al., 1991), 5-lipoxygenase (5-LO) inhibitors (Payne et al., 1988; Hui et al., 1990) and leukotriene (LT) antagonists (Gaddy et al., 1991) will meet this criterion. At the same time, the longitudinal impact of long-acting β-adrenoceptor agonists such as salmeterol (Larsson, 1990) which

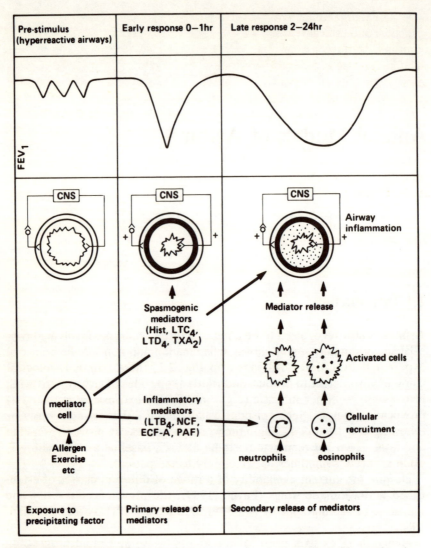

Fig. 2.1 Postulated pathopharmacological interactions in the early and late asthmatic response following exposure to precipitating factors (from Payne, 1989).

may have an anti-inflammatory as well as a bronchodilator action remains to be assessed.

2.2 Animal Models

Given the clinical requirement for new anti-asthmatic drugs, one is bound to consider the pathophysiological relevance and, by inference, the predictive value of animal models (Withnall and de Brito, 1990). For both practical and ethical reasons these will (at least for the foreseeable future) continue to have a role in the drug development process, not only for asthma but also in other research fields. In a recent report entitled 'Asthma – what are the important experiments' (Woolcock, 1988) the desirable characteristics of an animal model of asthma were listed.

Briefly, these were persistent BHR characterized by dose–response curves to inhaled histamine or cholinergic agonists with at least a 10-fold increase in sensitivity compared with control animals, bronchoconstrictor dose–response curves with increased reactivity (steep slope and increased maximal response), bronchoconstrictor responses to a wide range of provocation stimuli, and increases in residual volume during induced quasi-asthmatic attacks.

Few, if any, of those animal models of asthma currently in use meet all of the above criteria. However, providing that their inherent limitations are recognized (particularly when extrapolating results to the clinical scenario) animal models can prove of value in increasing the knowledge of under-lying pathophysiological mechanisms, establishing more conclusively the site of action of established anti-asthmatic drugs (e.g. cromoglycate, nedocromil, steroids), identifying new strategies for therapeutic interven-tion and facilitating pre-clinical evaluation of the therapeutic potential of new chemical entities.

For these purposes, which by necessity are interrelated, many different animal models of asthma have been developed in various species ranging in size from rats to horses (Payne *et al.*, 1989; Smith, 1989).

Most animal models are focused on allergen provocation and depend on classical type 1 immediate-type hypersensitivity reactions. In some cases a naturally occurring immunity to environmental antigens can be exploited (e.g. to *Ascaris suum* in dogs, monkeys and sheep). Alternatively, animals can be either actively or passively sensitized (e.g. to ovalbumin), with or without adjuvants as appropriate. It is important to note that the predomi-nant antibody type can vary depending on the sensitization procedure (route of antigen presentation, neonatal as opposed to adult sensitization, use or not of secondary 'booster' sensitization). This consideration can influence the modulation by drugs of the pulmonary response to antigen challenge.

Apart from *in vivo* models, *in vitro* models of pulmonary anaphylaxis are also employed (Ogunbiyi and Eyre, 1985). Primarily as a result of the increasing focus on BHR, many other 'non-immunological' animal models of asthma have been developed in which the manifestation and modulation of the possibly linked processes of BHR and inflammation has been ex-plored (Sheppard, 1989). Some of the various advantages and disadvan-tages of present day animal models of asthma are summarized in Table 2.1.

Table 2.1   Advantages and disadvantages of animal models of asthma

Advantages	Disadvantages
Documented aetiology	Usually relatively acute
Therapeutically naive	Species/breed idiosyncracies
Expendable	Different spectrum of mediators
Parallel histology	Often highly constrained
Availability	Different drug metabolism
Pre-determined time course	Relevance often uncertain

Early Response

The immediate fall in lung function (early asthmatic response) provoked in extrinsic asthmatics by inhalation of allergen can be readily assessed non-invasively by a marked drop in forced expiratory volume in 1 (FEV_1). This measurement, of course, involves a degree of active cooperation by the subject, which is rarely found in animals. Hence lung function measurements in animal models tend to be more invasive and are often performed in anaesthetized, mechanically ventilated preparations.

Probably the most extensively used animal model of the early response is that in sensitized guinea-pigs. In addition to marked allergic bronchoconstriction following allergen (i.v. or aerosol) challenge (see for example Payne and de Nucci, 1987) the pathology of the pulmonary response in this species is a reasonable counterpart to that of human asthma (Kallos and Kallos, 1984). As early as 10 min after exposure to a sublethal dose of aerosolized antigen there is histological evidence of the peribronchial vessels being infiltrated by granulocytes. After repeated challenge, cough and hypersecretion of mucus is apparent as would be the case in man. There are, however, some important differences between experimental asthma in guinea-pigs and the corresponding clinical situation. First the predominant homocytotropic antibody in this species is usually immunoglobulin (Ig)G, rather than IgE, and secondly histamine is the predominant mediator responsible for the immediate bronchoconstriction. The comparative lack of effect of anti-histamines in clinical asthma is well documented although some evidence of a protective effect against the immediate drop in FEV_1 following antigen challenge has been noted (Howarth and Holgate, 1985).

Nevertheless, guinea-pig models of the early asthmatic response continue to be used because of their expendability and also flexibility in that the functional response to antigen challenge can be pharmacologically modulated (Daffonchio et al., 1989) to focus on individual anaphylactic mediators, for example eicosanoids. It should, however, be noted that, except under specialized sensitization conditions, clinically used agents such as disodium cromoglycate and glucocorticoids are ineffective in the guinea-pig early response model.

Other, mostly long-established, animal models of the early asthmatic response include rats, rabbits, monkeys, sheep, dogs and cats (see Payne *et al.*, 1989, for references). In some of these models it is also possible to elicit late responses (see below).

Late Response

Approximately 50% of asthmatics who develop an early response to allergen challenge may exhibit total or partial resolution of the initial fall in lung function prior to a subsequent more protracted (lasting 24 h or more) airway narrowing termed the late asthmatic response (O'Byrne *et al.*, 1987). Conceptually this late response is associated with an inflammatory lesion within the airways rather than contraction of airway smooth muscle as, more often than not, it is refractory to the action of bronchodilators.

In recent years much effort has been directed towards developing animal models of the late response in which to investigate the attendant pathophysiology and to evaluate the therapeutic potential of new drugs targeted towards lung inflammation. Animal models that have been used in this respect include sheep (Abraham *et al.*, 1983), rabbits (Shampain *et al.*, 1982) and guinea-pigs (Hutson *et al.*, 1988). Of these models, that in sheep has probably produced the most data (Smith, 1989), although the relevance of such data to clinical asthma is equivocal. Whilst some studies have been performed on late responses in monkeys naturally sensitive to *Ascaris* (McFarlane *et al.*, 1987), underlying spontaneous changes in antigen sensitivity and BHR complicate their usage.

Nevertheless some elegant studies have been carried out in this species, most notably of late that of investigating the role of adhesion molecules (Wegner *et al.*, 1990, this volume). The possible role of endothelial and epithelial cell adhesion molecules in lung pathology has been recently reviewed (Albelda, 1991).

Bronchial Hyperreactivity

In addition to preventing the early and late asthmatic response, the reversal of BHR remains an important therapeutic target (O'Donnel and Payne, 1991).

Many studies in different animal models have been carried out in order to investigate the postulated link between airway inflammation and BHR (O'Byrne, 1986; Fitzgerald and Whittle, 1989; Sheppard, 1989). While

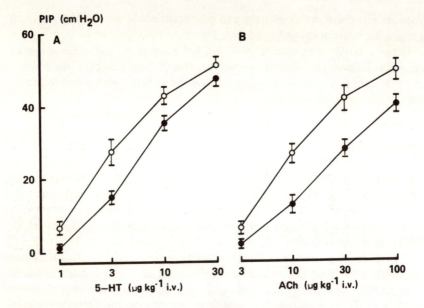

Fig. 2.2   Dose–response curves to the bronchoconstrictor effect of i.v. (A) 5-HT and (B) acetylcholine in anaesthetized pump-ventilated sensitized guinea-pigs 1 h after challenge with either saline (0.9%; 5 s) or antigen (ovalbumin; 0.3 mg ml^{-1}). PIP, pulmonary inflation pressure, an index of intrathoracic airway calibre; $n = 6–8$ in each case. Dose ratios were 1.7 and 2.5 ($p < 0.05$) for 5-HT and ACh respectively. From Daffonchio *et al.* (1989).

there is general consensus that the two phenomena are associated, a firm causal relationship has yet to be clearly established (Payne and Cheng, 1990; Simpson *et al.*, 1991). Indeed, in man airway inflammation can be evident without co-existing BHR (Gibson *et al.*, 1989). Furthermore, it is important to note that while BHR is more commonly associated with the late response, it can occur soon after the early response, in both animal models (Fig. 2.2) and man (Durham *et al.*, 1988). Thus BHR may contribute to, rather than be a resultant of, the late response.

2.3 Use of Animal Models for Drug Evaluation

As noted previously, sensitized guinea-pigs are a popular laboratory model of allergic asthma, and rightly or wrongly have been used extensively in the pre-clinical evaluation of new anti-asthma drugs.

By example, the effects of a series of hydroxamic acid 5-LO inhibitors (e.g. BW A4C) developed at the Wellcome Research Laboratories have been investigated in a pharmacologically constrained variant of this model (Fig. 2.3). By pre-treatment with an anti-histamine (mepyramine) and a

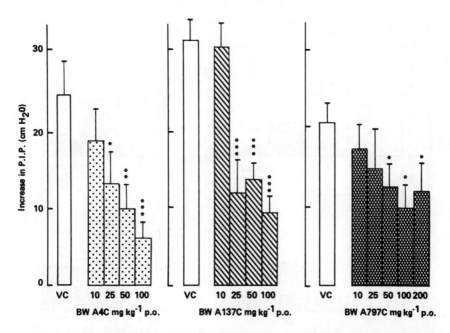

Fig. 2.3 Effect of hydroxamic acid 5-LO inhibitors of leukotriene biosynthesis on 'leukotriene-dependent' anaphylactic bronchospasm in anaesthetized pump-ventilated sensitized guinea-pigs. Each compound was given orally 1 h prior to challenge with antigen (ovalbumin) aerosol. Columns represent the mean increase in pulmonary inflation pressure (PIP) and vertical bars s.e. mean; *, $p < 0.05$; **, $p < 0.01$; ***, $p < 0.005$ versus vehicle (polyethylene glycol) control (VC); $n = 6–8$. From Payne et al. (1988).

cyclooxygenase inhibitor (indomethacin) the anaphylactic response to inhaled antigen is 'leukotriene (products of the 5-LO pathway)-dependent' (Payne et al., 1988).

The degree of inhibition of 'leukotriene-dependent' bronchospasm by these compounds was of the same order as that obtained with a leukotriene-receptor antagonist (FPL 55712). As leukotrienes may be important mediators of human asthma (Lewis, 1985) 5-LO inhibitors such as these have obvious clinical potential. Follow-up compounds to BW A4C, such as BW B70C (a hydroxyurea), with a longer duration of action were similarly tested in comparison with a related hydroxyurea A64077.

Figure 2.4 shows that, when administered orally to conscious animals at doses of 2–50 mg kg^{-1}, BW B70C and its separate enantiomers BW B70C (R) and BW B70C (S) each strongly inhibited 'leukotriene-dependent' bronchospasm when the animals were anaesthetized and challenged with antigen aerosol 6 h later. Furthermore, both BW B70C (R,S) and BW B70C (S) were more potent than A64077. It still remains to be determined, however, whether these and/or other 5-LO inhibitors have real therapeutic value in clinical asthma (Hui et al., 1990).

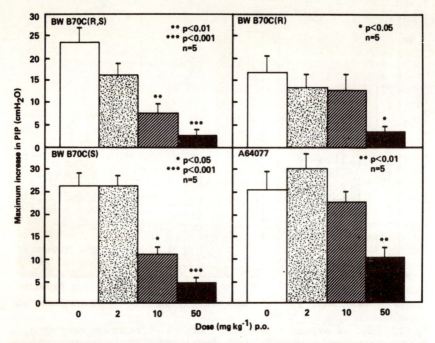

Fig. 2.4   Effect of hydroxyurea 5-LO inhibitors on 'leukotriene-dependent' anaphylactic bronchospasm in anaesthetized pump-ventilated sensitized guinea-pigs. Columns represent the mean increase in pulmonary inflation pressure (PIP) and vertical bars s.e. mean, n and p values as indicated.

For reviews of the profiling of other classes of potential anti-asthmatic drugs in animal models see Payne *et al.* (1989) and Smith (1989).

2.4 Conclusions

No animal model at present available shows all of the features characteristic of clinical asthma; in particular, most lack the element of chronicity. Hence the predictive value of animal models of asthma can only be established retrospectively.

In the final analysis, the true usefulness of a model should be judged on how well it answers the specific question it is being asked to answer, rather than how well it mimics the human disease. The recent development of transgenic animal models of human diseases (First and Haseltine, 1991), yet to be applied in regards to asthma, may open up new opportunities in this respect.

References

Abraham, W. M., Delehunt, J. C., Yerger, L. and Marchette, B. (1983). Characterization of a late phase pulmonary response after antigen challenge in allergic sheep. *Am. Rev. Respir. Dis.*, **128**, 839–44.

Albelda, S. M. (1991). Endothelial and epithelial cell adhesion molecules. *Am. J. Respir. Cell Mol. Biol.*, **4**, 195–203.

Daffonchio, L., Payne, A. N., Lees, I. W. and Whittle, B. J. R. (1989). Airway hyperreactivity follows anaphylactic microshock in anaesthetized guinea-pigs. *Eur. J. Pharmacol.*, **161**, 135–42.

Durham, S. R., Craddock, C. F., Cookson, W. O. and Berson, M. K. (1988). Increases in airway responsiveness to histamine precede allergen-induced late asthmatic responses. *J. Allergy Clin. Immunol.*, **82**, 764–70.

First, N. and Haseltine, F. P. (eds.) (1991). *Transgenic Animals*, Butterworth–Heineman, Boston, MA.

Fitzgerald, M. F. and Whittle, B. J. R. (1989). The involvement of inflammation in airway responsiveness. In Vane, J. R. and Higgs, G. A. (eds.), *Asthma: Basic Mechanisms and Therapeutic Perspectives*, Pythagora Press, Rome, 103–26.

Friday, G. A. and Fireman, P. (1988). Morbidity and mortality of asthma. *Pediatric Allergic Dis.*, **35**, 1149–62.

Gaddy, J., McCreedy, W., Margolskee, D., Williams, V. and Busse, W. (1991). A potent leukotriene D_4 (LTD_4) antagonist (MK-571) significantly reduces airway obstruction in mild to moderate asthma. *J. Allergy Clin. Immunol.*, **87**, 308.

Gibson, P. G., Dolovich, J., Denburg, J., Ramsdale, E. H. and Hargreave, F. E. (1989). Chronic cough: eosinophilic bronchitis without asthma. *Lancet*, **I**, 1346–8.

Gundel, R. H., Desai, S., Torcellini, C. C., Clarke, C. C., Honon, C. A., Letts, L. G. and Wegner, C. D. (1991). The PAF receptor antagonist WEB-2170 inhibits antigen-induced mediator release and late-phase bronchoconstriction in primates. *J. Allergy Clin. Immunol.*, **87**, 308.

Howarth, P. H., and Holgate, S. T. (1985). Astemizole, an H_1 antagonist in allergic asthma. *J. Allergy Clin. Immunol.*, **75**, 1–16.

Hui, K. P., Taylor, I. K., Barnes, N. C. and Barnes, P. J. (1990). Effect of a 5-lipoxygenase inhibitor, A64077 on allergen induced early and late asthmatic responses. *Am. Rev. Respir. Dis.*, **141**, A32.

Hutson, P. A., Church, M. K., Clay, T. P., Miller, P. and Holgate, S. T. (1988). Early and late-phase bronchoconstriction after allergen challenge of nonaesthetized guinea-pigs. *Am. Rev. Respir. Dis.*, **137**, 548–57.

Kallos, P. and Kallos, L. (1984). Experimental asthma in guinea-pigs revisited. *Int. Arch. Allergy Appl. Immunol.*, **73**, 77–85.

Larsson, S. (1990). Long term studies on long acting sympathomimetics. *Lung*, **168**, S22–S24.

Lewis, R. A. (1985). A presumptive role for leukotrienes in obstructive airway disease. *Chest*, **88**, 98s–102s.

McFarlane, C. S., Hamel, R. and Ford-Huchinson, A. W. (1987). Effect of a 5-lipoxygenase inhibitor (L-651,392) on primary and late pulmonary response to ascaris antigen in the squirrel monkey. *Agents Actions*, **22**, 63–8.

O'Byrne, P. M. (1986). Airway inflammation and airway hyperresponsiveness. *Chest*, **90**, 575–7.

O'Byrne, P. M., Dolovich, J. and Hargreave, F. E. (1987). Late asthmatic responses. *Am. Rev. Respir. Dis.*, **136**, 740–51.

O'Donnell, M. and Payne, A. N. (1991). Therapeutic approaches to reduce airway inflammation. In Ackerman, N. R., Bonney, R. J. and Welton, A. F. (eds.),

Progress in Inflammation Research and Therapy. Agents and Action, Supplements, **35**, 151–8.

Ogunbiyi, P. O. and Eyre, P. (1985). Pharmacological studies of pulmonary anaphylaxis *in vitro*. *Agents Actions*, **17**, 158–74.

Payne, A. N. (1989). Pharmacological prevention of bronchospasm. In Vane, J. R. and Higgs, G. A. (eds.), *Asthma: Basic Mechanisms and Therapeutic Perspectives*, Pythagora Press, Rome, 151–82.

Payne, A. N. and Cheng, J. B. (1990). PMNs and airway inflammation/hyperreactivity. *Agents Actions*, **29**, 181–3.

Payne, A. N. and de Nucci, G. (1987). Anaphylaxis in guinea-pigs induced by ovalbumin aerosol: *in vivo* and *in vitro* methods. *J. Pharm. Methods*, **17**, 83–90.

Payne, A. N., Garland, L. G., Lees, I. W. and Salmon, I. A. (1988). Selective inhibition of arachidonate 5-lipoxygenase by novel acetohydroxamic acids: effects on bronchial anaphylaxis in anaesthetized guinea-pigs. *Br. J. Pharmacol.*, **94**, 540–6.

Payne, A. N., de Nucci, G. and Pettipher, E. R. (1989). Experimental models of pulmonary and joint inflammation and their relevance to man. In Church, M. and Robinson, C. (eds.), *Eicosanoids in Inflammatory Conditions of the Lung, Skin and Joints*, MTP Press, Lancaster, 191–216.

Shampain, M. P., Behrens, B. L., Larsen, G. L. and Henson, P. M. (1982). An animal model of late pulmonary responses to Alternaria challenge. *Am. Rev. Respir. Dis.*, **126**, 493–8.

Sheppard, D. (1989). Airway hyperresponsiveness: mechanism in experimental models. *Chest*, **96**, 1165–8.

Simpson, J. F., Butterfield, M. J., Lefferts, P. L., Dyer, E. L., Snapper, J. R. and Meyrick, B. (1991). Role of pulmonary inflammation in altered airway responsiveness in three sheep models of acute lung injury. *Am. Rev. Respir. Dis.*, **143**, 585–589.

Smith, H. (1989). Animal models of asthma. *Pulm. Pharmacol.*, **2**, 59–74.

Wegner, C. D., Gundel, R. H., Reilly, P., Haynes, N., Letts, L. G. and Rothlein, R. (1990). Intercellular adhesion molecules (ICAM-1) in the pathogenesis of asthma. *Science*, **247**, 456–9.

Withnall, M. T. and De Brito, F. B. (1990). Asthma as an inflammatory disease: are animal models relevant? *Agents Actions*, **31**, 36–8.

Woolcock, A. J. (1988). Asthma—what are the important experiments? *Am. Rev. Respir. Dis.*, **138**, 730–4.

3

The Rat as Experimental Model of Airway Hyperresponsiveness

R. Pauwels, G. Joos and J. Kips

Abstract

The mechanisms involved in acute airway narrowing depend on the agonist. Some agonists act mainly on airway smooth muscle cells, while others activate different cell types including neurons and inflammatory cells. The rat, with the many inbred strains available, offers the possibility of investigating the mechanisms involved in the acute airway narrowing and the genetic influences on airway responsiveness. Both direct and indirect airway responsiveness are controlled by genetic factors. Exposure to aerosolized endotoxin increases non-specific airway responsiveness. This increase is not related to the influx of neutrophils but can, at least partially, be explained by the local secretion of tumour necrosis factor. The inhalation of human rTNF induces airway hyperresponsiveness.

A single exposure to aerosolized antigen in sensitized rats causes an increase in airway responsiveness but chronic antigen inhalation is not followed by a further increase. Both the endotoxin and the inhaled antigen model suggest the existence of a mechanism that prevents further increase in airway responsiveness in the rat.

3.1 Introduction

These studies were performed using inbred rat strains, i.e. each strain represents a very homogeneous genetic background and significant differences between inbred strains are therefore suggestive of a genetic control of the characteristic that is found to be different between strains (Hedrich, 1990). Further evidence can then be derived from breeding studies. We have chosen the rat as an animal model because the immunological system of this species is rather well defined, including the availability of monoclonal antibodies to the different immunoglobulin classes and subclasses, and because the size of the animal allows reproducible measurements of airway and lung function. The gestation period is sufficiently short to allow breeding studies for the investigation of genetic influences.

3.2 Non-allergenic Airway Responsiveness

In our *in vivo* rat model, we have observed bronchoconstrictor reactions to various agonists, including 5-hydroxytryptamine (5HT), carbachol, adenosine and tachykinins. The rat airways are almost non-reactive to histamine, PAF and leukotriene D4. We observed an important genetic influence on airway responsiveness to these different agonists (Pauwels *et al.*, 1985).

5HT is in the rat the major bronchoconstrictory mediator released from mast cells and acts mainly directly on the airway smooth muscle. We found significant differences in airway responsiveness to 5HT in inbred rat strains (Pauwels *et al.*, 1985). By crossing a low responder strain with a high responder strain and back-crossing the F1 hybrids with the parental strains we could demonstrate that the inheritance of 5HT-airway responsiveness follows the mendelian laws, high responsiveness being recessive. *In vitro* studies have confirmed the significant difference between inbred rat strains in the responsiveness of airway smooth muscle (Badier *et al.*, 1988). Carbachol, a muscarinic agonist, causes also bronchoconstriction in the rat by a direct action on airway smooth muscle. Inbred rat strains differ significantly in their airway responsiveness to carbachol, but we found no relationship between airway responsiveness to 5HT and to carbachol in the rat strains that we have studied.

Many of the bronchoconstrictor stimuli that cause an acute bronchoconstriction in asthma do not act directly on the airway smooth muscle but cause airway narrowing through activation of local or central nervous reflexes. Both purines such as adenosine and neuropeptides such as neurokinin A and substance P are thought to play a role in the neurally mediated airway narrowing. In studying the acute effect of adenosine on the airway calibre of rats, we again observed significant differences in airway respon-

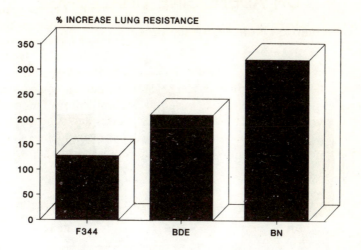

Fig. 3.1   Mean increase in total lung resistance in three different inbred rat strains ($n = 12$ for each strain), following intravenous challenge with 0.1 μmol NECA (5'-N-ethyl-carboxamido-adenosine).

siveness to adenosine between various inbred rat strains (Fig. 3.1) (Pauwels and Van Der Straeten, 1987). We also found significant differences in airway responsiveness to tachykinins such as substance P and neurokinin A between inbred rat strains (Joos *et al.*, 1986). However, no relationship was observed between the responsiveness to adenosine and to neuropeptides in the different inbred rat strains that were tested. This lack of relationship can be explained by the observation that the mechanisms of adenosine- and neuropeptide-induced bronchoconstriction differ between inbred rat strains as will be documented in the following experiments.

We have used the rat model for further investigation of the mechanisms involved in the neuropeptide- and adenosine-induced airway narrowing. We used the anaesthetized, ventilated rat and challenged the animals intravenously. Total lung resistance was measured to monitor airway calibre and immediately following challenge we performed bronchoalveolar lavage. We measured 5HT or histamine in the supernatant of the lavage fluid. Both mediators are present in rat mast cells and released upon cell activation. The airway smooth muscle of rats, however, does not have histamine receptors so that 5HT is the main bronchoconstrictor mast cell mediator.

We performed challenge studies with neurokinin A (NKA) and adenosine (5'-N-ethoxycarboxy-adenosine or NECA) and investigated the pro-

PROTECTIVE EFFECT OF VARIOUS DRUGS ON ADENOSINE CHALLENGE

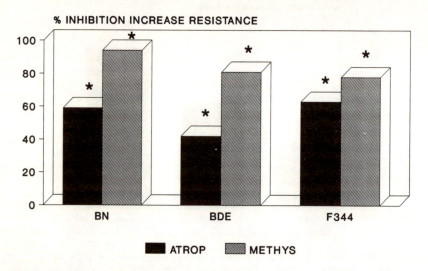

STRAIN DIFFERENCES

Fig. 3.2 Protective effect of atropine (atrop) (10 mg/kg) and methysergide (methys) (1 mg/kg) on the bronchoconstriction induced by challenge with NECA ($n = 9$ per group).

tective effect of atropine, a specific muscarinic receptor antagonist, and of methysergide, a 5HT-antagonist, in three inbred strains: BN, F344 and BDE. Methysergide inhibited in all strains the adenosine-induced bronchoconstriction, suggesting that mast cell activation and 5HT release was responsible for part of the adenosine-induced bronchoconstriction. Similarly, atropine significantly inhibited the adenosine-induced bronchoconstriction (Fig. 3.2). Further experiments proved indeed that adenosine activates postganglionic vagal nerve endings. Methysergide and atropine also significantly inhibited the adenosine-induced release of mast cell mediators in the airways, demonstrating that adenosine induces in the airways the release of mast cell mediators and that this release is further enhanced by the released 5HT and by the simultaneously released acetylcholine. The released mast cell mediator and neurotransmitter have a positive feedback effect on mast cell mediator release.

The picture is still more complex for the NKA-induced bronchoconstriction (Fig. 3.3). The effect of NKA in F344 rats is comparable with the adenosine-induced activation: simultaneous activation of mast cells and postganglionic nerve endings and positive feedback on mediators release.

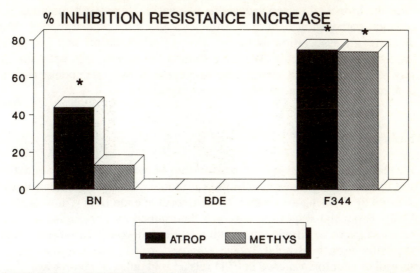

EFFECT OF VARIOUS DRUGS ON NEUROKININ A CHALLENGE

STRAIN DIFFERENCES

Fig. 3.3 Protective effect of atropine (atrop) (10 mg/kg) and methysergide (methys) (1 mg/kg) on the bronchoconstriction induced by challenge with NKA ($n = 9$ per group).

The NKA-induced bronchoconstriction in BDE rats is not influenced by either methysergide or atropine, suggesting that NKA acts directly on the airway smooth muscle of this strain. The bronchoconstriction induced by NKA in BN rats is partially inhibited by atropine but not by methysergide.

3.3 Airway Inflammation and Airway Hyperresponsiveness

It is now generally accepted that airway inflammation may play an important role in the pathogenesis of asthma and we have been particularly interested in the interaction between airway inflammation and non-allergic or non-specific airway responsiveness. Non-specific bronchial responsiveness in an individual is not invariable and various exogenous factors have been shown to modify the non-specific bronchial responsiveness and there is strong evidence that the changes in airway responsiveness are related to the presence of airway inflammation. The role of inflammation in the pathogenesis of bronchial hyperresponsiveness is suggested by the following observations:

factors known to increase bronchial responsiveness such as viral infections, exposure to air pollutants, allergens or occupational agents are known to induce airway inflammation; steroids, potent anti-inflammatory agents reduce the bronchial responsiveness in asthmatics; airway inflammation is a common pathological feature in asthmatics and some animal models demonstrate an association between airway inflammation and increased bronchial responsiveness. We have studied the relationship between airway inflammation and airway responsiveness in two rat models: the endotoxin model and the chronic antigen exposure model.

Endotoxin Model

We therefore investigated the relationship between airway inflammation and bronchial responsiveness in the rat model. Airway inflammation was induced by exposing the animals to an aerosol of endotoxin (Pauwels *et al.*, 1990). Bronchial responsiveness was determined by performing a dose–response curve to intravenous or inhaled bronchoconstrictor agents. Subsequently bronchoalveolar lavage was performed. The exposure to an aerosol of endotoxin caused in F344 rats a rapid influx of neutrophils in the airways. The neutrophils persisted up to 24 h after exposure. The exposure to the endotoxin aerosol was followed, 1–2 h later, by a significant increase in the airway responsiveness to 5HT. However, the increase in responsiveness disappeared and 9–12 h following the end of the exposure a significant decrease in airway 5HT-responsiveness was observed at a moment that more than 80% of the cells contained in the bronchoalveolar fluid were neutrophils. The hyperresponsiveness, observed 1–2 h after endotoxin exposure, was non-specific since a similar increase in airway responsiveness to carbachol, adenosine, NKA and vagal stimulation was observed.

We also compared the effect of endotoxin inhalation in five different inbred rat strains. The aerosol exposure induced in all five strains a comparable neutrophil influx in the airways but only four of the five strains became hyperresponsive to 5HT, 90 min after the end of the endotoxin exposure (Fig. 3.4). It was therefore obvious that there was no absolute relationship between the presence of neutrophils in the airways and changes in airway responsiveness.

The mechanisms involved in the endotoxin-induced airway responsiveness were further investigated in a serious of pharmacological experiments. Various pharmacological agents were administered before the exposure to endotoxin and their effects on airway inflammation and airway responsiveness were assessed. Methylprednisolone, indomethacine and theophylline significantly inhibited the endotoxin-induced increase in airway responsiveness. Theophylline also partially inhibited the influx of neutrophils in the airways. Pretreatment with cromoglycate, nedocromil, ketotifen, terbuta-

ENDOTOXIN AND AIRWAY RESPONSIVENESS STRAIN DIFFERENCES

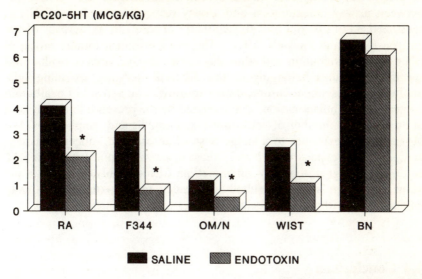

Fig. 3.4   Bronchial responsiveness to 5HT in different rat strains ($n = 9$ for each group), 90 min following exposure to either saline or endotoxin (100 µg/ml).

line or the PAF antagonist WEB 2086 had no significant influence on the increase in airway responsiveness following endotoxin exposure (Kips and Pauwels, in press).

Endotoxin is known to induce the secretion of various proinflammatory and inflammatory mediators. We therefore investigate the role of TNF-α in the endotoxin-induced increase in airway responsiveness and airway inflammation (Kips *et al.*, 1991). The exposure of rats to endotoxin aerosol induced a secretion of TNF into their airways. Pretreatment of rats with rabbit polyclonal anti-human TNF significantly inhibited the endotoxin-induced increase in airway responsiveness and also partially inhibited the influx of neutrophils into the airways. Exposure of rats to an aerosol of recombinant human TNF increased their airway responsiveness to 5HT. A significant shift of the dose–response curve to the left was observed. We therefore conclude that TNF is at least partially responsible for the endotoxin-induced increase in airway responsiveness.

Antigen Model

A second rat model that we have used to investigate the relationship between airway inflammation and airway responsiveness is the BN rat, sensitized to ovalbumin and subsequently exposed to an aerosol of the antigen (Kips and Pauwels, 1991). The intraperitoneal immunization of BN rats with ovalbumin and adjuvants causes the synthesis of ovalbumin-specific antibodies belonging to the different isotypes, including IgE-antibodies. Subsequent chronic daily exposure to an aerosol of ovalbumin induces airway inflammation, characterized by the presence in the airways of an increased number of neutrophils, eosinophils and lymphocytes. We observed that exposure to a single dose of aerosolized antigen is associated, 24 h after exposure, with an increase in airway responsiveness to 5HT and a minor degree of airway inflammation. Chronic daily exposure to the same ovalbumin aerosol resulted in a much more pronounced airway inflammation without an associated change in airway responsiveness.

3.4 Conclusions

Inflammatory mechanisms are thought to play a major role in the pathogenesis of asthma. Experimental studies in the rat demonstrate that inflammation is involved in the acute airway narrowing following challenge with adenosine and tachykinins, possible neurotransmitters of the non-adrenergic, non-cholinergic autonomic nervous system in the airways. The endotoxin model suggests that local production and secretion of TNF in the airways may contribute to the increase in airway responsiveness associated with airway inflammation. The antigen model proves that the relationship between chronic airway inflammation and increase in airway responsiveness is certainly not simple and that further physiopathological and pharmacological studies will be needed for a better understanding of the complex interaction of inflammatory mechanisms and airway responsiveness.

References

Badier, M., Soler, M., Mallea, M., Delpierre, S. and Orehek, J. (1988). Cholinergic responsiveness of respiratory and vascular tissues in two different rat strains. *J. Appl. Physiol.*, **64**, 323–8.

Hedrich, H. J. (ed.) (1990). *Genetic Monitoring of Inbred Strains of Rats*, Gustav Fischer, Stuttgart, 1–539.

Joos, G., Kips, J., Pauwels, R. and Van Der Straeten, M. (1986). The effect of tachykinins on the conducting airways of the rat. *Arch. Int. Pharmacodyn.*, Suppl., 176–90.

Kips, J. and Pauwels, R. (1991). In press.

Kips, J., Tavernier, J. and Pauwels, R. (1992). The rat as experimental model of airway hyperresponsiveness. *Am. Rev. Respir. Dis.*, **145**, 332–6.

Pauwels, R. and Van Der Straeten, M. (1987). An animal model for adenosine-induced bronchoconstriction. *Am. Rev. Respir. Dis.*, **136**, 374–8.

Pauwels, R., Van Der Straeten, M., Weyne, J. and Bazin, H. (1985). Genetic factors in non-specific bronchial reactivity in rats. *Eur. J. Respir. Dis.*, **66**, 98–104.

Pauwels, R., Kips, J., Peleman, R. and Van Der Straeten, M. (1990). The effect of endotoxin inhalation on airway responsiveness and cellular influx in rats. *Am. Rev. Respir. Dis.*, **141**, 540–5.

4

Allergen-induced Airway Changes in Conscious Guinea Pigs

J. G. Varley, M.-C. Seminario, M. G. Campos and M. K. Church

4.1 Introduction

Experimentally induced early and late asthmatic responses (EAR and LAR) are considered useful tools in the elucidation of the pathogenesis of asthma. Indeed, several features of the experimentally induced LAR have led researchers to suggest that this phase of the allergic response is analogous to chronic asthma for which patients seek medical advice (Gleich, 1982). First, the airway obstruction during the LAR may be more prolonged and severe than that associated with the EAR (Hargreave, 1989). Second, glucocorticosteroids, which reduce the chronic bronchial inflammation associated with asthma, reduce the LAR, whilst the $\beta2$-adrenoceptor stimulants, which do not affect the underlying inflammatory state, have little effect on the LAR. The converse is so for the EAR where $\beta2$-adrenoceptor stimulants, but not glucocorticosteroids, are effective (Barnes, 1989). Third, the pattern of bronchial oedema, inflammatory cell infiltration into the airways and the neutrophil-rich mucus within the airway during the LAR are all reminiscent of clinical asthma. Fourth, the airway reactivity to non-specific bronchial provocation is enhanced for possibly prolonged periods following allergen challenge of sufficient severity to induce an LAR. The presence of such hyperreactivity may explain the link between the frequency of asthma attacks and the incidence of the LAR (Warner, 1976).

In order to understand more fully the mechanisms underlying allergic

36

lung disease, animal models have been developed. Initially, these could only model early phase responses by assessing airways function in anaesthetized animals following intravenous or inhalation challenge with allergen. More recently these models have become more sophisticated using conscious animals and extending the measurements to include late phase airways changes. However, such developments have met with variable success, particularly in terms of reproducibility and the presence of LPR. It is now clear that, within any given species, the outcome of provocation will depend on the strain and age of the animal, sensitization regime, challenge route, aerosol particle size, duration of exposure and method of respiratory measurement. We have tried to minimize the effect of some of these variables by automating the airways function measuring equipment, redesigning the plethysmograph, and introducing allergen directly onto the airways through an endotracheal tube.

During the mid to late 1980s, a guinea pig model of allergic airways disease was investigated by our group (Hutson *et al.*, 1988), in which conscious free breathing guinea pigs were sensitized and challenged to inhaled aerosolized ovalbumin (OA). Measurement of airways function by whole body plethysmography resulted in airway calibre changes consistent with the presence of an early phase reaction (EPR), late phase reaction (LPR) and a second late LPR. The time scales were different to those seen with humans, the EPR peaking at 2 h, the LPR at 17–24 h and the later LPR at 72 h after challenge (Hutson *et al.*, 1988).

The pathological appearance of the guinea pig lungs is consistent with the pattern of chronic eosinophilia seen in the LAR in human asthma (DeMonchy *et al.*, 1985). Cellular infiltration into the tissues surrounding the airways following aerosol challenge in systematically sensitized guinea pigs is evident within 8 min with the appearance of granulocytes in the blood vessels surrounding the airways (Dunn *et al.*, 1988). The cells were drawn through the submucosa and mucosa towards the lumen of the airway until granulocytes were evident in mucus plugs within the airways. Quantitation of eosinophilic infiltration in tissues surrounding the major bronchi revealed that there was a single broad peak between 17 and 48 h after challenge (Frew *et al.*, 1990). The presence of a granulocytic infiltration into the airway lumen, quantified by histology of cells recovered by bronchoalveolar lavage, showed neutrophil numbers to reach a maximum at 17 h whereas eosinophil numbers continued to increase for up to 72 h after challenge (Hutson *et al.*, 1988). Subsequently, reports have shown different responses (Frew *et al.*, 1990; Walls *et al.*, 1991). In addition, we have demonstrated an infiltration into the airways of T lymphocytes (Frew *et al.*, 1990), cells which have been suggested as orchestrators of allergic inflammation (Walker *et al.*, 1991). Allergen inhalation led to an elevation of T lymphocyte numbers in both the bronchial mucosa and adventitia, but interestingly not in the bronchial lumen. Subset analysis of these cells revealed them to be CD8 negative (a putative T helper subset) (Frew *et al.*, 1990). The observation that T lymphocyte numbers changed little in the guinea pig airway lumen is in keeping with human studies where T lymphocytes are thought to enter the tissues from the lumen following allergen challenge, presumably responding to the increased expression of adhesion proteins and chemoattractants (Smith *et al.*, 1991). Investigation of the guinea pig airway epithelium by electron microscopy revealed the discharge of goblet cells and evidence of oedema after allergen challenge. However, other changes were not regularly observed particularly in the more distal airways. While these changes are indicative of an allergen-induced airways response, it soon became evident that they were variable both in their magnitude and, on occasions, by their presence or absence. For a model of airways responsiveness to allergen challenge to be useful either for the study of mechanisms of airway inflammation or for the assessment of drug modulation of the response, it must be readily reproducible. From our own data, using standard statistical criteria for accepting changes from baseline airways resistance in guinea pigs sensitized and challenged as previously described (Hutson *et al.*, 1988), the incidences of EPR, LPR and EPR + LPR were 14%, 27% and 12% respectively. This is in agreement with Johns *et al.* (1990) who detected an LPR in 28% of guinea pigs sensitized and challenged by the same method although using a different method of measurement. As a consequence we have had to redesign our guinea pig model in order to fulfil the requirements of reproducible allergen-induced changes.

4.2 Development of Automated Plethysmography

Two aspects of the manual plethysmograph used in the studies of Hutson *et al.* (1988) and Frew *et al.* (1990) were regarded by us to need attention. These were the design of the nose cone which isolates the nares of the animal from the rest of the plethysmograph and the manual method for calculating airways parameters. The nose cone used by Hutson *et al.* (1988) was essentially a cone-shaped funnel narrowing to a tube onto which could be fitted the pneumotachograph. Inside this funnel was fitted an inflatable rubber membrane which effected the seal with the nares. There were two major problems with this. First, the circular cross-section formed an incomplete seal even when inflated to a high pressure. This resulted in an overestimation in thoracic gas volume (TGV). Second, the high pressure on the nose area stimulated reflexes which influenced breathing patterns, usually in an inhibitory manner. As a consequence, we redesigned the nose mask by using casts of guinea pig heads. In addition, use of lubricating gel on the fur of the nose in conjunction with a larger seal area allowed a low pressure seal to be made which was much more effective than the high pressure one. This single change resulted in the estimate of TGV being reduced from 25 ml to 13 ml for guinea pigs of the 700–750 g range. Other changes made to the plethysmograph to increase the ease of handling of, and to reduce stress to, the animals included supporting tray, fresh air to the nose, adjustible collar and a lower resistance pneumotachograph.

The second major change in the plethysmograph was its automation. Computer-controlled valves replaced manual clamping of tubes to seal the plethysmograph and to activate the shutter at the airway opening. The manual system of calculating airway function from a chart recorder was subject to a variety of problems. The peak-to-peak measurements which this method necessitated meant that calculations were subject to 'temperature–humidity' artifacts (Agrawal, 1981) and potential problems with difference in phase between the signals generated by the guinea pig. Furthermore, the measurement of such charts was tedious, time consuming and subject to operator error or bias. A more traditional approach for airways resistance measurement would be to measure the slope subtended by the plethysmograph pressure and airway flow signals at zero flow from an oscilloscope. However, variation in the ability of different operators to interpret slopes derived from humans has been reported (Lord, 1977). The new program incorporated a different approach to signal analysis by measuring the maximum differentials of each individual signal (Lorino *et al.*, 1980) and applied these to the equations described originally by Dubois *et al.* (1956a, b), in effect abolishing the effect of temperature–humidity artifact and phase differences (Varley *et al.*, 1991a). This is an adaptation of a method which has been used in our clinical laboratories for the past 10 years (Shah *et al.*, 1980). The reproducibility of the new computer method has been compared simultaneously with our initial chart method (Hutson *et al.*, 1988) and our modification of this method (Frew *et al.*, 1990), using equations originally described by Dubois *et al.* (1956a, b). Four measurements of airways resistance (Raw), TGV and specific airways conductance (sGaw) derived by the three methods were taken at each of four time points during one day. From these data the overall coefficient of variation (CV%) was calculated as a measure of 'within guinea pig' reproducibility. The results (Table 4.1) show that the computer-derived Raw and sGaw are significantly more reproducible than those derived from the other two methods (Varley *et al.*, 1991b).

To investigate whether the new automated system is more sensitive to changes in airway calibre, the three methods of signal analysis were compared following allergen challenge. Guinea pigs were sensitized by intraperitoneal injection to ovalbumin (Andersson, 1980). They were challenged 14 days later with aerosolized ovalbumin (2% w/v, 0.9% saline) for 5 min. Specific airways conductance changes were followed for up to 6 h (Fig. 4.1). The results show that the computer method is more sensitive in

Table 4.1 Comparison of values of coefficient of variation for assessing within guinea pig variation for airways resistance, thoracic gas volume and specific airways conductance by different methods of signal analysis

Method	n	TGV	Raw	sGaw
Computer	4	4.5 (2.8–7.7)	8.1 (4.8–12.2)	8.3 (3.9–12.3)
Chart	4	6.4 (3.1–15.3)	11.6 (6.0–15.1)	9.2 (5.3–14.2)
Hutson	4	6.4 (3.1–15.3)	13.2 (9.6–18.9)	11.0 (8.0–18.5)

Values are median coefficient of variation (CV%) with range. Raw, airways resistance; TGV, thoracic gas volume; sGaw, specific airways conductance. Data from 10 guinea pigs with n repeats per time point.

specific airways conductance (sGaw)

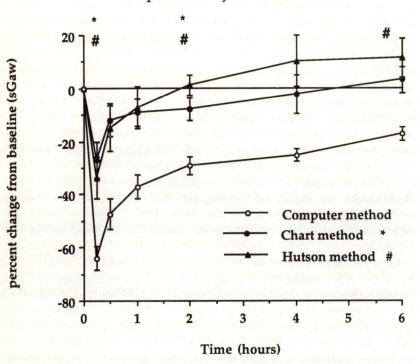

Fig. 4.1 Comparison of the ability of three different methods to detect change in guinea pig airways calibre (specific airways conductance, sGaw) with time after aerosol allergen challenge. 'Computer' method (○), modified 'chart' method (●) and 'Hutson chart' method (▲). Mean ± SEM, n = 11. Tested at the times indicated, statistically significant differences between the 'computer' method and modified chart method (*) and Hutson chart method (#) are thus marked.

picking up changes at 15 min, the earliest time point assessed. Similar results were seen at 2 h (Varley *et al.*, 1991b). Hence computerization of the guinea pig plethysmograph increased reproducibility and sensitivity in addition to removing artifacts and possible bias.

4.3 Aerosol Distribution in the Airway

The inhaled route of allergen delivery is the most applicable to animal models of allergic airways disease as it is the route of allergen penetration into the airways in asthma. However, in man, allergen may gain access to the lung particularly when breathing through the mouth when the nasal filtration and humidification systems are bypassed. This is not possible in the majority of small animals including guinea pigs because they are obligate nose breathers. Furthermore, the nose is an extremely efficient filter, as demonstrated by the studies of Raabe *et al.* (1988) in which it was shown that a particle size of less than 1 μm was able to pass through the nose and deposit in the lower airways. An increase in particle size led to an increased retention in the nasal passages.

To assess the relative deposition of particles within the lungs and nose of our guinea pigs, we generated a radio-aerosol of DTPA Tc-99m with mass median diameter (MMD) of 1.5 μm using a Wright nebulizer and settling chamber. This was inhaled by free-breathing guinea pigs restrained in the plethysmograph to prevent environmental contamination. Aerosol distribution and activity were measured with a gamma camera and analysed with a VAX computer. 30% of the aerosol delivered to the animal was retained in the airways, of which 80% was deposited in the nose and 12% in the lungs (Varley *et al.*, 1991c). Even less lung deposition would have been expected with the aerosol of 4 μm MMD used by Hutson *et al.* (1988). These results may explain the weak and inconsistent changes seen by electron microscopic examination of the airways.

There are two ways to overcome the problem of nasal deposition. The first is to generate particles of less than 0.5 μm which are able to pass through the nose. This is difficult, expensive and still results in some nasal deposition. The second way is to deliver the aerosol directly to the lower airways by bypassing the upper airways following endotracheal intubation. We have adopted this latter system in which animals are sedated with Hypnorm (Janssen, UK), anaesthetized with Metofane (C-Vet, UK) and a 12G cannula (Angiocath, Becton Dickinson, UK) is introduced through the mouth into the trachea with the aid of a modified laryngoscope and introducer. When they have recovered from the anaesthetic, but are still sedated, the animals are exposed to the aerosol. Following exposure, the tube is removed and the mildly sedated animals are returned to the cage or placed in the plethysmograph for airways function measurements. Analysis of aerosol distribution using this system revealed that 7% of the aerosol delivered to the guinea pig was retained in the airways of which 88% was in the lungs with the remainder in the trachea or on the fur around the nose (Varley *et al.*, 1991c).

4.4 Airways Function Tests and Pathology

To assess the effect of the new plethysmograph and, in particular, aerosol delivery via the endotracheal tube we have performed sensitization and challenge experiments using a protocol similar to that described by Hutson *et al.* (1988). Briefly, guinea pigs of 450–500 g were sensitized by exposure to a 1% aerosol of ovalbumin inhaled through the endotracheal (ET) tube for 3 min on two occasions one week apart. Seven days later, they were similarly exposed to a 2% ovalbumin aerosol for 5 min while under cover of mepyramine maleate, 10 mg/kg given intraperitoneally.

Changes in sGaw, derived from data previously described (Seminario *et al.*, 1991), showed that the early response was maximal at the first time point of measurement, 15 min (Fig. 4.2) rather than at 2 h as described previously. Furthermore, the magnitude of the response was greater than when a similar aerosol was inhaled through the nose as was the case with the experiments of Hutson *et al.* (1988). The fall in sGaw decayed rapidly over the following 2 h, returning to baseline by 6 h (Fig. 4.2). There was no evidence of LPRs seen at 17 or 72 h suggesting there to be no discrete LPR with this sensitization and challenge protocol.

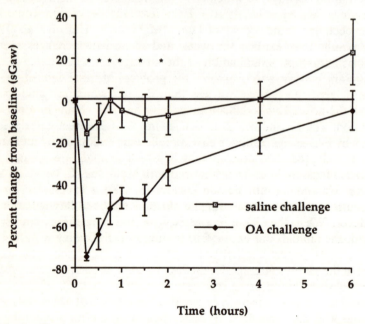

specific airways conductance (sGaw)

Fig. 4.2 Specific airways conductance (sGaw) changes with time in guinea pigs after sensitization and challenge with either aerosol allergen (◆) or saline (□) breathed through an endotracheal tube. Mean ± SEM, $n = 22$–8. Statistically significant differences between the allergen and saline group are denoted by (*).

The nose may represent the largest resistance component within the airways (Amdur and Mead, 1958; Holroyde and Norris, 1988) and is a major contributor to the allergen-induced alteration in airways resistance in rats (Bellofiore *et al.*, 1987) and guinea pigs (Johns *et al.*, 1990). However, Bellofiore *et al.* (1987) have demonstrated that rats sensitized systemically and exposed to aerosolized allergen via a tracheostomy did not exhibit significant changes in the upper airways resistance whereas the response in the lower airways after nasal exposure was, in part, mediated by cholinergic reflex changes induced by the upper airways (Bellofiore *et al.*, 1987). For these reasons we believe that the changes in airways function recorded in our guinea pigs represent changes in the lungs rather than the nose even though measurement was made through the two organs in series.

Eosinophil leukocyte infiltration is perhaps the most prominent feature of the airway mucosa in asthma (Djukanovic *et al.*, 1990) and the early recruitment of eosinophils into the airways is associated with late phase asthmatic reactions (Rossi *et al.*, 1991). The inflammatory cell infiltrate after ET challenge with aerosolized ovalbumin has been measured in bronchoalveolar lavage fluid (BAL). Cell numbers were measured up to 24 h. Saline induced a relatively small response in neutrophil numbers and a rise in eosinophil numbers. In the OA challenged group, neutrophil counts increased to a maximum at 6 h, falling away by 24 h, and were significantly higher than the saline group at all time points (Seminario *et al.*, 1991). After ET challenge, eosinophil numbers rose gradually and were still rising by 24 h, although the differences between the saline and allergen group were significant only at 15 min and 24 h. The inflammatory cell influx in the saline group may have been associated with the procedure; either physical trauma or the effect of saline reaching the lower airways directly.

While histology can give evidence of the presence of eosinophils in the bronchial tissues and lumen, it gives little or no indication of their activation. A knowledge of activation is important because, while allergen-induced eosinophilia may be associated with pulmonary inflammation, chronic eosinophilia in mice induced by interleukin-5 (IL-5), which does not induce cell activation in the lung, is not accompanied by inflammatory changes (Dent *et al.*, 1990). In order to assess eosinophilic activation we have made monoclonal antibodies to guinea pig eosinophil major basic protein (MBP) from which we have developed an ELISA for estimation of its concentration in biological fluids (Campos *et al.*, 1992).

After aerosolized allergen challenge in free-breathing guinea pigs, MBP significantly increased above control levels in the BAL fluid between 6 and 12 h, remaining elevated for up to 72 h (Campos *et al.*, 1992). Using BAL fluid from guinea pigs investigated previously (Walls *et al.*, 1991), a correlation between eosinophil numbers and MBP concentration was observed, although this was not statistically significant ($r = 0.616$), indicat-

Table 4.2   Major basic protein concentration in bronchoalveolar lavage fluid from ovalbumin sensitized guinea pigs according to exposure method 24 h after saline or allergen challenge

Method	n	Saline	n	Ovalbumin
Free breathing	6	117 ± 60	6	318 ± 142
Endotracheal	8	244 ± 15	7	1643 ± 60

Data represent mean ± SEM in ng ml^{-1} from n guinea pigs.

ing that MBP may reflect not only the activation of eosinophils recovered in BAL fluid, but also their destruction, and, possibly, MBP released into the airways from activated tissue eosinophils. A significant eosinophilic influx into the lumen of the airways has been reported 17 h after nasal (Hutson *et al.*, 1988) and 24 h after endotracheal (Seminario *et al.*, 1991) exposure. Therefore we have compared the MBP concentration in BAL fluid from both groups of animals 24 h after challenge with either saline or allergen. The MBP concentration from endotracheally challenged animals was significantly higher than that from nasally challenged animals (Table 4.2).

4.5 Local Sensitization of Guinea Pig Airways

In humans, allergic disorders are associated with raised levels of allergen-specific immunoglobulin E (IgE) which mediate the responses. The predominant anaphylactic antibody in guinea pigs is IgG1 (Ovary *et al.*, 1963). Nevertheless, IgE has been shown to mediate responses *in vitro* (Regal, 1985; Ito *et al.*, 1984; Graziano *et al.*, 1984) and *in vivo* (Iijima *et al.*, 1987; Andersson *et al.*, 1988) in guinea pigs, the latter two groups concluding that allergen-specific IgE was responsible for the LPR following challenge. However, systemic sensitization together with the use of adjuvants are required to stimulate IgE synthesis. To try to mimic asthma as closely as possible, we have used aerosol sensitization without concomitant adjuvants. For animals sensitized both by inhalation of allergen through the nose (Hutson *et al.*, 1988) and through the ET tube (Seminario *et al.*, 1991) we have estimated allergen-specific immunoglobulin levels in the BAL and circulation using an ELISA to estimate allergen specific IgG and its isotypes IgG1 and IgG2, and passive cutaneous anaphylaxis to estimate IgE levels.

Although aerosol sensitization of free-breathing guinea pigs did not establish an IgE mediated response, sensitization of guinea pigs by the ET aerosol route resulted in significantly raised serum IgG and IgG1 but not IgG2 levels above saline sensitized or naive animals (Varley *et al.*, 1991d). IgE mediated anaphylaxis following OA inhalation in guinea pigs has been

Table 4.3 Allergen-specific IgG levels in the circulation and BAL and Schultz–Dale responses of isolated lung tissue from guinea pigs sensitized by different routes

Sensitization route	Serum IgG	BAL IgG	Schultz–Dale response
Free breathing	+	+	±
Endotracheal	++	+++	+++
Systemic	++++	ND	++++

Relative allergen-specific IgG levels in serum and BAL and relative airway tissue responses to allergen challenge of Schultz–Dale preparations from guinea pigs sensitized by exposure to aerosol while either breathing freely (nasal) or through an endotracheal tube or sensitized by intraperitoneal injection. Range of IgG levels from low (+) to high (++++). Range of Schultz–Dale responses from weak or no response (±) to strong (++++) response. Note serum diluted 1/40 and BAL fluid used undiluted.

shown to be blocked by IgG2 antibodies (Yamauchi et al., 1986). Since IgG2 is not elevated in our aerosol sensitized animals (and is elevated in serum from systemically sensitized guinea pigs), aerosol exposure to allergen may produce a more marked response to challenge. IgG levels in the BAL fluid of ET aerosol sensitized guinea pigs were significantly higher than in BAL from nasally sensitized animals (Table 4.3). The relatively small difference in serum levels of immunoglobulin between routes of sensitization and the larger difference between nasally and ET sensitized IgG in BAL suggests local synthesis. There may be an advantage with restricting the aerosol deposition to the lungs, since down regulation of IgE production in rats and mice has been shown to be associated with lymph nodes which drain the respiratory tract and, in particular, the oronasal cavity (Sedgewick and Holt, 1985).

Schultz–Dale preparation of airway tissue elicited small responses in only some tissues from free-breathing aerosol sensitized guinea pigs (Varley et al., 1990) whereas large changes were observed in all tissues from ET sensitized guinea pigs (Table 4.3). These were similar to responses observed in tissues from systemically sensitized guinea pigs. Despite the relatively low levels of allergen-specific IgG in the serum from aerosol sensitized guinea pigs when compared with systemically sensitized guinea pigs, the responses evoked by allergen challenge in vitro are similar. These data reinforce the hypothesis that ET sensitization results in the local generation of anaphylactic antibodies.

4.6 Conclusions

Hutson et al. (1988) described a model of allergen-induced airway obstruction and inflammation which demonstrated both early and late phase responses. However, this model was too variable for routine use. We have, therefore, modified this model by redesigning and automating the pleth-ysmograph, improving the methods for data aquisition and calculation and using an endotracheal tube for the sensitization and challenge of the animals. With this system, which sensitizes the lungs locally, we have obtained consistent early phase responses and, less consistently, prolonga-tion of airway obstruction for up to 6 h. We have not demonstrated obvious late phase reactions despite having evidence of inflammatory cell influx. In contrast, others (Wieslander *et al.*, 1985; Iijima *et al.*, 1987; Iwama *et al.*, 1991) have reported the presence of LPR using other sensitization and challenge procedures. From this we may conclude that the ability of a guinea pig to respond with late phase reactions is highly dependent on the route and dose of allergen sensitization and challenge. In our model we suggest that, whereas local antibody production in the lung is sufficient to mediate a large early phase response, the induction of a late phase re-sponse requires either a higher local concentration of antibody or the influx of systemic antibody from the circulation to arm the invading inflammatory cells thus allowing them to interact with the allergen in the airways. In addition, the presence of antigen-specific IgE may be a necessary precipi-tating factor.

Acknowledgements

J.G.V. was supported by a program grant from the Medical Research Council, M.-C.S. by a grant from Pfizer (UK) Ltd and M.G.C. by a grant from Rhone Poulenc Rorer (UK) Ltd.

References

Agrawal, K. P. (1981). Specific airway conductance in guinea pigs: normal values and histamine induced fall. *Respir. Physiol.*, **43**, 23–30.
Amdur, M. O. and Mead, J. (1958). Compliance and lung resistance in guinea pigs. *J. Physiol.*, **192**, 364–8.
Andersson, P. (1980). Antigen induced bronchial anaphylaxis in actively sensitized guinea pigs. Pattern of response in relation to immunization regimen. *Allergy*, **35**, 65–71.
Andersson, P., Brange, C., Kogerer, B. von, Sonmark, B. and Stahre, G. (1988). Effect of glucocorticosteroid treatment on ovalbumin-induced IgE-mediated im-mediate and late allergic response in guinea pig. *Int. Arch. Allergy Appl. Im-munol.*, **87**, 32–9.
Barnes, P. J. (1989). A new approach to the treatment of asthma. *N. Engl. J. Med.*, **321**, 1517–27.
Bellofiore, S., DiMaria, G. U. and Martin, J. G. (1987). Changes in upper and

lower airway resistance after inhalation of antigen in sensitized rats. *Am. Rev. Respir. Dis.*, **144**, 379–83.

Campos, M. G., Summers, J. A., Hunt, T. C., Rimmer, S. J., Sturton, R. G., Palsai, S. and Church, M. K. (1992). Measurement by ELISA of eosinophil major basic protein in bronchoalveolar lavage fluid from allergen challenged guinea pigs. *Clin. Exp. Allergy*, **22**, 131 (abstract P31).

De Monchy, J. G. R., Kauffman, H. F., Venge, P., Koëter, G. H., Jansen, H. M., Sluiter, H. J. and De Vries, K. (1985). Bronchoalveolar eosinophilia during allergen induced late asthmatic reactions. *Am. Rev. Respir. Dis.*, **131**, 373–6.

Dent, L. A., Strath, M., Mellor, A. L. and Sanderson, C. J. (1990). Eosinophilia in transgenic mice expressing interleukin 5. *J. Exp. Med.*, **172**, 1425–31.

Djukanovic, R., Wilson, J. W., Britten, K. M., Wilson, S. J., Walls, A. F., Roche, W. R., Howarth, P. H. and Holgate, S. T. (1990). Quantitation of mast cells and eosinophils in the bronchial mucosa of symptomatic atopic asthmatics and healthy control subjects using immunohistochemistry. *Am. Rev. Respir. Dis.*, **142**, 863–71.

Dubois, A. B., Bothelo, S. Y., Bedell, G. N., Marshall, R. and Comroe, J. H., Jr (1956b). A rapid plethysmographic method for measuring thoracic gas volume: a comparison with a nitrogen washout method for measuring functional residual capacity in normal subjects. *J. Clin. Invest.*, **35**, 322–6.

Dubois, A. B., Bothelo, S. Y. and Comroe, J. H., Jr (1956a). A new method for measuring airway resistance in man using a body plethysmograph: values in normal subjects and in patients with respiratory disease. *J. Clin. Invest.*, **35**, 327–35.

Dunn, C. J., Elliot, G. A., Oostven, J. A. and Richards, I. M. (1988). Development of a prolonged eosinophil-rich inflammatory leukocyte infiltration in the guinea pig asthmatic response to ovalbumin inhalation. *Am. Rev. Respir. Dis.*, **137**, 541–7.

Frew, A. J., Moqbel, R., Azzawi, M., Hartnell, A., Barkans, J., Jeffery, P. K., Kay, A. B., Scheper, R. J., Varley, J., Church, M. K. and Holgate, S. T. (1990). T lymphocytes and eosinophils in allergen-induced late phase asthmatic reactions in the guinea pig. *Am. Rev. Respir. Dis.*, **141**, 407–13.

Gleich, G. J. (1982). The late phase of the immunoglobulin E-mediated reaction: a link between anaphylaxis and common allergic disease. *J. Allergy Clin. Immunol.*, **70**, 160–9.

Graziano, F. M., Gunderson, L., Larson, L. A., Harley, P. and Buckner, C. K. (1984). Receptor specific mediation by immunoglobulin E of antigen-induced contraction of tracheal and lung parenchymal strips isolated from the guinea pig. *J. Clin. Invest.*, **73**, 1215–22.

Hargreave, F. E. (1989). Late phase asthmatic responses and airway inflammation. *J. Allergy Clin. Immunol.*, **83**, 525–7.

Holroyde, M. C. and Norris, A. A. (1988). The effect of ozone on reactivity of upper and lower airways in guinea pigs. *Br. J. Pharmacol.*, **94**, 938–46.

Hutson, P. A., Church, M. K., Clay, T. P., Miller, P. and Holgate, S. T. (1988). Early and late phase bronchoconstriction after allergen challenge of non anaesthetised guinea pigs. 1. The association of disordered airway physiology to leukocyte infiltration. *Am. Rev. Respir. Dis.*, **137**, 548–57.

Iijima, H., Ishii, M., Yamauchi, K., Chao, C.-L., Kimura, K., Shimura, S., Shindoh, Y., Inuoe, H., Mue, S. and Takishima, T. (1987). Bronchalveolar lavage and histologic characterisation of late asthmatic response in guinea pigs. *Am. Rev. Respir. Dis.*, **136**, 922–9.

Ito, K., Ohta, K., Yamauchi, N., Suko, M., Hayakawa, T., Suzuki, S. and

Miyamoto, T. (1984). Contractions of guinea pig trachea with antibodies to guinea pig IgE. An *in vitro* model for asthma. II. Reactivity of guinea pig tracheas to anti IgG1 and anti IgG2 in comparison with anti IgE. *Ann. Allergy*, **52**, 375–8.

Iwama, T., Shikada, K., Yamamoto, A., Sakashita, M., Hibi, M. and Tanaka, S. (1991). Effect of NZ-107 on late phase airway responses and airway hyperreactivity in guinea pigs. *Eur. J. Physiol.*, **199**, 271–8.

Johns, K., Sorkness, R., Graziano, F., Castleman, W. and Lemanske, R. F. (1990). Contribution of upper airways to antigen-induced late airway obstruction in guinea pigs. *Am. Rev. Respir. Dis.*, **142**, 138–42.

Lord, P. W., Brooks, A. G. F. and Edwards, J. M. (1977). Variation between observers in the estimation of airway resistance and thoracic gas volume. *Thorax*, **32**, 67–70.

Lorino, H., Harf, A., Atlan, G., Brault, Y., Lorino, A. M. and Laurent, D. (1980). Computer determination of thoracic gas volume using plethysmographic "thoracic flow". *J. Appl. Physiol.*, **48**, 911–16.

Ovary, Z., Benacerraf, B. and Bloch, K. J. (1963). Properties of 7S antibodies. II. Identification of antibodies involved in passive cutaneous and systemic anaphylaxis. *J. Exp. Med.*, **117**, 951–64.

Raabe, O. G., Al-Bayati, M. A., Teague, S. V. and Rasolt, A. (1988). Regional deposition of inhaled monodisperse coarse and fine aerosol particles in small laboratory animals. *Ann. Occup. Hyg.*, **32**, 53–63.

Regal, J. F. (1985). IgG vs IgE: mediators of antigen-induced guinea pig lung parenchymal strip. *Immunopharmacology*, **10**, 137–46.

Rossi, G. A., Crimi, E., Lantero, S., Gianiorio, P., Oddera, S., Crimi, P. and Brusasco, V. (1991). Late phase asthmatic reaction to inhaled allergen is associated with early recruitment of eosinophils in the airways. *Am. Rev. Respir. Dis.*, **144**, 379–80.

Sedgewick, J. D. and Holt, P. G. (1985). Induction of IgE secreting cells and IgE isotype-specific suppressor T cells in the respiratory lymph nodes of rats in response to antigen challenge. *Cell Immunol.*, **94**, 182–94.

Seminario, M. C., Varley, J. G., Holgate, S. T. and Church, M. K. (1991). Aerosol challenge through an endotracheal tube in guinea pigs. *Eur. Resp. J.*, **4**, 595s.

Shah, J., Keeping, I. M. and Jackson, I. L. (1980). A simple numerical analysis of whole body plethysmograph data. *Clin. Sci.*, **59**, 29p.

Smith, L., Gratziou, C., Carroll, M., Wilson, S., Howarth, P. and Holgate, S. T. (1991). Bronchial lavage and biopsies after local allergen challenge in atopic asthmatic patients. *Am. Rev. Respir. Dis.*, **143**, A802.

Varley, J. G., Featherstone, R. L., Walls, A. F., Church, M. K. and Holgate, S. T. (1990). Local antibody production in aerosol sensitised guinea pigs. *J. Allergy Clin. Immunol.*, **85**, 299.

Varley, J. G., Heath, J. R., Bacon, R., Holgate, S. T. and Church, M. K. (1991a). Pulmonary function values using a new guinea pig body plethysmograph. *Am. Rev. Respir. Dis.*, **143**, A354.

Varley, J. G., Heath, J. R., Bacon, R., Holgate, S. T. and Church, M. K. (1991b). Reproducibility of a new automated body plethysmograph. *Am. Rev. Respir. Dis.*, **143**, A353.

Varley, J. G., Perring, S., Seminario, M.-C., Fleming, J., Holgate, S. T. and Church, M. K. (1991c). Aerosol deposition in the guinea pig. A comparison of two methods of exposure. *Am. Rev. Respir. Dis.*, **143**, A708.

Varley, J. G., Deller, M., Walls, A. F., Church, M. K. and Holgate, S. T. (1991d). Antibody production in guinea pigs sensitised by different routes; systemic and aerosol. *Clin. Exp. Allergy*, **22**, 123 (abstract P07).

Walker, C., Virchow, J.-C., Jr, Bruijnzeel, P. L. B. and Blaser, K. (1991). T cell subsets and their soluble products regulate eosinophilia in allergic and non allergic asthma. *J. Immunol.*, **146**, 1829–35.

Walls, A. F., Rhee, Y. K., Gould, D. J., Walters, C., Robinson, C., Church, M. K. and Holgate, S. T. (1991). Inflammatory mediators and cellular infiltration of the lungs in a guinea pig model of the late asthmatic reaction. *Lung*, **169**, 227–40.

Warner, J. O. (1976). Significance of late reactions after bronchial challenge with house dust mite. *Arch. Dis. Child.*, **51**, 905–11.

Wieslander, E., Andersson, P., Linden, M., Axelsson, B., Källstöm, L., Brattsand, R. and Paulsson, I. (1985). Importance of particulate antigen for the induction of dual bronchial reaction in guinea pigs. *Agents Actions*, **16**, 37–8.

Yamauchi, N., Ito, K., Suko, M., Ishii, A. and Miyamoto, T. (1986). IgG2 antibodies block IgE antibody induced asthma in guinea pigs. *Int. Arch. Allergy Appl. Immunol.*, **80**, 76–80.

5

Pharmacologic Modulation of Antigen-induced Airway Eosinophilia and Hyperresponsiveness in Guinea Pigs

R. R. Schellenberg

5.1 Introduction

The phenomenon of airway hyperresponsiveness to numerous different smooth muscle contractile agonists is a hallmark of human bronchial asthma. The mechanisms by which this condition occurs are unknown and may be multiple. However, increased responsiveness has been demonstrated after antigen exposure in the laboratory (Cockcroft and Murdock, 1987; Cockcroft et al., 1977) and after seasonal pollen exposure (Boulet et al., 1983). Many investigators have suggested that airway hyperresponsiveness is brought about secondary to factors inducing late asthmatic responses and may be coupled with the eosinophilia noted in the airway which is prominent at this time course. A causal relationship between the airway eosinophilia and airway hyperresponsiveness remains to be defined despite the appeal of circumstantial evidence. It remains equally plausible that similar factors or divergent factors are involved in the simultaneous production of airway eosinophilia and mechanisms inducing airway hyperresponsiveness. In an attempt to link more clearly eosinophilia with airway hyperrresponsiveness, or to dissociate these two factors, we have chosen to develop a guinea pig model of airway eosinophilia and hyperresponsiveness following repeated antigen challenge. We hypothesized that repeated exposure to antigen with the concomitant release of mediators was required to induce sustained airway hyperresponsiveness. In fact, we have

50

clearly demonstrated that sensitization alone without repeated challenges fails to induce airway hyperresponsiveness, despite the ability of isolated airway tissues from these animals to release mast cell mediators and to induce acute smooth muscle contractile activity following antigen challenge (Ishida *et al.*, 1989). In addition to the development of airway eosinophilia, we wished to demonstrate that the hyperresponsiveness induced by repeated antigen challenge lasted for a number of days rather than being a transient response which could be attributed to changes in vascular permeability and airway wall oedema. The final goal in developing a model was our desire to demonstrate changes in airway smooth muscle function since we (Schellenberg and Foster, 1984; Schellenberg *et al.*, 1985) and others (DeJongste *et al.*, 1987) have demonstrated increased isometric contractile responses of human asthmatic bronchial smooth muscle when compared with non-asthmatic tissues.

To date, a number of specific pharmacologic agents have been evaluated for their effects upon both the airway eosinophilia and airway hyperresponsiveness. This discussion will deal specifically with the evaluation of pharmacologic manipulations including the antagonism of platelet activating factor, depletion of neuropeptides by capsaicin treatment, and treatment with nedocromil sodium.

5.2 Features of Guinea Pig Model of Airway Hyperresponsiveness

A schematic representation of the methodology employed to sensitize and challenge the guinea pigs repeatedly is shown in Fig. 5.1. Cam-Hartley female guinea pigs were sensitized to ovalbumin (OA) by inhalation of an aerosolized solution of 1% OA and 4% heat-killed *Bordatella pertussis* vaccine for an exposure period of 10 min (Ishida *et al.*, 1989).

Acute Bronchoconstriction

To assess the effects of acute antigen challenge, sensitization of guinea pigs by this method was confirmed with a single challenge with 0.5% OA aerosol one week later. Animals were then studied three days following. Diphenhydramine 0.2 ml of 40 mg/ml, i.p., saline solution was given 1 h before antigen challenge. Animals were anaesthetized by inhalation with 4% halothane and a carotid artery catheter was inserted by a mid-neck incision. After the animals awakened from the anaesthesia, acute antigen challenge was performed by exposure to 0.5% OA aerosol by a DeVilbiss nebulizer for 1 min. Arterial blood gas samples were taken prior to and 1, 4

[PROTOCOL]

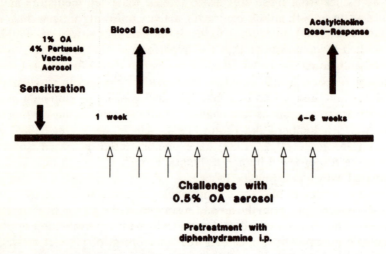

Fig. 5.1   Schematic diagram of protocol for inducing airway hyperresponsiveness utilizing repeated aerosolized antigen challenge twice weekly for 4–6 weeks following initial sensitization (OA, ovalbumin).

and 10 min after the beginning of the antigen exposure. Figure 5.2 demonstrates the dramatic changes in arterial oxygenation following antigen exposure which did not occur with the same antigen exposure in non-sensitized controls. In addition to the drop in the arterial blood oxygen pressure (pO_2), there was a significant increase of arterial blood carbon dioxide pressure (pCO_2) in sensitized animals. These acute responses had returned to normal in 20 to 30 min post-antigen challenge.

Airway Hyperresponsiveness

For development of hyperresponsiveness, animals were exposed to aerosolized 0.5% OA solution twice weekly for 4–6 weeks. Control animals received saline challenges in identical fashion. Airway responsiveness to acetylcholine (ACh) was assessed three days following the last antigen challenge. Animals were anaesthetized, tracheostomized and placed in a body plethysmograph. Following installation of an oesophageal balloon, animals were connected to a ventilator and paralysed. Measurements of volume, transpulmonary pressure and flow were recorded and pulmonary resistance was calculated from these signals using the method of von Neergaard and Wirz (1927) by a computer program developed in our laboratory (Hulbert *et al.*, 1985). Figure 5.3 shows the changes in pulmon-

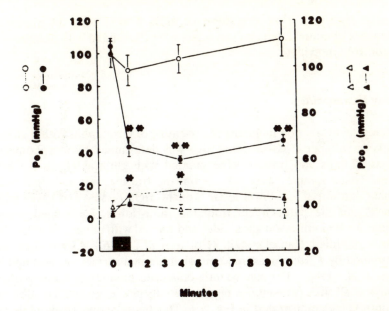

Fig. 5.2 Changes in arterial blood gases (pO_2 and pCO_2) after a 1 min exposure to aerosolized ovalbumin 0.5%. Data are the means ± SE for six guinea pigs previously sensitized to OA (closed symbols) and five unsensitized controls (open symbols). *$p < 0.05$, **$p < 0.01$ (from Ishida et al., 1989).

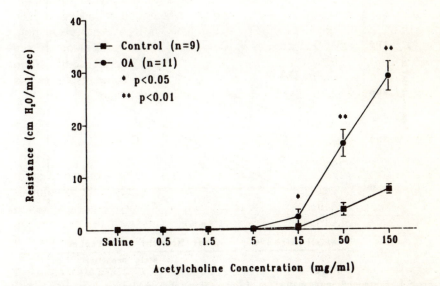

Fig. 5.3 Pulmonary resistance changes to increasing ACh concentrations (mg/ml) in guinea pigs sensitized to OA and repeatedly challenged to aerosolized OA (•, $n = 11$), or unsensitized and challenged with aerosolized saline (■, $n = 9$). Data are the means ± SE for each group. **$p < 0.01$ (from Ishida et al., 1989).

ary resistance with increasing doses of ACh. The striking differences in
resistances obtained from animals repeatedly challenged with antigen versus control are evident.

Airway Eosinophilia

Histological evaluation including the counting of eosinophils within airway
compartments per cross-sectional area was determined by morphometric
analysis. Lungs and trachea were inflated with glutaraldehyde 2.5% in
buffer. Tissue samples were taken from the trachea, left and right main
bronchi, left upper and lower lobar bronchi, right middle and lower lobar
bronchi and the parenchyma from the same lobes. Embedded plastic
sections were mounted on glass slides and stained with either toluidine blue
O or a modified Hansel's stain (Nolan *et al.*, 1986). Airway size was
determined by P_i, the measured epithelial luminal surface, as outlined by
James *et al.* (1988). The significantly enhanced number of eosinophils in
airways of all sizes from guinea pigs repeatedly challenged with ovalbumin
vs controls is demonstrated in Fig. 5.4. This figure shows eosinophils per
millimetre squared epithelial area, but increased numbers were also noted
in the subepithelial mucosa.

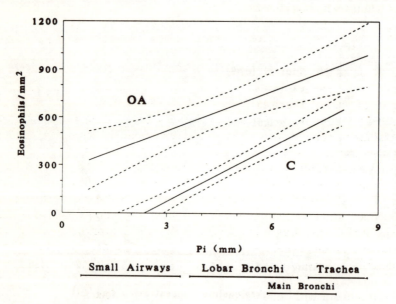

Fig. 5.4   Eosinophils in the epithelium of airways from saline-challenged controls (C) ($n = 5$)
and from OA-challenged guinea pigs ($n = 3$). Absolute eosinophil counts per mm^2 of
epithelial area are expressed for airways of all sizes defined by their internal perimeter (P_i).
Regression lines and 95% confidence intervals are shown for the two groups. (Data derived
from Ishida *et al.* (1989).)

In Vitro *Smooth Muscle Responses*

To evaluate whether there were alterations in the mechanics of guinea pig airways from those animals demonstrating *in vivo* airway hyperresponsiveness following repeated antigen challenge, we assessed the isobaric and isovolumetric responses of tracheal tube preparations. The schematic diagram in Fig. 5.5 shows the experimental set-up, which allows for the assessment of passive pressure–volume characteristics and active pressure changes produced at any given transmural pressure as well as changes in volume produced at any given transmural pressure following stimulation with an electrical field or a smooth muscle contractile agonist such as histamine. It can be appreciated that both the changes in pressure and the changes in volume following electrical field stimulation were greater in tissues from animals demonstrating *in vivo* hyperresponsiveness following repeated antigen challenge. More recently, isolated tracheal smooth muscle from these two groups of guinea pigs has confirmed these findings by showing both enhanced isometric and isotonic responses in tissues from the hyperresponsive guinea pigs. These findings suggest that the repeated release of mediators following antigen stimulation over this longer time course is capable of inducing alterations in smooth muscle itself or in components affecting smooth muscle contractile responses by altering the load against which it must contract.

5.3 Role of Platelet Activating Factor

Although platelet activating factor (PAF) has been postulated to play a significant role in many facets of bronchial asthma, an increasing number of studies in humans as well as animals has failed to support the initial enthusiasm (Cuss *et al.*, 1986), especially regarding its role in acute bronchoconstriction and as an eosinophil chemotactic factor. To evaluate this in our guinea pig model, we utilized the PAF antagonist SDZ 64–412 (Sandoz, East Hanover, NJ), an agent shown to inhibit the hypotension, bronchoconstriction and platelet aggregation produced by PAF (Handley *et al.*, 1988). This drug was administered orally 2 h prior to each of the multiple ovalbumin challenges using an identical protocol as that previously described. Further experimental details are provided in the manuscript by Ishida *et al.* (1990b).

Pretreatment with the PAF antagonist had no effect on the severity of hypoxemia produced by a 1-min exposure to aerosolized antigen. This suggested that other mediators in the acute response are of more importance in the induction of acute bronchoconstriction than is PAF.

Despite its lack of activity upon antigen-induced bronchoconstriction, it

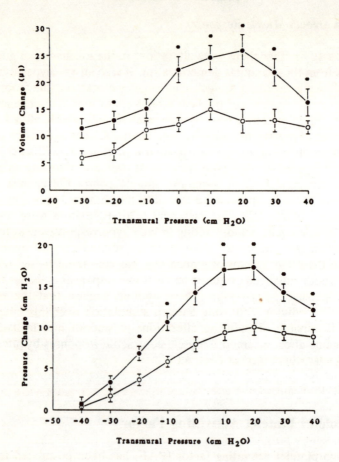

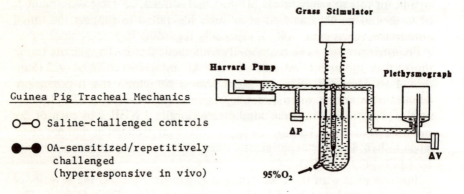

Fig. 5.5 Effects of electrical field stimulation upon tracheal preparations obtained from saline-challenged controls (○, $n = 14$) and from OA-sensitized and repeatedly challenged guinea pigs (●, $n = 14$). A schematic of the experimental set-up is provided. For both isobaric responses (upper graph) and isovolumetric responses (lower graph) tracheal preparations from antigen-challenged hyperresponsive animals demonstrated significantly greater changes (*$p < 0.05$). (Data from Ishida *et al.* (1990a).)

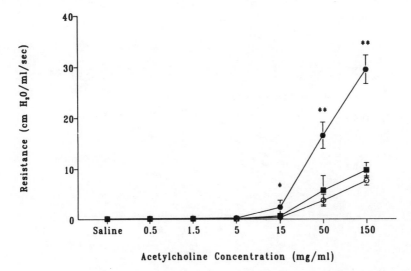

Fig. 5.6 Pulmonary resistance changes (mean ± SE) to ACh of controls (○) and OA-sensitized and repeatedly challenged guinea pigs with (■) or without (●) pretreatment with the PAF antagonist SDZ 64–412. (p^* < 0.05, $^{**}p$ < 0.01 different from controls and SDZ 64–412 treated groups) (from Ishida et al., 1990b).

showed amazing efficacy in the inhibition of airway hyperresponsiveness as demonstrated in Fig. 5.6 where it can be appreciated that pretreatment with the PAF antagonist completely inhibited antigen-induced hyperresponsiveness.

Unlike its effects on airway hyperresponsiveness, this PAF antagonist had absolutely no effect upon the degree of eosinophilic infiltration into airway tissues as demonstrated in Fig. 5.7. These data suggest that either airway hyperresponsiveness is not linked to the eosinophilia, or that the eosinophils are the major source of the platelet activating factor which subsequently produces alterations leading to airway hyperresponsiveness.

Preliminary results utilizing a chemically dissimilar PAF antagonist have shown it to produce no significant effect on airway hyperresponsiveness, raising the possibility that differing PAF antagonists may operate via different PAF receptors on target cells involved in airway hyperresponsiveness. These results may help explain the failure of WEB 2086 to alter the acute increases and airway hyperresponsiveness following antigen challenge in human asthmatics (Freitag et al., 1991).

5.4 Effects of Neuropeptide Depletion

Neuropeptide-containing nerves have been demonstrated to inervate the airways (Lundberg et al., 1983; Uddman and Sundler, 1987). Treatment

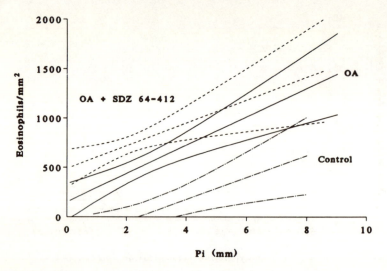

Fig. 5.7 Epithelial eosinophils of airways from saline-challenged controls ($n = 5$), OA-challenged hyperresponsive guinea pigs ($n = 6$) and SDZ 64–412 pretreated, OA-challenged guinea pigs ($n = 3$). Regression lines with 95% confidence intervals are shown for the three groups over the range of airway sizes. P_i values are comparable with those shown for Fig. 5.4. (Data from Ishida *et al.* (1990b).)

with capsaicin has been shown to deplete substance P and other neurokinins found in airway tissues (Lundberg *et al.*, 1983; Gamse *et al.*, 1980; Buck and Burks, 1986). Since neurokinins appear to play an important role in the airway hyperresponsiveness induced by toluene diisocyanate (Thompson *et al.*, 1987; Sheppard and Scypinski, 1988), we evaluated whether depletion of neurokinins with capsaicin treatment following sensitization of guinea pigs to antigen, but prior to their repeated challenges with aerosolized antigen, would alter airway hyperresponsiveness and/or eosinophilia. Capsaicin treatment had no effect upon reaginic antibody titres to the antigen and did not alter the production of lipoxygenase products produced by antigen challenge of isolated bronchial tissue *in vitro* (Matsuse *et al.*, 1991). However, it had a striking effect upon airway hyperresponsiveness as demonstrated in Fig. 5.8. Despite this effect, it did not alter the degree of eosinophilic infiltration within the epithelium in animals repeatedly challenged with antigen. These results are shown in Fig. 5.9. These results argue against a role for neuropeptides in eosinophil recruitment, but do not preclude a role for the eosinophil in the development of hyperresponsiveness. It remains possible that a factor released from eosinophils may trigger neuropeptide release or that neuropeptides are the primary stimulus for the release of an eosinophil-derived factor causing airway hyperresponsiveness, since substance P has been demonstrated to cause the release of eosinophil peroxidase from guinea pigs eosinophils (Kroegel *et al.*, 1990).

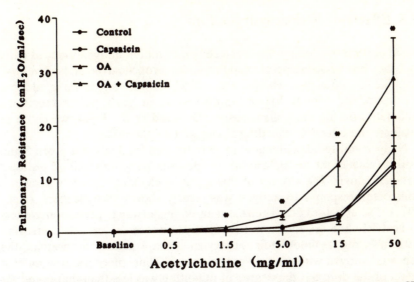

Fig. 5.8   Effect of capsaicin upon pulmonary resistance to ACh. Values are means ± SE. Repeatedly OA-challenged guinea pigs ($n = 6$) showed significantly greater ($p < 0.05$) responses than did capsaicin-pretreated, repeatedly OA-challenged guinea pigs ($n = 4$), capsaicin-treated and saline-challenged animals ($n = 4$) or saline-challenged controls ($n = 4$). (Data from Matsuse et al. (1991).)

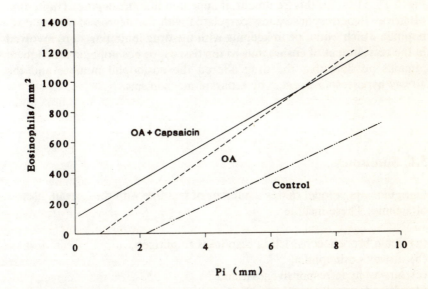

Fig. 5.9 Regression lines for epithelial eosinophils within airways from saline-challenged controls ($n = 9$), OA-challenged hyperresponsive guinea pigs ($n = 8$) and capsaicin-treated, OA-challenged guinea pigs ($n = 4$). Internal perimeter (P_i) values are comparable with those of Fig. 5.4. (Data from Matsuse et al. (1991).)

5.5 Effects of Nedocromil Sodium

Since nedocromil sodium has been shown to inhibit antigen-induced early
and late bronchoconstrictor responses plus bronchoalveolar lavage eosinophilia in guinea pigs (Hutson *et al.*, 1988; Crimi *et al.*, 1989) in addition
to decreasing airway hyperresponsiveness in grass pollen-sensitized
asthmatics during the pollen season (Dorward *et al.*, 1986), we chose to
evaluate the effects of this drug in our guinea pig model.

Nedocromil sodium 10 mg/ml by nebulization for 3 min was given 5 min
prior to each of the multiple antigen exposures using our standard protocol
detailed above. The efficacy of this agent in blocking the acute bronchoconstrictor response to antigen was clearly shown (Schellenberg *et al.*,
1991). The effects of drug pretreatment on the airway hyperresponsiveness
to acetylcholine are shown in Fig. 5.10. Responses of animals pretreated
with this drug lay intermediate between controls and those receiving the
repeated antigen without drug pretreatment. Thus, there was a significant
effect of the drug but the degree of inhibition was less than that noted for
either pretreatment with the PAF antagonist, SDZ 64–412, or capsaicin
depletion of neuropeptides.

This treatment was the only producing depletion of eosinophils within
airways. The degree of eosinophil depletion was also intermediate between
the controls and the non-drug treated antigen challenged group as shown in
Fig. 5.11. Thus, for this treatment, it appeared that the degree of inhibition
of airway hyperresponsiveness correlated with the degree of airway eosinophilia which would be in keeping with the drug inhibiting steps involved
in the recruitment of eosinophils to the tissues, or eosinophilic function. It
remains possible that the drug altered the eosinophil number and the
airway hyperresponsiveness by separate mechanisms.

5.6 Summary

Our guinea pig model shares a number of features with the human disease
of asthma. These include

(a) acute bronchoconstriction responses to antigen,
(b) airway eosinophilia,
(c) airway hyperresponsiveness, and
(d) altered smooth muscle mechanics.

To date, we are unable to determine whether the airway eosinophilia is
causally linked with the airway hyperresponsiveness. Although both the

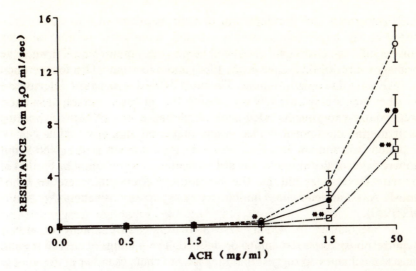

Fig. 5.10 Changes in pulmonary resistance with increasing doses of ACh in saline-challenged controls ($\square$, $n = 21$), in guinea pigs receiving repeated OA challenges with ($\bullet$, $n = 10$) nebulized nedocromil sodium 10 mg/ml pretreatment or without ($\circ$, $n = 36$) pretreatment. $*p < 0.05$, $**p < 0.01$ different from OA without drug pretreatment. Both groups were significantly different at the 5 mg/ml dose. (Data from Schellenberg *et al.* (1991).)

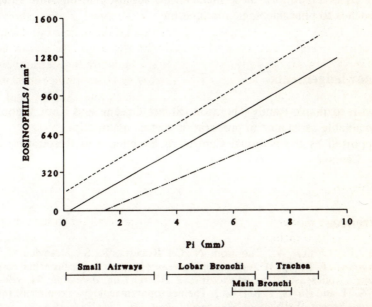

Fig. 5.11 Regression lines for epithelial eosinophils from airways of guinea pigs receiving repeated OA challenges with (——) or without (– – –) nedocromil sodium pretreatment for airways of all sizes (P_i values comparable with Fig. 5.4). Lowest regression line represents saline-challenged controls. Differences in airway epithelial cells for the two groups were most prominent in smaller airways. (Data from Schellenberg *et al.* (1991).)

PAF antagonist and the depletion of neuropeptides with capsaicin inhibited airway hyperresponsiveness virtually completely without altering eosinophils, the eosinophil could still be playing a major role if it were the primary source of PAF (Lee *et al.*, 1984) and if its stimulation for secretion of PAF were due to neurokinins. The most definitive means of determining whether eosinophils are actively causing the airway hyperresponsiveness will require experiments adequately depleting eosinophils or preventing their migration. Recent evidence has suggested that eosinophils can be depleted utilizing an anti-IL-5 antibody (Gulbenkian *et al.*, 1991), but airway hyperresponsiveness was not evaluated in these animals. Studies in primates have suggested that the inhibition of eosinophil migration by an anti-ICAM-1 antibody does inhibit airway hyperresponsiveness (Wegner *et al.*, 1990).

The mechanism by which these mediators induce a state of airway hyperresponsiveness remains to be defined. The findings of altered smooth muscle mechanics do suggest that they lead to changes either in the smooth muscle cells themselves, possibly by modulating intracellular biochemical steps which would be common to all receptor-mediated agonists, or by altering structural components within muscle cells or between muscle cells which provide a load against which the smooth muscle must contract. A better understanding of these mechanisms should provide more rational approaches to pharmacologic modulation.

Acknowledgements

We wish to thank Randy Thomson, Stuart Greene and Kent Webb for their valuable assistance in preparation of this manuscript.

Supported by the National Centres of Excellence in Respiratory Diseases, Canada.

References

Boulet, L., Cartier, A., Thomson, N. C., Roberts, R. S., Dolovich, J. and Hargreave, F. E. (1983). Asthma and increases in non-allergic bronchial responsiveness from seasonal pollen exposure, *J. Allergy Clin. Immunol.*, **71**, 399–406.
Buck, S. H. and Burks, T. F. (1986). The neuropharmacology of capsaicin: review of some recent observations. *Pharmacol. Rev.*, **38**, 179–226.
Cockcroft, D. W. and Murdock, K. Y. (1987). Comparative effects of inhaled salbutamol, sodium cromoglycate, and beclomethasone dipropionate on allergen-induced early asthmatic responses and increased bronchial responsiveness to histamine. *J. Allergy Clin. Immunol.*, **79**, 734–40.
Cockcroft, D. W., Ruffin, R. E., Dolovich, J. and Hargreave, F. E. (1977).

Allergen-induced increase in non-allergic bronchial reactivity. *Clin. Allergy*, **7**, 503–13.

Crimi, E., Brusasco, V. and Crimi, P. (1989). Effect of nedocromil sodium on the late asthmatic reaction to bronchial antigen challenge. *J. Allergy Clin. Immunol.*, **83**, 985–90.

Cuss, F. M., Dixon, C. M. S. and Barnes, P. J. (1986). Effect of inhaled platelet activating factor on pulmonary function and bronchoresponsiveness in man. *Lancet*, **2**, 189–92.

De Jongste, J. C., Mons, H., Bonta, I. L. and Kerrebijn, K. F. (1987). *In vitro* responses of airways from an asthmatic patient. *Eur. J. Respir. Dis.*, **71**, 23–9.

Dorward, A. J., Roberts, J. A. and Thomas, N. C. (1986). Effect of nedocromil sodium on histamine airway responsiveness in grass-pollen sensitive asthmatics during the pollen season. *Clin. Allergy*, **16**, 309–15.

Freitag, A., Watson, R. M., Matsos, G., Eastwood, C. and O'Byrne, P. M. (1991). The effect of treatment with an oral platelet activating factor antagonist (WEB 2086) on allergen induced asthmatic responses in human subjects. *Am. Rev. Respir. Dis.*, **143**, A157 (Abstract).

Gamse, R., Holzer, P. and Lembeck, F. (1980). Decrease of substance P in primary afferent neurones and impairment of neurogenic plasma extravasation by capsaicin. *Br. J. Pharmacol.*, **68**, 207–13.

Gulbenkian, A. R., Egan, R. W., Fernandez, X., Jones, H., Kreutner, W., Kung, T., Payyandi, F., Sullivan, L., Zurcher, J. A. and Watnick, A. S. (1991). IL-5 modulates eosinophil accumulation in allergic guinea pig lung. *J. Allergy Clin. Immunol.*, **87**, 206 (Abstract 265).

Handley, D. A., Van Valen, R. G., Melden, M. K., Houlihan, W. J. and Saunders, R. N. (1988). Biological effects of the orally active platelet activating factor receptor antagonist SDZ 64–412. *J. Pharmacol. Exp. Ther.*, **247**, 617.

Hulbert, W. C., McLean, T., Wiggs, B., Paré, P. D. and Hogg, J. C. (1985). Histamine dose–response curves in guinea pigs. *J. Appl. Physiol.*, **58**, 625–34.

Hutson, P. A., Holgate, S. T. and Church, M. K. (1988). Inhibition by nedocromil sodium of early and late phase bronchoconstriction and airway cellular infiltration provoked by ovalbumin inhalation in conscious sensitized guinea pigs. *Br. J. Pharmacol.*, **94**, 6–8.

Ishida, K., Kelly, L. J., Thomson, R. J., Beattie, L. L. and Schellenberg, R. R. (1989). Repeated antigen challenge induces airway hyperresponsiveness with tissue eosinophilia in guinea pigs. *J. Appl. Physiol.*, **67**, 1133–9.

Ishida, K., Paré, P. D., Thomson, R. J. and Schellenberg, R. R. (1990a). Increased *in vitro* responses of tracheal smooth muscle from hyperresponsive guinea pigs. *J. Appl. Physiol.*, **68**, 1316–20.

Ishida, K., Thomson, R. J., Beattie, L. L., Wiggs, B. and Schellenberg, R. R. (1990b). Inhibition of antigen-induced airway hyperresponsiveness, but not acute hypoxia nor airway eosinophilia, by an antagonist of platelet-activating factor. *J. Immunol.*, **114**, 3907–11.

James, A. L., Dirks, P., Ohtaka, H., Schellenberg, R. R. and Hogg, J. C. (1987). Airway responsiveness to intravenous and inhaled acetylcholine in the guinea pig after cigarette smoke exposure. *Am. Rev. Respir. Dis.*, **136**, 1158–62.

James, A. L., Paré, P. D. and Hogg, J. C. (1988). Effects of lung volume, bronchoconstriction and cigarette smoke on morphometric airway dimensions. *J. Appl. Physiol.*, **64**, 913–19.

Lee, T.-C., Lenihan, D. J., Malone, B., Roddy, L. L. and Wasserman, S. I. (1984). Increased biosynthesis of platelet-activating factor in activated human eosinophils. *J. Biol. Chem.*, **259**, 5526–30.

Lundberg, J. M., Brodin, E. and Saria, A. (1983). Effects and distribution of vagal capsaicin-sensitive substance P neurons with special reference to the trachea and lungs. *Acta Physiol. Scand.*, **119**, 243–52.

Matsuse, T., Thomson, R. J., Chen, X.-R., Salari, H. and Schellenberg, R. R. (1991). Capsaicin inhibits airway hyperresponsiveness but not lipoxygenase activity or eosinophilia after repeated aerosolized antigen in guinea pigs. *Am. Rev. Respir. Dis.*, **144**, 368–72.

Nolan, C. R., Anger, M. S. and Kelleher, S. P. (1986). Eosinophilia – a new method of detection and definition of the clinical spectrum. *N. Engl. J. Med.*, **315**, 1516–19.

Schellenberg, R. R. and Foster, A. (1984). *In vitro* responses of human asthmatic bronchial airway and pulmonary vascular smooth muscle. *Int. Arch. Allergy Appl. Immunol.*, **75**, 237–41.

Schellenberg, R. R., Duff, M. F., Foster, A. and Paré, P. D. (1985). Asthmatic bronchial reactivity *in vitro*. *Clin. Invest. Med.*, **8**, A-202 (Abstract).

Schellenberg, R. R., Ishida, K. and Thomson, R. J. (1991). Nedocromil sodium inhibits airway hyperresponsiveness and eosinophilic infiltration induced by repeated antigen challenge in guinea pigs. *Br. J. Pharmacol.*, **103**, 1842–6.

Sheppard, D. and Scypinski, L. (1988). A tachykinin receptor antagonist inhibits and an inhibitor of tachykinin metabolism potentiates toluene diisocyanate-induced airway hyperresponsiveness in guinea pigs. *Am. Rev. Respir. Dis.*, **138**, 547–51.

Thompson, J. E., Scypinski, L. A., Gordon, T. and Sheppard, D. (1987). Tachykinins mediate the acute increase in airway responsiveness caused by toluene diisocyanate in guinea pigs. *Am. Rev. Respir. Dis.*, **136**, 43–9.

Uddman, R. and Sundler, F. (1987). Neuropeptides in the airways: a review. *Am. Rev. Respir. Dis.*, **136** (Suppl: 3–8).

von Neergard, K. and Wirz, K. (1927). Die messung der Stromungseviderstande in den Atemwegen des Menschen, insbesondere bei Asthma und Emphysem. *Z. Klin. Med.*, **105**, 51–82.

Wegner, C. D., Gundel, R. H., Reilly, P., Haynes, N., Lets, L. G. and Rothlein, R. (1990). Intercellular adhesion molecule-1 (ICAM-1) in the pathogenesis of asthma. *Science*, **247**, 456–9.

6

Experimental Lung Hyperreactivity: Pharmacological Control and Possible Role of Cytokines

M. Pretolani, J. Lefort and B. B. Vargaftig

6.1 Introduction

Asthma is a chronic and disabling disease, characterized rather by unspecific bronchopulmonary hyperresponsiveness (HR) and by delayed reactions than by only acute reversible bronchoconstriction, as was considered in the past. Since the *in vivo* experimental models for HR, based on the ability of antigen (Murphy *et al.*, 1986) or platelet-activating factor (PAF-acether) (Vargaftig *et al.*, 1983) to enhance the responses to standard bronchoconstrictor mediators are difficult to explore from the point of view of its physiopathology, the isolated guinea-pig lung as a model for studying HR was introduced. The isolated lung preparation allows the study of bronchoconstriction, vascular permeability and the release of mediators after administration of various agonists, the donor animals can be sensitized by different procedures or treated with drugs and their cells can be depleted, to analyse their role in the *ex vivo* lung responses.

When studying the mechanisms of HR, we observed that isolated perfused lungs from actively sensitized guinea-pigs respond to PAF-acether with an enhanced bronchoconstriction, form larger amounts of thromboxane $(TX)B_2$, leukotriene (LT) C_4-like material and 6-keto-$PGF_{1\alpha}$ and are turned into histamine-releasing tissues (Pretolani *et al.*, 1988, 1989a), as compared with lungs from non-immunized or from passively sensitized animals. Since enhanced responses were also observed when LTD_4, arachidonic acid or histamine were used as triggering agents (Pretolani *et al.*, 1988), it is clear that immunization modifies the lung reactivity to mediators, both quantitatively and qualitatively.

The kinetics of the development of HR to PAF-acether showed that the increased lung response appeared between 2 and 4 days after the booster injection of the antigen, which was performed 2 weeks after the first sensitizing injection. HR then reached a plateau 7 days after the booster injection and persisted for at least 3 months. Interestingly, the lung response to antigen challenge increased also a couple of days after the booster injection of antigen, but then decreased steadily (Pretolani *et al.*, 1988). This allowed us to dissociate HR and hypersensitivity since the booster injection of antigen determines HR, which is independent of hypersensitivity *per se*. We hypothesized that the booster injection, probably acting as a micro-shock, leads to airways inflammation, characterized by the migration of inflammatory cells into the lung tissue. These cells might become new targets for the different agonists and thus amplify the lung response. Indeed, we have shown that actively sensitized guinea-pigs exhibit an increased number of eosinophils in the bronchoalveolar lavage fluid (Pretolani *et al.*, 1990a) and in the bone-marrow (Pretolani *et al.*, 1991), as compared with non-immunized or non-boosted animals.

6.2 Participation of Cytokines in Lung Hyperresponsiveness to PAF-acether

Lung responses to exogenous stimuli may be enhanced because resident cells are primed by cytokines generated after the booster injection of the antigen. Indeed, more recently it has become apparent that cytokines, secreted by helper T cells in response to antigenic stimulation, may play a role in pulmonary eosinophilia and lung inflammation and in the consequent HR (Gonzales *et al.*, 1987; Frew *et al.*, 1990). The cytokines mainly involved are interleukins: IL-5 and IL-3 and granulocyte–macrophage colony stimulating factor (GM-CSF), which support eosinophil proliferation and differentiation from their bone-marrow precursors (Coffman *et al.*, 1988; Miyajima *et al.*, 1988) and prime target cells (Silberstein *et al.*, 1986; Dahinden *et al.*, 1989; Bischoff *et al.*, 1990a; Bischoff *et al.*, 1990b). Nevertheless, since very large doses of rhIL-3, or rhGM-CSF or tumor necrosis factor α administered to non-sensitized guinea-pigs induce an increased eosinophilia in the bronchoalveolar lavage fluid (Kings *et al.*, 1990; Sanjar *et al.*, 1990), but no HR, pulmonary eosinophilia and cytokines alone cannot account for HR. The data discussed above, showing that mediators show a different profile when administered to lungs from actively sensitized as opposed to non-immunized or passively sensitized animals (Pretolani *et al.*, 1988), led us to compare the effect of the *in vitro* intra-pulmonary administration of recombinant human (rh) IL-5 on PAF-acether-induced bronchoconstriction and mediator release from lungs from non-sensitized guinea-pigs or from animals immunized by different procedures. The intra-tracheal administration of 100 or 300 ng of rhIL-5 to isolated perfused lungs from guinea-pigs actively sensitized to ovalbumin triggers a marked dose-dependent HR to the subsequent (10 min) intra-arterial injection of PAF-acether. This phenomenon, which is characterized by an enhanced bronchoconstriction and an increased release of TXB_2 and histamine in the effluent, occurs markedly in lungs from guinea-pigs used 2 or 7 days after the booster injection of the antigen, and to a lower extent in those from animals actively sensitized by a single antigen administration, the booster injection of the antigen being omitted. By contrast, rhIL-5 does not modify the lung response to PAF-acether in lungs from passively sensitized or from adjuvant-treated guinea-pigs, suggesting the participation of the immune system in this process. HR to PAF-acether reaches a plateau 10 min after the administration of rhIL-5, and persists for at least 30 min, whereas no significant increase of the response is observed after 2 min. The enhancement of the lung response to PAF-acether induced by rhIL-5 is concomitant with eosinophil invasion into the airways. Indeed, as compared with non-sensitized animals, the number of eosinophils in the bronchoalveolar lavage fluid is markedly increased in guinea-pigs sacrificed 2 or 7 days after the booster injection of the antigen and, to a lower extent, when the booster was omitted (Fig. 6.1). Bronchoconstriction to serotonin was unaffected by rhIL-5, indicating an effect of the cytokine against those mediators which act through the activation of pro-inflammatory cells rather than on smooth muscle. These results suggest that probably eosinophils, which are present in the lung only after the booster injection of the antigen, could be the targets for rhIL-5.

6.3 Pharmacological Modulation of Lung Hyperresponsiveness

The differences between lungs from sensitized and boosted as compared with non-immunized or non-boosted guinea-pigs extend to the effectiveness of inhibitors and antagonists of recognized mediators. Indeed, cyclooxygenase inhibitors block bronchoconstriction by PAF-acether injected intra-arterially to lungs from non-immunized guinea-pigs (Lefort *et al.*, 1984), but become inactive in those from sensitized animals, even though suppression of the formation of TXB_2 and 6-keto-$PGF_{1\alpha}$ is maintained. The anti-histamine drug mepyramine, alone or in combination with aspirin, only slightly decreased bronchoconstriction and histamine release by PAF-acether, whereas a mixed cyclooxygenase and lipoxygenase inhibitor,

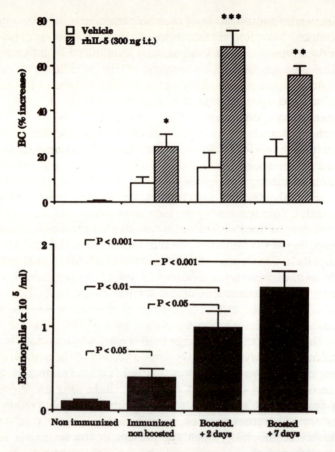

Fig. 6.1 Bronchoconstriction (BC, upper panel) induced by the intra-arterial administration of 1 ng PAF-acether into isolated guinea-pig lungs 10 min after an intra-tracheal (i.t.) injection of 100 μl saline (vehicle) or 300 ng rhIL-5. Bronchoconstriction was expressed as percentage of the area of the tracing measured over the basal resistance to inflation for 10 min. Results are expressed as mean ± SEM of 5 or 6 experiments. *$P < 0.05$, **$P < 0.01$, ***$P < 0.001$. The lower panel represents the eosinophil content of bronchoalveolar lavage fluid obtained from anaesthetized guinea-pigs. Bronchoalveolar cells were collected in 10 successive lavages and differentiated by May–Grünwald–Giemsa staining. Results are expressed as absolute number of eosinophils/ml. Data are expressed as mean ± SEM of 8–10 experiments. In both cases, i.e. for the study on the effect of rhIL-5 on PAF-acether-induced bronchoconstriction and for the eosinophil determinations in the bronchoalveolar lavage fluid, the experiments were performed on non-immunized guinea-pigs or on animals actively sensitized by a first injection of 10 μg ovalbumin in 1 mg of the adjuvant, i.e. Al(OH)$_3$, and used either 2 days after a s.c. injection of the adjuvant alone (group 'immunized non-boosted'), or 2 or 7 days after a booster injection of the antigen (groups 'boosted + 2 days' and 'boosted + 7 days' respectively).

compound BW755C, inhibited the enhanced responsiveness to PAF-acether, histamine secretion being again unaffected (Pretolani *et al.*, 1988). Bronchoconstriction on the one hand and histamine secretion on the other are thus separate events and lipoxygenase metabolites may be important for the expression of lung HR to PAF-acether. In confirmation, an enhanced PAF-acether-induced release of LTC_4-like material started 2–4 days after the booster injection of antigen (Pretolani et al., 1989a), as if a 'physiological' cyclooxygenase-dependent phase were replaced by a 'pathological' lipoxygenase-dependent one.

PAF-acether antagonists are widely used to study the participation of this phospholipid mediator in various physiopathological events, particularly at the lung level. When studying the effect of drug modulation in the ex vivo model of lung HR, we observed that concentrations of PAF-acether antagonists up to 10–100-fold above those which are effective against PAF-acether in control lungs failed to impair bronchoconstriction and release of LT-like material and histamine in lungs from actively sensitized guinea-pigs (Pretolani et al., 1989b). By contrast, the increased lung wet weight, an index of œdema formation, was inhibited, showing that failure to block the effects of PAF-acether with its otherwise specific antagonists is limited to those effects which are new 'acquisitions', whereas antagonism is maintained with respect to resident targets, such as the endothelial cells which are mainly involved with œdema formation. These observations further support the suggestion that the lung behaviour following active immunization is profoundly modified.

Nedocromil sodium, a pulmonary anti-inflammatory agent, inactive on arachidonate metabolism, was used to support the concept that isolated lungs from sensitized and boosted guinea-pigs may be used as a model for the in vivo situation. Nedocromil sodium failed to inhibit HR to PAF-acether or bronchoconstriction and mediator release in response to antigen challenge when it was added directly into the perfusion buffer at concentrations up to 0.1 mM. By contrast, when nedocromil sodium was administered in vivo daily, from the day of the booster injection of the antigen until the day of the experiment, bronchoconstriction, release of histamine, LTC_4 and TXB_2 in response to PAF-acether were markedly decreased (Pretolani et al., 1990a). The target of nedocromil sodium was not identified precisely, but since the increased number of eosinophils observed in the bronchoalveolar lavage fluid of the boosted animals was also reduced, and the inhibition of cell recruitment may account for the protection. In contrast to nedocromil sodium, which prevents the establishment of HR and fails to interfere directly with it, azelastine was effective in downregulating PAF-acether-induced release of histamine and of LTC_4 from lungs from sensitized and boosted guinea-pigs, using a protocol where its recognized anti-histamine properties were minimized (Pretolani et al., 1990b).

6.4 Conclusions

The bulk of these results indicate that our *ex vivo* model allows us to study the lung reactivity in term of variations in bronchial resistance on the one hand and the release of secondary mediators, which reflects the activation of the resident and invasive cells, on the other hand. Furthermore, since the lung response to the antigen and hyperresponsiveness appear to be dissociated in time and pharmacologically, the model parallels the human situation in which atopic patients are continuously exposed to an allergen thus perpetuating the recruitment and activation of inflammatory cells. The ability of IL-5 to enhance the lung response to PAF-acether in lungs from actively sensitized guinea-pigs only further strengthens the importance of the booster injection and suggests that the interaction between this and other cytokines on the one hand, and lipid mediators on the other, may represent a further approach for understanding the mechanisms of the development of bronchopulmonary hyperresponsiveness.

References

Bischoff, S. C., Brunner, T., De Weck, A. L. and Dahinden, C. A. (1990a). Interleukin-5 modifies histamine release and leukotriene generation by human basophils in response to diverse agonists. *J. Exp. Med.*, **172**, 1577–82.

Bischoff, S. C., De Weck, A. L. and Dahinden, C. A. (1990b). Interleukin-3 and GM-CSF render human basophils responsive to low concentrations of the complement component C3a. *Proc. Natl. Acad. Sci. USA*, **87**, 6813–17.

Coffman, R. L., Seymour, B. W. P., Lebman, D. A., Hiraki, D. D., Christiansen, J. A., Shrader, B., Cherwinski, H. M., Savelkoul, H. F. J., Finkelman, F. D., Bond, M. W. and Mosmann, T. R. (1988). The role of helper T cell products in mouse B cell differentiation and isotype regulation. *Immunol. Rev.*, **102**, 5–28.

Dahinden, C. A., Kurimoto, Y., De Weck, A. L., Lindley, B., Dewald, B. and Baggiolini, M. (1989). The neutrophil-activating peptide NAF/NAP-1 induces histamine and leukotriene release by interleukin-3-primed basophils. *J. Exp. Med.*, **170**, 1787–92.

Frew, A. J., Moqbel, R., Azzawi, M., Hartnell, A., Barkans, J., Jeffery, P. K., Kay, A. B., Scheper, R. J., Varley, J., Church, M. K. and Holgate, S. T. (1990). Lymphocytes and eosinophils in allergen-induced late-phase asthmatic reactions in the guinea pig. *Am. Rev. Respir. Dis.*, **141**, 407–13.

Gonzales, M. C., Diaz, P., Galleguillos, F. R., Ancic, P., Cromwell, O. and Kay, A. B. (1987). Allergen-induced recruitment of bronchoalveolar helper (OKT4) and suppressor (OKT8) T-cells in asthma. *Am. Rev. Respir. Dis.*, **136**, 600–4.

Kings, M. A., Chapman, I., Kristersson, A., Sanjar, S. and Morley, J. (1990). Human recombinant lymphokines and cytokines induce pulmonary eosinophilia in the guinea-pig which is modified by ketotifen and AH 21–132. *Int. Arch. Allergy Appl. Immunol.*, **91**, 354–61.

Lefort, J., Rotilio, D. and Vargaftig, B. B. (1984). The platelet-independent release of thromboxane A2 by PAF-acether from guinea-pig lungs involves mechanisms distinct from those of leukotrienes. *Br. J. Pharmacol.*, **82**, 565–75.

Miyajima, A., Miyatake, S., Schreurs, J., De Vries, J., Arai, N., Yokota, T. and Arai, K. (1988). Coordinate regulation of immune and inflammatory responses by T cell-derived lymphokines, *Faseb J.*, **2**, 2462–73.

Murphy, K. R., Wilson, M. C., Irvin, C. G., Glezen, L. S., Marsh, W. R., Haslett, C., Henson, P. M. and Larsen, G. L. (1986). *Am. Rev. Respir. Dis.*, **134**, 62–8.

Pretolani, M., Lefort, J. and Vargaftig, B. B. (1988). Active immunization induces lung hyperresponsiveness in the guinea pig. Pharmacological modulation and triggering role of the booster injection. *Am. Rev. Respir. Dis.*, **138**, 1572–8.

Pretolani, M., Lefort J., Dumarey, C. and Vargaftig, B. B. (1989a). Role of lipoxygenase metabolites for the hyperresponsiveness to platelet-activating factor of lungs from actively sensitized guinea-pigs. *J. Pharmacol. Exp. Ther.*, **248**, 353–9.

Pretolani, M., Lefort, J. and Vargaftig, B. B. (1989b). Limited interference of specific PAF antagonists with hyperresponsiveness to PAF itself of lungs from actively sensitized guinea-pigs. *Br. J. Pharmacol.*, **97**, 433–42.

Pretolani, M., Lefort, J., Silva, P., Malanchère, E., Dumarey, C., Bachelet, M. and Vargaftig, B. B. (1990a). Protection by nedocromil sodium of active immunization-induced bronchopulmonary alterations in the guinea pig. *Am. Rev. Respir. Dis.*, **141**, 1259–65.

Pretolani, M., Lefort, J. and Vargaftig, B. B. (1990b). Inhibition by azelastine of *in vitro* lung hyperreactivity in the guinea-pig. *Eur. J. Pharmacol.*, **183**, 216–17.

Pretolani, M., Lefort, J., Boukili, M. A., Bachelet, C. M. and Vargaftig, B. B. (1991). Potential involvement of eosinophils and of rh interleukin-5 (rhIL-5) in the *ex vivo* lung hyperresponsiveness in the guinea-pig. *Am. Rev. Respir. Dis.*, **143**, A14.

Sanjar, S., Smith, D., Kings, M. A. and Morley, J. (1990). Pretreatment with rh-GM-CSF, but not rh-IL-3, enhances, PAF-induced eosinophil accumulation in guinea-pig airways. *Br. J. Pharmacol.*, **100**, 399–400.

Silberstein, D. S. Owen, W. F., Gasson, J. C., DiPersio, J. F., Golde, D. W., Bina, J. C., Soberman, R., Austen, K. F. and David, J. R. (1986). Enhancement of human eosinophil cytotoxicity and leukotriene synthesis by biosynthetic (recombinant) granulocyte-macrophage colony-stimulating factor. *J. Immunol.*, **137**, 3290–4.

Vargaftig, B. B., Lefort, J. and Rotilio, D. (1983). Route dependent interactions between PAF-acether and guinea-pig bronchopulmonary smooth muscle: relevance of cyclooxygenase mechanisms. In Benveniste, J. and Arnoux, B. (eds.), *Platelet-Activating Factor, INSERM Symposium*, Vol. 23, Elsevier, Amsterdam, 307–17.

7

Properties of Human Lung Mast Cells

F. L. Pearce

7.1 Introduction

Asthma may be most simply defined as a reversible obstruction of the intrathoracic airways. The characteristic hallmarks of the disease are smooth muscle contraction, a non-specific increase in bronchial reactivity to diverse stimuli, mucosal oedema, inflammation of the airways and an accumulation of mucus. The latter can be the result of both glandular secretion of mucus glycoproteins and an increased movement of interstitial fluid into the airway lumen. This complex pathological profile is now recognized to involve a diversity of inflammatory cells, mediators and neuronal mechanisms (Barnes, 1987; Kay, 1987).

The involvement of mast cells in airway responses will depend on the range of chemical mediators that they produce and the mechanisms by which they may be activated. It has now been recognized for some years that mast cells from different locations may be functionally heterogeneous. This phenomenon is especially apparent in the gastrointestinal tract of the rat where two subpopulations, namely mucosal mast cells (MMCs) and connective tissue mast cells (CTMCs), may be identified. These phenotypes differ in their size, granule content of proteoglycans and neutral proteases, and in their responsiveness to a range of secretagogues and antiallergic agents (Befus *et al.*, 1982; Enerbäck, 1981; Pearce *et al.*, 1982). In the human, the difference between mast cell subsets seems to be more subtle and complex but two phenotypes have been designated on the basis of their granule protease content, namely TC mast cells (MC_{TC}) which contain the enzymes tryptase and chymase and T mast cells (MC_T) which contain tryptase alone (Irani *et al.*, 1986). In the lung, mast cells in the epithelium and in the lumen of the bronchioles and bronchi are almost exclusively of the MC_T phenotype while both populations occur in the subepithelium. However, the functional properties of these populations and their particular role in the asthmatic process have yet to be determined. For this reason, we have now recovered mast cells from the luminal surface of the airways by bronchoalveolar lavage (BAL) and from the lung parenchyma by enzymic dispersion of the intact tissue (dispersed lung (DL) cells). The superficially located BAL cells might be expected to participate in the earliest stages of the asthmatic response, with the DL cells becoming progressively more involved in the chronic disease as breakdown of the surface respiratory epithelium allows increased ingress of inhaled allergens.

7.2 Morphology and Histochemistry of Human Lung Mast Cells

Mast cells constitute 0.1–0.3% of the total nucleated population recovered by BAL and up to 5% of cells from dispersed lung (Pearce *et al.*, 1987; Walls *et al.*, 1990). The histamine content of the BAL cell (1.2 ± 0.3 pg) is significantly less than that of the DL cell (2.6 ± 0.1 pg) (Pearce *et al.*, 1987). Both populations stain with alcian blue dye, but do not counterstain with safranin O, a property that seems to be characteristic of most human mast cells. The majority of the cells are also sensitive to formaldehyde-based fixatives (Liu *et al.*, 1991; Walls *et al.*, 1990), a criterion which has been used as a diagnostic marker for the MMC phenotype in the rodent (Enerbäck, 1981). Interestingly, the numbers of formaldehyde-sensitive cells are significantly enhanced in the BAL fluid in a variety of disease states, suggesting that this population may expand under these conditions (Walls *et al.*, 1990).

The ultrastructure of the human parenchymal cell is dominated by secretory granules that can exhibit a range of ultrastructural patterns. The most common granule type contains cylindrical scrolls, which may be characteristic of the MC_T phenotype (Craig and Schwartz, 1990), while other mast cells contain granules whose matrices appear as highly ordered crystals or electron-dense particles. In addition, the cells also contain cytoplasmic lipid bodies.

The BAL cell broadly resembles that from the lung parenchyma. However, there are generally fewer granules, some of which are characteristically 'basket shaped' or partially disrupted, and numerous lipid bodies and cytoplasmic folds and projections. Overall, the cell appears to be in a partially activated state.

7.3 Bronchoalveolar Lavage in Extrinsic Asthma

The BAL fluid of asthmatic subjects contains considerably increased numbers of both eosinophils and mast cells compared with normal controls (Casale *et al.*, 1987; Flint *et al.*, 1985b; Wardlaw *et al.*, 1987). Strikingly, there is a highly significant correlation between the percentage of mast cells in the lavage and the severity of the disease as measured by spirometric indices of both airway obstruction and hyperresponsiveness (Flint *et al.*, 1985b). There is also an increased amount of free histamine in the BAL fluid of asthmatic subjects (Casale *et al.*, 1987), indicating that such individuals may have ongoing pulmonary mast cell degranulation (see also below). Consistently, the potent histamine H_1-receptor antagonist terfenadine produces a significant increase in baseline pulmonary function in these cases (Finnerty *et al.*, 1989). Antigen challenge in asthmatic subjects leads to a further bronchial eosinophilia and to a recovery of degranulated mast cells and eosinophils in the BAL fluid (Wardlaw *et al.*, 1987). While the above data would appear to implicate the BAL mast cell in the pathogenesis of asthma it should, however, be noted that similar increases in mast cell numbers have been observed in a diversity of other pulmonary disorders (Walls *et al.*, 1990).

7.4 Immunological and Pharmacological Activation of Human Lung Mast Cells

Stimulation of both BAL and DL mast cells with anti-human IgE produces a dose-dependent release of histamine, leukotriene C_4 (LTC_4), and prostaglandin D_2 (PGD_2) (Table 7.1). The antiserum is more effective in inducing PGD_2 production than histamine release and maximal amounts of the prostanoid are generated at lower concentrations of antibody. Higher concentrations of anti-IgE are required to evoke the *de novo* production of LTC_4. The spontaneous release of all three mediators is greater for the BAL than for the DL cells. In our hands, PGD_2 is the predominant eicosanoid produced by both cell populations and exceeds the amount of LTC_4 formed by about one order of magnitude. However, a comparable production of the two mediators has been reported by other workers (Fox *et al.*, 1985).

The spontaneous release of histamine from the BAL cells of extrinsic asthmatic patients (Flint *et al.*, 1985b) is significantly greater than that of normal controls (Fig. 7.1). The BAL cells of asthmatic subjects then appear to be inherently unstable, which is in accord with the finding of increased amounts of free histamine in the lavage fluid of such individuals and the clinical benefit afforded by histamine H_1-receptor antagonists (see

Table 7.1 Immunologically induced release of mediators from BAL and dispersed lung (DL) cells

Anti-IgE (dilution)	Histamine (% release)		LTC$_4$ (ng/10^6 mast cells)		PGD$_2$ (ng/10^6 mast cells)	
	BAL	DL	BAL	DL	BAL	DL
100	39.0 ± 6.2	49.5 ± 6.5	18.2 ± 3.5	16.1 ± 5.0	242 ± 50	145 ± 49
300	34.8 ± 5.7	41.0 ± 9.0	10.5 ± 3.5	11.8 ± 3.2	251 ± 60	139 ± 39
1000	31.9 ± 4.9	31.7 ± 7.3	7.0 ± 2.5	8.8 ± 2.9	219 ± 47	142 ± 30
10000	17.1 ± 10.2	10.0 ± 5.0	2.2 ± 1.2	2.9 ± 1.8	127 ± 34	63 ± 20
100000	0 ± 2.0	0.5 ± 0.5	—	0.6 ± 0.3	61 ± 33	36 ± 20

All values are means ± SEM for 10 (BAL) or 8 (DL) experiments and are corrected for the spontaneous releases in the absence of inducer. Spontaneous releases for the BAL and DL cells respectively were as follows: histamine, 11.5 ± 2.0 and 4.4 ± 1.4; LTC$_4$, 11.0 ± 7.3 and 1.8 ± 0.6; PGD$_2$, 55 ± 10 and 20 ± 14. From Leung et al. (1987), with permission.

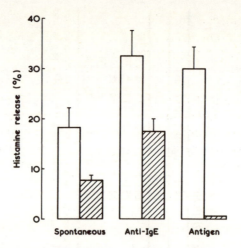

Fig. 7.1 Histamine release from BAL mast cells from asthmatic subjects (open bars) and normal controls (hatched bars) in the absence of any stimulus (spontaneous release) or following challenge with anti-human IgE (300-fold dilution) or specific antigen to house dust mite (10 µg/ml). All differences were statistically significant ($P < 0.05$).

above). Most interestingly, the BAL cells from asthmatics are also hyper-responsive to immunological activation with anti-IgE (Fig. 7.1) and respond to challenge with specific antigen while control cells do not (Flint *et al.*, 1985b).

Human lung mast cells may also be activated pharmacologically by the calcium ionophores A23187 and ionomycin but are totally refractory to a range of polycations including compound 48/80, polylysine, polyarginine, morphine, codeine and substance P (Tainsh *et al.*, 1991). The latter observation may have important implications for neurogenic models of inflammation in which the antidromic release of sensory neuropeptides such as substance P is suggested to lead to mast cell activation. Such models are largely based on studies in human skin (Foreman and Jordan, 1984). However, the human cutaneous mast cell is uniquely responsive to basic neuropeptides (Tainsh *et al.*, 1991) and the complete lack of effect of these agents on the lung cell suggests that such neurogenic mechanisms do not operate in the airways.

7.5 Hyperosmolar-induced Histamine Release

Exercise-induced asthma (EIA) is the term used to describe the broncho-constriction which occurs in some 70–80% of the asthmatic population following a period of strenuous activity. The mechanisms involved in EIA have been the subject of much debate. For some time it was assumed that the precipitating event was cooling of the airways brought about by the increase in respiratory heat exchange caused by hyperventilation. Airway cooling might then *per se* contract bronchial smooth muscle or, alternatively, lead to mast cell activation in a fashion similar to that observed in cold-induced urticaria. However, more recent observations have suggested that loss of water, rather than or in addition to loss of heat, from the bronchial mucosa can initiate EIA. This latter effect would act to increase the osmolarity of the periciliary fluid which in turn could lead to the activation of pulmonary mast cells. Consistently, increases in circulating levels of mast cell markers including histamine have been demonstrated during EIA (Lee *et al.*, 1984), and incubation in a hyperosmolar medium *in vitro* both produces a modest release of histamine from DL mast cells and strikingly augments their response to anti-IgE (Eggleston *et al.*, 1984).

To test this hypothesis further, we examined the effect of hyperosmolar buffer solutions on both BAL and DL cells (Flint *et al.*, 1985a). This experiment seemed to be particularly relevant since it is the lumenal BAL, rather than the tissue DL, cell that would be exposed to the proposed hyperosmolar environment. In each case, raising the osmolarity of the incubation medium from 280 to 1270 mOsm/kg by adding increasing concentrations of mannitol (0.1–1 M) led to a dose-dependent release of histamine. The kinetics of the process was complex: there was an initial, fairly rapid release of the amine which reached a plateau after 10–20 min. Thereafter, the release increased progressively and slowly over a 60 min period. Strikingly, after 10 min of incubation, the BAL cells were very much more reactive than the DL cells, the two populations giving optimal releases of histamine of 12.1 ± 1.2% and 2.7 ± 0.5% respectively.

7.6 Inhibition of Histamine Release from Pulmonary Mast Cells

Disodium cromoglycate was introduced into clinical practice in the United Kingdom in 1967 for the management and prophylaxis of human bronchial asthma. At that time, this activity was essentially ascribed to its ability to prevent the release of inflammatory mediators from mast cells. While it is now recognized that the mode of action of the compound is probably considerably more complex than first envisaged (Pearce, 1989), there persists considerable interest in mast cell stabilizing drugs. We have therefore examined the effect of a number of anti-asthmatic compounds on BAL and DL cells (Pearce *et al.*, 1987; Leung *et al.*, 1988). The former cells are of particular interest in this respect since they are located on the lumenal surface of the airways and will come into direct and immediate contact with

Table 7.2   Effect of various anti-asthmatic drugs on histamine release from BAL
and dispersed lung (DL) mast cells

Drug	$IC_{30}{}^*$ (μM)	
	BAL	DL
Salbutamol	0.02	0.1
Theophylline	500	300
Sodium chromoglycate	3	200
Nedocromil sodium	0.3	5

$IC_{30}{}^*$ denotes the concentration of drug required to produce 30% inhibition of histamine release induced by anti-human IgE.

inhaled drugs. A comparison of the two cell types is of further relevance since cromoglycate-like compounds are well known to exhibit a high degree of species and tissue selectivity in their action (Foreman and Pearce, 1988).

Histamine release from both the BAL and DL cells is comparably inhibited by the B_2-adrenoceptor agonist salbutamol and the phosphodiesterase inhibitor theophylline (Table 7.2). However, both sodium cromoglycate and its more potent congener nedocromil sodium are strikingly more active against the BAL cell than the DL cell, and nedocromil sodium is about one order of magnitude more effective than sodium cromoglycate against both cell types (Table 7.2). In addition, tachyphylaxis to the chromone and the pyranoquinoline is observed with the DL but not with the BAL cell (Leung *et al.*, 1988). The latter observation is, of course, more in keeping with the prophylactic clinical utility of the drugs.

7.7 The Role of Mast Cells in Human Bronchial Asthma

Human bronchial asthma is a highly complex, multi-factorial disease. Attempts to assign a specific role to any given inflammatory cell type within this process are highly problematical. However, mast cell products are capable of producing many of the hallmarks of the disease. Thus, histamine, leukotrienes and PGD_2 are all able to evoke smooth muscle contraction, mucus hypersecretion and oedema formation (Peters, 1990). Tryptase and chymase may regulate neuropeptide activity, bronchomotor tone and submucosal gland secretion (Caughey, 1989).

Current evidence indicates that the immediate bronchoconstrictor response to inhaled allergens is largely mediated by mast cell products. In particular, the effect is dramatically attenuated by pretreatment with potent, specific H_1-antihistamines (Wood-Baker and Church, 1990) and the available data suggest that about one-half of the constriction is due to histamine and the remainder to arachidonic acid metabolites.

The role of the mast cell in the development of bronchial hyperreactivity and airway inflammation, which are probably more relevant to the situation in chronic clinical asthma, is more controversial. However, it has recently been shown that murine mast cell lines are able to secrete a wide range of cytokines (Gordon *et al.*, 1990). If a similar activity is expressed by human lung mast cells, their activation could recruit, prime and stimulate neutrophils, macrophages, basophils and eosinophils, increase immunoglobulin secretion and regulate the proliferation and phenotype of other mast cells. As such, the human pulmonary mast cell would once again be firmly implicated in the ongoing inflammatory events of chronic asthma.

Acknowledgements

Work from the author's laboratory was supported by grants from the National Asthma Campaign, Fisons plc and the Wellcome Trust.

References

Barnes, P. J. (1987). Inflammatory mediator receptors and asthma. *Am. Rev. Respir. Dis.*, **135**, S26–S31.

Befus, A. D., Pearce, F. L., Gauldie, J., Horsewood, P. and Bienenstock, J. (1982). Mucosal mast cells. I. Isolation and functional characteristics of rat intestinal mast cells. *J. Immunol.*, **128**, 2475–80.

Casale, T. B., Wood, D., Richerson, H. B., Trapp, S., Metzger W. J., Zavala, D. and Hunninghake, G. W. (1987). Elevated bronchoalveolar lavage fluid histamine levels in allergic asthmatics are associated with methacholine bronchial hyperresponsiveness. *Clin. Invest.*, **79**, 1197–203.

Caughey, G. H. (1989). Roles of mast cell tryptase and chymase in airway function. *Am. J. Physiol.*, **257**, L39–L46.

Craig, S. S. and Schwartz, L. B. (1990). Human MC_{TC} type of mast cell granule: the uncommon occurrence of discrete scrolls associated with focal absence of chymase. *Lab. Invest.*, **63**, 581–5.

Egglestone, P. A., Kagey-Sobotka, A., Schleimer, R. P. and Lichtenstein, L. M. (1984). Interaction between hyperosmolar and IgE-mediated histamine release from basophils and mast cells. *Am. Rev. Respir. Dis.*, **130**, 86–91.

Enerbäck, L. (1981). The gut mucosal mast cell. *Monogr. Allergy*, **17**, 222–32.

Finnerty, J. P., Wilmot, C. and Holgate, S. T. (1989). Inhibition of hypertonic saline-induced bronchoconstriction by terfenadine and flurbiprofen. Evidence for the predominant role of histamine. *Am. Rev. Respir. Dis.*, **140**, 593–7.

Flint, K. C., Hudspith, B. N., Leung, K. B. P., Pearce, F. L., Brostoff, J. and Johnson, N. McI. (1985a). The hyperosmolar release of histamine from bronchoalveolar mast cells and its inhibition by sodium cromoglycate. *Thorax*, **40**, 717.

Flint, K. C., Leung, K. B. P., Hudspith, B. N., Brostoff, J., Pearce, F. L. and

Johnson, N. McI. (1985b). Bronchoalveolar lavage in extrinsic asthma: a mechanism for the initiation of antigen specific bronchoconstriction. *Br. Med. J.*, **291**, 923–6.

Foreman, J. C. and Jordan, C. C. (1984). Neurogenic inflammation. *Trends Pharmacol. Sci.*, **5**, 116–19.

Foreman, J. C. and Pearce, F. L. (1988). Cromolyn. In Middleton, E., Reed, C. E., Ellis, E. F., Adkinson, N. F., and Yunginger, J. W. (eds.), *Allergy: Principles and Practice*, C. V. Mosby, St. Louis, MO, 744–81.

Fox, C. C., Kagey-Sobotka, A., Schleimer, R. P., Peters, S. P., MacGlashan, D. W. and Lichtenstein L. M. (1985). Mediator release from human basophils and mast cells from lung and intestinal mucosa. *Int. Arch. Allergy Appl. Immunol.*, **77**, 130–6.

Gordon, J. R., Burd, P. R. and Galli, S. J. (1990). Mast cells as a source of multifunctional cytokines. *Immunol. Today*, **11**, 458–64.

Irani, A. A., Schechter, N. M., Craig, S. S., DeBlois, G. and Schwartz, L. B. (1986). Two types of human mast cells that have distinct neutral protease compositions. *Proc. Natl. Acad. Sci. USA*, **83**, 4464–8.

Kay, A. B. (1987). Inflammatory cells in acute and chronic asthma. *Am. Rev. Respir. Dis.*, **135**, S63–S66.

Lee, T. H., Nagakura, T., Papageorgiou, N., Cromwell, O., Iikura, Y. and Kay, A. B. (1984). Mediators in exercise-induced asthma. *J. Allergy Clin. Immunol.*, **73**, 634–9.

Leung, K. B. P., Flint, K. C., Hudspith, B. N., Brostoff, J., Johnson, N. M, Seager, K., Hammond, M. D. and Pearce, F. L. (1987). Some further properties of human pulmonary mast cells recovered by bronchoalveolar lavage and enzymatic dissociation of lung tissue. *Agents Actions*, **20**, 213–15.

Leung, K. B. P., Flint, K. C., Brostoff, J., Hudspith, B. N., Johnson, N. McI., Lau, H. Y. A., Liu, W. and Pearce, F. L. (1988). Effects of sodium cromoglycate and nedocromil sodium on histamine secretion from human lung mast cells. *Thorax*, **43**, 756–61.

Liu, W. L., Boulos, P. B., Lau, H. Y. A. and Pearce, F. L. (1991). Mast cells from human gastric mucosa: a comparative study with lung and colonic mast cells. *Agents Actions*, **33**, 13–15.

Pearce, F. L. (1989). Mast cells: function, differentiation and activation. *Curr. Opinion Immunol.*, **1**, 630–6.

Pearce, F. L., Befus, A. D., Gauldie, J. and Bienenstock, J. (1982). Mucosal mast cells. II. Effect of anti-allergic compounds on histamine secretion by isolated intestinal mast cells. *J. Immunol.*, **128**, 2481–6.

Pearce, F. L., Flint, K. C., Leung, K. P. B., Hudspith, B. N., Seager, K., Hammond, M. D., Brostoff, J., Geraint-James, D. and Johnson, M. McI. (1987). Some studies on human pulmonary mast cells obtained by bronchoalveolar lavage and by enzymic dissociation of whole lung tissue. *Int. Arch. Allergy Appl. Immunol.*, **82**, 507–12.

Peters, S. P. (1990). Mast cells and histamine in asthma. *J. Allergy Clin. Immunol.*, **86**, 642–6.

Tainsh, K. R., Lau, H. Y. A., Liu, W. L. and Pearce, F. L. (1991). The human skin mast cell: a comparison with the human lung cell and a novel mast cell type, the uterine mast cell. *Agents Actions*, **33**, 16–19.

Walls, A. F., Roberts, J. A., Godfrey, R. C., Church, M. K. and Holgate, S. T. (1990). Histochemical heterogeneity of human mast cells: disease related differences in mast cell subsets recovered by bronchoalveolar lavage. *Int. Arch. Allergy Appl. Immunol.*, **92**, 223–41.

Wardlaw, A. J., Collins, J. V. and Kay, A. B. (1987). Mechanisms in asthma using the technique of bronchoalveolar lavage. *Int. Arch. Allergy Appl. Immunol.*, **82**, 518–25.

Wood-Baker, R. and Church, M. K. (1990). Histamine and asthma. *Allergy Clin. N. Am.*, **10**, 329–36.

8

Antigenic and Peptidergic Pathways of Mast Cell Activation

C. Bronner, A. Vallé and Y. Landry

8.1 Introduction

Two pathways of mast cells activation are now well characterized. The antigenic pathway involves the preliminary binding of immunoglobulin E (IgE) to specific high affinity receptors, called FcεRI, and the subsequent cross-linking of bound IgE molecules by specific antigens (allergens). This mechanism, related to allergic diseases, account for the activation of basophils and of the different types of mast cells. In contrast, the second pathway of mast cell activation occurs only in the so-called serosal, typical or connective tissue mast cells (see Chapter 7 in this book) which models are rat peritoneal mast cells and human skin mast cells. A number of items of evidence reported by our group and largely confirmed by others show that this pathway involves the activation of trimeric GTP-dependent proteins (G proteins) by peptides and polyamines through a receptor-independent mechanism. The physiological relevance of this mechanism of mast cell activation is discussed below.

8.2 The Antigenic Pathway of Mast Cell Activation

Molecular Characterization of the High Affinity Receptor for IgE: FcεRI

The first attempts to purify FcεRI using classical affinity chromatography yielded only one polypeptide (Conrad and Froese, 1976). Molecular weight studies with mild detergent showed that this receptor contains more than one single polypeptide (Perez-Montfort et al., 1983). FcεRI is at least a tetrameric complex of one α subunit, one β subunit and two γ subunits (αβγ2). As reviewed by Kinet (1990) and by Ravetch and Kinet (1991), complementary DNAs for each subunit have been isolated from three different species: mouse, rat and human. The cloning of the human β chain is not yet published but will be described soon (J. P. Kinet, personal communication). With the exception of FcεRII/CD23, the low affinity receptor for IgE which is homologous to lectin binding proteins (reviewed by Conrad, 1990), the receptors of the different immunoglobulins (Fc receptors) belong to the immunoglobulin superfamily. Molecular charac-terization of Fcγ receptors for IgG through their molecular cloning (FcγRI/ CD64, FcγRII/CD32 and FcγRIII/CD16) led to considerable progress in defining the heterogeneity of Fc receptors, FcεRI for IgE and FcγRIII-A for IgG are now known to be multimeric complexes of non-covalently associated subunits. FcεRI is the most complicated of cellular Fc receptors so far identified, and it may represent a model structure of other Fc receptors.

The α Subunit is the IgE Binding Subunit

This subunit of FcεRI is homologous to FcγRs binding proteins (IgG) and to the recently identified IgA binding protein (Malizewski et al., 1990). The extracellular segment of these receptors contains homologous immunoglobulin-related domains defined by characteristic loops between two cysteine residues. Detailed gene analysis indicated that these Fc recep-tors have evolved from a common precursor through gene duplication (Ravetch and Kinet, 1991). These binding subunits are structurally related but differ in their transmembrane and intracellular domains which presum-ably mediate intracellular signalling.

The β Subunit

The β subunit contains four presumptive transmembrane domains and has cytoplasmic amino and carboxy terminals. It shares homology with Ly-44/ CD20 (Hupp et al., 1989). Cotransfection studies indicated that this sub-unit is not absolutely necessary in human for expression of high affinity binding of human immunoglobulin E (Miller et al., 1989; Blank et al., 1989). Such β, or β-like, proteins may be associated with other Ig super-family members such as FcγRs for IgG.

The γ Subunit is Expressed as a Disulphide-linked Dimer

Comparison between the gene structure of the γ chain of the receptor and of the ζ (zeta) chain of the T cell receptor (TCR) indicates that these genes have evolved from a common ancestor by gene duplication and define a new gene family (Küster *et al.*, 1990). A third member of the same family is the TCR η chain which is generated by alternate splicing from the same gene as the TCR ζ chain (Jin *et al.*, 1990). These chains are essential for surface expression of their receptors (Blank *et al.*, 1989; Küster *et al.*, 1990). Furthermore, the ζ chain can substitute γ subunits of FcεRI in assembly (Howard *et al.*, 1990). These chains are expressed as disulphide-linked dimers in FcεRI but may be also expressed as heterodimers (Orlof *et al.*, 1990; Letourneur *et al.*, 1991). The mouse FcγRIIa and its human homologue (FcγRIII-A) of macrophages and natural killer cells share such disulphide-linked dimers, as well as a mouse T cell line (CTLL) as part of the T cell receptor complex (Orlof *et al.*, 1990). This is of interest since CD3 negative natural killer cells express ζ TCR chain or FcεRI γ chain as part of a novel molecular complex (Anderson *et al.*, 1989; Lanier *et al.*, 1989). The γ chain is required for surface expression of the receptor (Blank *et al.*, 1989; Küster *et al.*, 1990) but the extracellular domain of α subunit alone is sufficient for high affinity IgE binding (Hakimi *et al.*, 1990). These subunits of FcεRI do not display tyrosine kinase activity by themselves but β and γ chains are quickly and transiently phosphorylated upon antigenic stimulation (Paolini *et al.*, 1991).

The IgE-mediated Transducing Events, an Overview

Since the pionering studies of Ishizaka's group on the IgE-mediated intracellular signalling in mast cells some progress has been made in the understanding of the sequence of biochemical events following the IgE receptor of high affinity (FcεRI). Numerous interesting reports have shown that several other actors than those proposed initially by Ishizaka's group are involved and have indicated that the activation of FcεRI exhibits a complexity higher than that expected. The first proposed series of intracellular events occurring after the stimulation of FcεRI included phospholipid methylations, calcium entry, activation of phospholipase A_2 and of adenylate cyclase (extensively reviewed in Siraganian (1983) and Ishizaka (1982). However, none of these events can totally account for the secretory effect. The putative candidates involved in the early stage following FcεRI activation are summarized below.

Is There Any Role for a G Protein in the FcεRI Transducing Events?

A diverse range of cellular functions in eukariotic cells are regulated by proteins that undergo a cycle of GTP binding and hydrolysis. These G proteins are located on the inner face of the plasma membrane and are linked to the membrane by two types of lipid modifications, myristoylation and isoprenylation (reviewed in Spiegel et al., 1991). G proteins are heterotrimeric and couple many monomeric surface receptors with seven transmembrane domains to their effectors. These G proteins exhibit a high molecular weight ($\sim$ 90 kDa) when compared with the vast range of monomeric GTP-binding proteins of low molecular mass (20–25 kDa). The small G proteins show clear sequence homology to the α subunit of trimeric G proteins and to the proteins encoded by ras oncogenes (reviewed in Downward, 1990; Balch, 1990). However, in mast cells, little is known about the nature and structure of the G proteins involved in stimulus–secretion coupling events. Two types of trimeric G proteins have been suggested to exist in mast cells, one coupled to phospholipase C and another distal to this enzyme (Cockcroft et al., 1987). Activation of pertussis toxin-sensitive G_i-like proteins has been proposed to be one of the early events occurring during peptidergic activation of mast cells (Bueb et al., 1990b; see also below). However, it is now clear that the IgE-dependent histamine release from rat peritoneal mast cells (Saito et al., 1989; Bronner et al., 1990) and from rat basophilic leukaemia cells (RBL), subline 2H3 (Wilson et al., 1991), is insensitive to pertussis toxin. Therefore, it is unlikely that G_i-like proteins are involved in FcεRI activation. Nevertheless, other G proteins might be involved but depending on mast cell heterogeneity. A cholera-sensitive G protein potentiates IgE-dependent histamine release from RBL 2H3 by enhancing $[Ca^{2+}]_i$ (Wilson et al., 1991; Nakashima, 1991; McCloskey, 1988) but is without effect on that induced in bone marrow-derived mouse mast cells (Saito et al., 1988). $GDP_\beta S$, an inhibitor of G proteins, inhibits in a dose-dependent manner the IgE-mediated histamine release from rat peritoneal mast cells but not that from bone marrow-derived mast cells (Saito et al., 1989). Together these results show that the role of G proteins for FcεRI-mediated events strongly depends on the mast cell model. Trimeric and/or small G proteins may be involved in a step distal to the early signalling process, but the direct coupling of FcεRI to trimeric G proteins seems unlikely.

Phospholipase C, Non-receptor Tyrosine Kinases and FcεRI

One important pathway activated after IgE-receptor cross-linking involves the hydrolysis of phosphatidylinositol bisphosphate by phospholipase C (Beaven et al., 1984), leading to the concomitant generation of diacylglycerol and inositol triphosphates, which mobilizes calcium from intracellular stores. The identity of these stores is not well defined in mast cells (Rossier *et al.*, 1989). Several putative types of phospholipase C might exist throughout the different types of mast cells or even in a single cell. Four subtypes of phospholipase C are known in mammalian tissues (α, β, γ and δ), all of which are single polypeptides, and the products of discrete genes (Rhee *et al.*, 1989; Ryu *et al.*, 1987). Molecular masses measured by SDS–PAGE are 62–68 kDa, 150–154 kDa, 145–148 kDa and 85–88 kDa for α, β, γ and δ respectively (Rhee *et al.*, 1989). The structures and functional domains of phospholipases C are reviewed in Rhee (1991). Phospholipase C can be activated by at least two different pathways, involving a trimeric G protein insensitive to pertussis toxin (Gq) (Strahtman and Simon, 1990) or via tyrosine and serine phosphorylation by receptor tyrosine kinases or non-receptor tyrosine kinases. The activation by Gq concerns the β_1 isoform but not the α_1 or δ_1 isoforms. The γ_1 isoform can be activated by receptors that contain tyrosine kinase activity such as PDGF (platelet-derived growth factor) and EGF (epidermal growth factor) receptors but also by non-receptor tyrosine kinases stimulated by the TCR (CD3) (reviewed in Rhee, 1991).

Antigen-mediated activation of phospholipase C in rat peritoneal mast cells or bone marrow-derived mouse mast cells does not involve a G protein (Saito *et al.*, 1989). However, in rat basophilic leukaemia cells some evidence suggests a coupling of phospholipase C to a G protein (Woldemussie *et al.*, 1987). Nevertheless, phosphorylation of phospholipase C through some indirect pathway seems a more reasonable mode of regulation by FcεRI. Tyrosine phosphorylation is an early event subsequent to FcεRI aggregation (Benhamou *et al.*, 1990; Connely *et al.*, 1991). The phosphotyrosine content of proteins of M_r = 139, 117, 84, 69, 66, 57 and 40 kDa was increased after IgE-dependent RBL stimulation (Connely *et al.*, 1991). Benhamou and coworkers (1990) found phosphotyrosine-containing proteins with a molecular mass of 83, 72, 62 and 57 kDa. FcεRI does not contain any tyrosine kinase domain in the protein sequence suggesting that the FcεRI might be associated with an intracellular tyrosine kinase, most likely to be a member of the *src* family of tyrosine kinases. Eiseman and Bolen (1990) showed that cross-linking of FcεRI activates *src* family members, *lyn* in the RBL cells and *yes* in the mouse mast cell line PT-18. Tyrosine phosphorylation by FcεRI has been found to be independent of protein kinase C activity, or calcium influx (Benhamou *et al.*, 1990) and of phospholipase C since inositol phospholipid breakdown is dramatically reduced in the absence of external calcium (Cunha-Melo *et al.*, 1987; Pribluda and Metzger, 1987) whereas tyrosine phosphorylation by FcεRI aggregation is calcium independent (Benhamou *et al.*, 1990). This shows that all the studied metabolisms are subsequent to the stimulation of a tyrosine kinase. It remains to determine whether one of the phosphotyrosine-containing proteins is a member of the phospholipase C family. Recently, it was shown that genistein, a protein tyrosine kinase inhibitor, inhibited antigen-induced phosphatidylinositol (PI) turnover in RBL cells (Deanin *et al.*, 1991). These authors suggested that the tyrosine kinase-dependent event is the activation of γ phospholipase C. Paolini *et al.* (1991) showed that tyrosine phosphorylation of FcεRI occurs within 5 s after adding the antigen and is quickly reversible. Thus, non-receptor tyrosine kinase activation might be the earliest event following the activation of FcεRI.

Phospholipase D, Phospholipase A2, Protein Kinase C and FcεRI

Studies during the last decade revealed that protein kinase C (PKC) may play a role in the signal transduction process in many receptor coupling events preceding mediator release, by interfering with several metabolisms, including PI metabolism (reviewed in Garcia-Sainz, 1991). PKC, a calcium- and phospholipid-dependent enzyme, is endogenously activated by diacylglycerol and can be experimentally stimulated by phorbol esters such as PMA (phorbol myristate acetate). The role of PKC in FcεRI-mediated processes is not yet clearly determined. Activation of PKC appears to be solely involved in the IgE-mediated histamine release from rat peritoneal mast cells (White *et al.*, 1989). The targets of PKC in mast cells are still unknown. Antigen-induced histamine release in PT-18 cells is associated with increased PKC activity in the plasma membrane (White *et al.*, 1985). PKC substrate proteins were identified in the cytosol of IgE-mediated stimulation of bone-marrow-derived mast cells. Three proteins of 45 kDa were described (White *et al.*, 1989). Other PKC substrates were reported, namely myosin heavy and light chains and a plasma membrane glycoprotein (Ludowyke *et al.*, 1989; Katz *et al.*, 1989).

The endogenous activator of PKC, diacylglycerol (DAG), is usually recognized to result from phosphatidylinositol breakdown catalysed by phospholipase C. However, recent studies pointed out that the major source of DAG is not phosphatidylinositol and that the major enzyme responsible for DAG synthesis is not phospholipase C. When DAG levels become maximal in IgE-dependent stimulation of mast cells, no more than 25% is derived from phosphatidylinositol whereas as much as 75% could come from phosphatidylcholine (Kennerly, 1990). The synthesis of DAG from phosphatidylcholine can result from two pathways. The first (direct) involves phospholipase C (PLC) with the concomitant release of phosphocholine and the second (indirect) would implicate phospholipase D (PLD) leading to the generation of phosphatidic acid and subsequently to DAG by phosphatidic acid hydrolase (Gruchalla *et al.*, 1990). IgE receptor cross-linking resulted in a 3- to 10-fold increase in PLD activity during the 10 min after stimulation (Gruchalla *et al.*, 1990). Further observations allowed Kennerly's group to suggest that the major mechanism of DAG formation during mast cell activation is phosphatidylcholine → phosphatidic acid → diacylglycerol. Similar results were obtained with the IgE-dependent stimulation of rat basophilic leukaemia cells (Lin *et al.*, 1991). Nevertheless, a recent report by Nakashima *et al.* (1991), showed that the phosphatidylcholine hydrolysis in rat basophilic leukaemia cells may be dependent on PKC and calcium. Therefore, phospholipase D activation would be secondary to phosphatidylinositolphosphate 2 (PIP_2) breakdown. On the other hand, antigen-induced activation of PLD in rat mast cells was found to be independent of PKC (Yamada *et al.*, 1991). The authors concluded that diacylglycerol, formed by PLC, can stimulate directly or indirectly PLD, independently of PKC.

The role of phospholipase A_2 (PLA_2) in IgE-mediated histamine is still unclear. Considering the studies mentioned above, the synthesis of arachidonic acid would result either from a combined effect of PLC–DAG lipase or PLD–PA hydrolase–DAG lipase since no lysophosphatidylcholine (lyso PC), a metabolite of PLA_2, could be detected in IgE-dependent stimulated RBL cells (Lin *et al.*, 1991). However, the authors could not totally rule out a role for PLA_2 since the synthesis of lyso PC could be masked by a rapid acylation. In contrast, it was shown that parabromophenacyl bromide, a selective inhibitor of PLA_2, inhibited antigen and IgE-dependent histamine release from rat peritoneal mast cells (Chand *et al.*, 1987; Bronner *et al.*, 1990) and from rat basophilic leukaemia cells (Givney *et al.*, 1981). Thus, the arachidonic acid metabolites generated by PLA_2 might be not only inflammatory mediators but also second messengers.

Conclusion

In conclusion, the first biochemical event following IgE receptor cross-linking by the antigen might be an interaction of FcεRI with a non-receptor tyrosine kinase which leads to the rapid phosphorylation of the receptor. The sequence of transducing events cannot yet be constructed but might involve the following: non-receptor tyrosine kinase activation → PLC_γ activation → (IP_3 + DAG) → (Ca^{2+} increase + PKC activation) → PLD–PLA_2 activation. The identification of the substrates of tyrosine kinase and of protein kinase C should help to identify further this sequence.

8.3 The Peptidergic Pathway of Mast Cell Activation

The activation of rat peritoneal mast cells by polyamines, and by various peptides, has been recognized for three decades as a non-lytic process depending on the active metabolism of the cells (for review see Lagunoff *et al.*, 1983). These observations have been extended to human skin mast cells (Church *et al.*, 1989) and might also apply to other human connective tissue mast cells. These sensitive mast cells represent a minor population of human lung mast cells but are largely represented in rodent lungs. A perivascular localization in the brain has also been proposed recently considering mast cells as a gate to the brain (Theoharides, 1990). Thus the peptidergic pathway of mast cell activation is putatively involved in many processes, such as skin sensitivity to venom peptides, urticaria, impairment of the blood–brain barrier and central inflammatory processes, peripheral neurogenous inflammation and the different inflammatory diseases involving the blood complement cascade.

The Triggers of the Peptidergic Pathway, Pathophysiological Relevance

The common point of the structure in these triggers is their cationic amphiphilic property. These triggers include (1) natural and synthetic polyamines such as spermine (Bueb *et al.*, 1991, 1992) and compound 48/80 (Mousli *et al.*, 1989, 1990b, c; Tomita *et al.*, 1991a), (2) venom peptides such as mastoparan from wasp venom and mast cell degranulating peptide (MCD) from bee venom (Mousli *et al.*, 1991; Fujimoto *et al.*, 1991; Tomita *et al.*, 1991b) and mellitin (Higashijima *et al.*, 1990), (3) neuropeptides such as substance P (Mousli *et al.*, 1990b, c) and dynorphin (Higashijima *et al.*, 1990), (4) peptidic hormones such as bradykinin, Lys-bradykinin (Bueb *et al.*, 1990a, b), ACTH and angiotensin II (Higashijima *et al.*, 1990), and (5) anaphylatoxins, which are components of the blood complement cascade that also belong to this family of mast cell triggers, as recently demonstrated in the case of C_{3a} (Mousli *et al.*, 1992b).

This list is not exhaustive since most of the cationic amphyphilic peptides, including for instance synthetic antagonists of substance P and bradykinin receptors, are known to stimulate mast cells and are candidates as triggers of this pathway. However, the concentration of trigger required to activate mast cells is usually high (10^{-6} to 10^{-3} M) and the physiological relevance of *in vitro* assays requires special attention. To be effective, a high concentration of trigger has to be expected near mast cells. This is easily conceivable in the case of venom peptides with a local effect but not in the case of drugs given by a systemic route of administration. For endogenous mediators we can reasonably expect high concentrations of neuropeptides in the vicinity of neuronal endings. This might be the case for substance P released by C-fibres which have been shown to be closely associated with mast cells. However, this remains speculative because the local levels of substance P have not yet been measured. Similarly, a high local concentration of bradykinin might be achieved in inflammatory tissues considering that tryptase released by the different types of mast cells can generate bradykinin from inactive precursors, kininogens. However, serosal mast cells, i.e. mast cells sensitive to peptides, also release chymase which is able to hydrolyse bradykinin. Thus, bradykinin effects on mast cells should be quite short but might potentiate IgE-dependent mast cell activation. To our knowledge, the anaphylatoxin C_{3a} is the unique trigger of the peptidergic pathway whose blood concentration reaches micromolar levels (Fukuoka and Hugli, 1990) in agreement with a secretory effect on mast cells (Mousli et al., 1992b). Considering the wide involvement of the complement in pathology, the interest in this pathway is largely justified.

Trimeric G Proteins in the Activation of the Peptidergic Pathway

Many attempts have been made to discover the receptors of the triggers of mast cells described above, considering that such receptors might be proteins of the plasma membrane as are most of the receptors of mediators. This was the case for compound 48/80, substance P (for review see Mousli et al., 1990a) and more recently for C_{3a} (Fukuoka and Hugli, 1990). However, no decisive evidence was obtained. This is quite in agreement with some indirect observations. For instance, in the case of substance P, membrane receptors are now well known. They belong to the superfamily of seven transmembrane domain-spanning receptors coupled to G proteins. These receptors are also stimulated by neurokinin A and neurokinin B, but mast cells are not sensitive to these peptides. These receptors are antagonized by well-known analogues of substance P, but these current antagonists also stimulate mast cells. Also, these receptors are sensitive to lower concentrations of substance P as referred to the concentrations required to stimulate mast cells. Similar observations also apply to other endogenous triggers such as bradykinin or C_{3a}.

An alternative needed to be found to the occurrence of selective membrane receptors for these triggers. This has been done from the demonstration by Higashijima et al. (1987, 1988) that the venom peptide mastoparan can activate purified trimeric G proteins. At that time we were demonstrating that mastoparan, substance P and compound 48/80 shares large similarity in their effect on mast cells (Mousli et al., 1989). These similarities include (1) rapid kinetics of histamine release, reaching a maximum at 10 s after the trigger was added, (2) similar ionic requirements for mast cell activation and a reduction in the sensitivity of mast cells to these triggers in the presence of millimolar Ca^{2+} concentrations, (3) desensitization of mast cells by pretreatment with neuraminidase, which removes sialic acid residues from the cell surface, (4) inhibition by the hydrophobic quaternary amine benzalkonium chloride, a selective inhibitor of G_i, and

(5) inhibition by pertussis toxin pretreatment and transient stimulation of polyphosphoinositide breakdown, demonstrating that a pertussis toxin-sensitive G protein and the activation of phospholipase C are involved in the activation of rat peritoneal mast cells by mastoparan, substance P and 48/80. Using G proteins purified from bovine brain, we showed that, like mastoparan, compound 48/80 and substance P are able to increase the binding of GTP to the α subunit and to increase its GTPase activity (Mousli et al., 1990b). The inhibitory effect of antibodies selective of the C-terminal sequence of the α subunit of the G proteins strongly suggested that compound 48/80, substance P and mastoparan interact with this end of the α subunit (Mousli et al., 1990c). Interestingly, this C-terminus has been shown to interact with receptors allowing us to consider that these cationic compounds mimic receptors coupled to G proteins. More recently we extended the activation of purified G proteins to bradykinin and analogues (Bueb et al., 1990a, b) to mast cell degranulating peptide (Mousli et al., 1991), to natural polyamine of the spermine family (Bueb et al., 1991, 1992) and to the anaphylatoxin C_{3a} and analogues (Mousli et al., 1992b). Other groups have confirmed this effect in the case of compound 48/80 (Aridor et al., 1990; Tomita et al., 1991a, b), substance P (Higashijima et al., 1990) and MCD (Fujimoto et al., 1991). Higashijima et al. (1990) also showed the activation of purified G proteins by angiotensin II, dynorphin, melittin and gramicidin S. However, there is a large gap between rat mast cell activation and the activation of G proteins purified from bovine tissues, but we showed that the GTPase activity of mast cell supernatant is sensitive to peptides (Bueb et al., 1990b). Based on the inhibitory effect of pertussis toxin-induced ADP-ribosylation, on the inhibitory effect of benzalkonium chloride and on the molecular mass of the ADP-ribosilated α subunits, the involved trimeric G proteins in peritoneal rat mast cells can be classified as belonging to the G_i subtype (Bueb et al., 1990b). Subsequent intracellular events include the activation of phospholipase C but also of phospholipase A_2 (Mousli et al., 1992a).

The Peptidergic Pathway: a Membrane-assisted Process

Altogether the above results strongly suggest that the α subunit of G_i-like proteins might be the direct target, or in other terms the binding site or the receptor, of active polyamines and peptides in mast cells. The effects of these drugs on mast cells and purified G proteins are nicely correlated considering their active concentrations and their net positive charges, as demonstrated for polyamines (Bueb et al., 1991, 1992) and anaphylatoxins (Mousli et al., 1992b). However, this does not mean that these triggers freely pass through the plasma membrane and reach G proteins in the cytosol. Indeed, peptides are currently considered to be unable to pass through membranes, but a few arguments have been developed to support the electrophoretic transfer of peptides across a lipid bilayer (Kaiser and Kezdy, 1983) or the insertion of peptides into membranes (Schwyzer, 1986, 1987). Whatever the case may be, it has to be noticed that the activation of purified G proteins related above has been observed in the presence of added lipids. Thus, both in intact mast cells and in purified G proteins experiments, a role for lipids in the stimulation of G proteins by polyamines and peptides cannot be excluded. We proposed a role for sialic acid residues of the cell surface considering that their removal by neuraminidase pretreatment of the cell inhibited the response to polyamines and peptides without altering the response to IgE-dependent stimulation or to calcium ionophores (see for instance Mousli *et al.*, 1989, 1990a; Bueb *et al.*, 1990b). The role of sialic acid residues, which are the negatively charged endings of membrane glycolipids and glycoproteins, might be a preliminary binding of drugs to the cell surface increasing their local level and allowing the drugs to pass the plasma membrane. The binding to lipids of peptides such as mastoparan has been widely reported (Higashijima *et al.*, 1983; Katsu *et al.*, 1990). Thus, we cannot exclude the possibility that lipids are required in the activation of mast cell G proteins. Whatever the case may be, the peptidergic pathway of mast cell activation is independent of selective peptide receptors but involves G_i-like proteins with either a direct peptide–G protein interaction or a lipid-assisted interaction.

References

Anderson, P., Caliguiri, M., Ritz, J. and Schlossman, S. E. (1989). CD3-negative natural killer cells express ζ TCR as part of a novel molecular complex. *Nature (London)*, **341**, 159–62.

Aridor, M., Traub, L. M. and Sagi-Eisenberg, R. (1990). Exocytosis in mast cells by basic secretagogues: evidence for direct activation of GTP-binding proteins. *J. Cell. Biol.*, **111**, 909–17.

Balch, W. E. (1990). Small GTP-binding proteins in vesicular transport. *Trends Biochem. Sci.*, **15**, 473–7.

Beaven, M. A., Moore, J. P., Smith, G. A., Hesketh, T. R. and Metcalfe, J. C. (1984). The calcium signal and phosphatidylinositol breakdown in 2H3 cells. *J. Biol. Chem.*, **259**, 7137–42.

Benhamou, M., Gutkind, J. S., Robbins, K. C. and Siragagnian, R. P. (1990). Tyrosine phosphorylation coupled to IgE receptor-mediated signal transduction and histamine release. *Proc. Natl. Acad. Sci. USA*, **87**, 5327–30.

Blank, U., Ra, C., Miller, L., White, K., Metzger, H. and Kinet, J. P. (1989). Complete structure and expression in transfected cells of high affinity IgE receptor. *Nature (London)*, **337**, 187–9.

Bronner, C., Cothenet, V., Monté, D., Joseph, M., Landry, Y. and Capron, A. (1990). Role of phospholipase A_2 and G-proteins in the IgE-dependent activation of mast cells and macrophages. *Agents Actions*, **30**, 95–7.

Bueb, J. L., Mousli, M., Landry, Y. and Bronner, C. (1990a). A pertussis toxin-sensitive G protein is required to induce histamine release from rat peritoneal mast cells by bradykinin. *Agents Actions*, **30**, 98–101.

Bueb, J. L., Mousli, M., Bronner, C., Rouot, B. and Landry, Y. (1990b). Activation of G_i-like proteins, a receptor-independent effect of kinins in mast cells. *Mol. Pharmacol.*, **38**, 816–22.

Bueb, J. L., Mousli, M. and Landry, Y. (1991). Molecular basis for cellular effects of naturally occurring polyamines. *Agents Actions*, **33**, 84–7.

Bueb, J. L., Da Silva, A., Mousli, M. and Landry, Y. (1992). Natural polyamines stimulates G proteins. *Biochem. J.*, **282**, 545–50.

Chand, N., Pillar, J., Diamantis, W. and Sofia, R. D. (1987). Inhibition of histamine release from rat peritoneal mast cells and rabbit leucocytes by p-bromophenacyl bromide, a phospholipase A_2 inhibitors. *Res. Commun. Chem. Pathol. Pharmacol.*, **55**, 17–24.

Church, M. K., Lowman, M. A., Pees, P. H. and Benyon, R. C. (1989). Mast cells, neuropeptides and inflammation. *Agents Actions*, **27**, 8–16.

Cockcroft, S., Howell, T. W. and Gomperts, B. D. (1987). Two G-proteins act in series to control stimulus–secretion coupling in mast cells: use of neomycin to distinguish between G-proteins controlling polyphosphoinositide phosphodiesterase and exocytosis. *J. Cell. Biol.*, **105**, 2745–50.

Connely, P. A., Farrell, C. A., Merenda, J. M., Conklyn, M. J. and Showell, H. J. (1991). Tyrosine phosphorylation is an early signaling event common to Fc receptor cross-linking in human neutrophils and rat basophilic leukemia cells (RBL-2H3). *Biochem. Biophys. Res. Commun.*, **177**, 192–201.

Conrad, D. H. (1990). FcεRII/CD23: the low affinity receptor for IgE. *Annu. Rev. Immunol.*, **8**, 623–45.

Conrad, D. H. and Froese, A. (1976). A characterization of the target cell receptor for IgE. II-D polyacrylamide gel analysis of the surface IgE receptor from normal rat mast cells and from rat basophilic leukemia cells. *J. Immunol.*, **116**, 319–26.

Cunha-Melo, J. R., Dean, N. M., Moyer, J. D., Maeyama, K. and Beaven, M. A. (1987). The kinetics of phosphoinositide hydrolysis in rat basophilic leukemia (RBL-2H3) cells varies with the type of IgE receptor cross-linking agent used. *J. Biol. Chem.*, **262**, 11455–63.

Deanin, G. G., Martinez, A. M., Pfeiffer, J. R., Gardner, M. E. and Oliver, J. M. (1991). Tyrosine kinase-dependent phosphatidylinositol turnover and functional responses in the FcεRI signalling pathway. *Biochem. Biophys. Res. Commun.*, **179**, 551–7.

Downward, J. (1990). The ras superfamily of small GTP-binding proteins. *Trends Biochem. Sci.*, **15**, 469–72.

Eiseman, E. and Bolen, J. B. (1990). src-related tyrosine protein kinases as signalling components in hematopoietic cells. *Cancer Cells*, **10**, 303–10.

Fujimoto, I., Ikenaka, K., Kondo, T., Aimoto, S., Kuno, M. and Mikoshiba, K. (1991). Mast cell degranulating (MCD) peptide and its optical isomer activate GTP binding protein in rat mast cells. *FEBS Lett.*, **287**, 15–18.

Fukuoka, Y. and Hugli, T. E. (1990). Anaphylatoxin binding and degradation by rat peritoneal mast cells. *J. Immunol.*, **145**, 1851–8.

Garcia-Sainz, J. A. (1991). Cell responsiveness and protein kinase C: receptors, G proteins, and membrane effectors. *News Physiol. Sci.*, **6**, 169–73.

Givney, A. M. C., Morita, Y., Crews, F. T., Hirata, F., Axelrod, J. and Siragagnian, R. P. (1981). Phospholipase activation in the IgE-mediated and Ca^{2+} ionophore A23187-induced release of histamine from rat basophilic leukemia cells. *Arch. Biochem. Biophys.*, **212**, 572–80.

Gruchalla, R. S., Dinh, T. T. and Kennerly, D. A. (1990). An direct pathway of receptor-mediated 1,2-diacylglycerol formation in mast cells. I. IgE receptor-mediated activation of phospholipase D[1]. *J. Immunol.*, **144**, 1334–42.

Hakimi, J., Seals, C., Kondas, J. A., Pettine, L., Danho, W. and Kochan, J. (1990). The α subunit of the human IgE receptor (FcεRI) is sufficient for high affinity IgE binding. *J. Biol. Chem.*, **265**, 22079–81.

Higashijima, T., Wakamatsu, K., Wakamatsu, M., Fujino, M., Nakajima, T. and Miyazawa, T. (1983). Conformational change of mastoparan from wasp venom on binding with phospholipid membrane. *FEBS Lett.*, **152**, 227–30.

Higashijima, T., Uzu, S., Nakajima, T. and Miyazawa, T. (1987). Mechanism of histamine-release by mastoparan. In T. Miyazawa (ed.), *Peptide Chemistry*, Protein Research Foundation, Osaka, 75–8.

Higashijima, T., Uzu, S., Nakajima, T. and Ross, E. M. (1988). Mastoparan, a peptide toxin from wasp venom, mimics receptors by activating GTP-binding regulatory proteins (G proteins). *J. Biol. Chem.*, **263**, 6491–4.

Higashijima, T., Burnier, J. and Ross, E. M. (1990) Regulation of G_i and G_o by mastoparan, related amphiphilic peptides, and hydrophobic amines. *J. Biol. Chem.*, **265**, 14176–86.

Howard, F. D., Rodewald, H.-R., Kinet, J.-P. and Reinherz, E. L. (1990). CD3 ζ subunit can substitute for the γ subunit of Fcε receptor type I in assembly and functional expression of the high-affinity IgE receptor: evidence for interreceptor complementation. *Proc. Natl. Acad. Sci. USA*, **87**, 7015–19.

Hupp, K., Siwarski, D., Mock, B. A. and Kinet, J. P. (1989). Gene mapping of the three subunits of the high affinity FcR for IgE to mouse chromosome 1 and 19. *J. Immunol.*, **143**, 3787–91.

Ishizaka, T. (1982). Biochemical analysis of triggering signals induced by bridging of IgE receptors. *Fed. Proc.*, **14**, 17–21.

Jin, Y. J., Clayton, L. K., Howard, F. D., Koyasu, S., Sieh, M., Steinbrich, R., Tarr, G. E. and Reinherz, E. L. (1990). Molecular cloning of the CD3η subunit identifies a CD3 ζ-related product in thymus-derived cells. *Proc. Natl. Acad. Sci. USA*, **87**, 3319–23.

Kaiser, E. T. and Kezdy, F. J. (1983). Secondary structures of proteins and peptides in amphiphilic environments (a review). *Proc. Natl. Acad. Sci. USA*, **80**, 1137–43.

Katsu, T., Kuroko, M., Morikawa, T., Sanchika, K., Yamanaka, H., Shinoda, S. and Fujita, Y. (1990). Interaction of wasp venom mastoparan with biomembranes. *Biochim. Biophys. Acta*, **1027**, 185–90.

Katz, H. R., Bension, A. C. and Austen, K. F. (1989). Activation- and phorbol ester-stimulated phosphorylation of a plasma membrane glycoprotein antigen expressed on mouse IL-3-dependent mast cells and serosal mast cells. *J. Immunol.*, **142**, 919–26.

Kennerly, D. A. (1990). Phosphatidylcholine is a quantitatively more important source of increased 1,2-diacylglycerol than is phosphatidylinositol in mast cells. *J. Immunol.*, **144**, 3912–19.

Kinet, J. P. (1990). The high-affinity receptor for IgE. *Curr. Opinion Immunol.*, **2**, 499–505.

Küster, H., Rodewald, H. R., Kinet, J. P. and Reinherz, E. L. (1990). CD3ζ subunit can substitute for the γ subunit of FCε receptor type I in assembly and functional expression of the high-affinity IgE receptor: evidence for interreceptor complementation. *Proc. Natl. Acad. Sci. USA*, **87**, 7015–19.

Lagunoff, D., Martin, T. W. and Read, G. (1983). Agents that release histamine from mast cells. *Annu. Rev. Pharmacol. Toxicol.*, **23**, 331–51.

Lanier, L. L., Yu, G. and Phillips, J. H. (1989). Co association of CD3ζ with a receptor (CD16) for IgG Fc on human natural killer cells. *Nature (London)*, **342**, 803–5.

Letourneur, O., Kennedy, I. C. S., Brini, A. T., Ortaldo, J. R., O'Shea, J. J. and Kinet, J. P. (1991). Characterization of the family of dimers associated with Fc receptor (FcεRI and FcγRIII). *J. Immunol.*, **147**, 2652–6.

Lin, P., Wiggan, G. A. and Gilfillan, A. M. (1991). Activation of phospholipase D in a rat mast (RBL-2H3) cell line. A possible unifying mechanism for IgE-dependent degranulation and arachidonic acid metabolite release. *J. Immunol.*, **146**, 1609–16.

Ludowyke, R. I., Peleg, I., Beaven, M. A. and Adelstein, R. S. (1989). Antigen-induced secretion of histamine and the phosphorylation of myosin by protein kinase C in rat basophilic leukemia cells. *J. Biol. Chem.*, **264**, 12492–501.

Maliszewski, C. R., March, C. J., Schoenborn, M. A., Gimpel, S. and Shen, L. (1990). Expression cloning of a human Fc receptor for IgA. *J. Exp. Med.*, **172**, 1665–72.

McCloskey, M. A. (1988). Cholera toxin potentiates IgE-coupled inositol phospholipid hydrolysis and mediator secretion by RBL-2H3 cells. *Proc. Natl. Acad. Sci. USA*, **85**, 7260–4.

Miller, L., Blank, U., Metzger, H. and Kinet, J. P. (1989). Expression of high-affinity binding of human immunoglobulin E by transfected cells. *Science*, **244**, 334–337.

Mousli, M., Bronner, C., Bueb, J. L., Tschirhart, E., Gies, J. P. and Landry, Y. (1989). Activation of rat peritoneal mast cells by substance P and mastoparan. *J. Pharmacol. Exp. Ther.*, **250**, 329–35.

Mousli, M., Bueb, J. L., Gies, J. P., Bronner, C., Rouot, B. and Landry, Y. (1990a). G protein activation: a receptor-independent mode of action for amphiphilic neuropeptides and venom peptides. *Trends Pharmacol. Sci.*, **11**, 358–62.

Mousli, M., Bronner, C., Landry, Y., Bockaert, J. and Rouot, B. (1990b). Direct activation of GTP-binding regulatory proteins (G proteins) by substance P and compound 48/80. *FEBS Lett.*, **259**, 260–2.

Mousli, M., Bronner C., Bockaert, J., Rouot, B. and Landry, Y. (1990c). Substance P, compound 48/80 and mastoparan interact with C-terminals of G proteins. *Immunol. Lett.*, **25**, 355–8.

Mousli, M., Bronner, C., Bueb, J. L. and Landry, Y. (1991). Evidence for the interaction of mast-cell-degranulating-peptide (MCD) with pertussis toxin-sensitive G proteins in mast cells. *Eur. J. Pharmacol. (Mol. Pharmacol. Sect.)*, **207**, 249–55.

Mousli, M., Fischer, T. and Landry, Y. (1992a). Role of phospholipase A2 and pertussis toxin-sensitive G proteins in histamine secretion induced by substance P. *Agents Actions* (in press).

Mousli, M., Hugli, T. E., Landry, Y. and Bronner, C. (1992b). A mechanism of action for anaphylatoxin C3a stimulation of mast cells. *J. Immunol.*, **148**, 2456–61.

Nakashima, S., Fujimiya, H., Miyata, H. and Nozawa, Y. (1991). Antigen-induced biphasic diacylglycerol formation in RBL-2H3 cells: the late sustained phase due to phosphatidylcholine hydrolysis is dependent on protein kinase C. *Biochem. Biophys. Res. Commun.*, **177**, 336–42.

Orloff, D. G., Ra. C., Frank, S. J., Klausner, R. D. and Kinet, J. P. (1990). Family of disulphide-linked dimers containing the ζ and η chains of the T-cell receptor and the γ chain of Fc receptors. *Nature (London)*, **347**, 189–91.

Paolini, R., Jouvin, M. H. and Kinet, J. P. (1991). *In vivo* phosphorylation and dephosphorylation of the high affinity receptor for immunoglobulin E immediately follow receptor engagement and disengagement, *Nature* (*London*), **353**, 855–8.

Perez-Montfort, R., Kinet, J. P. and Metzger, H. (1983). A previously unrecognized subunit of the receptor for immunoglobulin E. *Biochemistry*, **22**, 5722–8.

Pribluda, V. S. and Metzger, H. (1987). Calcium-independent phosphoinositide breakdown in rat basophilic leukemia cells. *J. Biol. Chem.*, **262**, 11449–54.

Ravetch, J. V. and Kinet, J. P. (1991). Fc receptors. *Annu. Rev. Immunol*, **9**, 457–92.

Rhee, S. G. (1991). Inositol phospholipid-specific phospholipase C: interaction of the γ isoform with tyrosine kinase. *Trends Biochem. Sci.*, **16**, 297–301.

Rhee, S. G., Suh, P. G., Ryu, S. H. and Lee, S. Y. (1989). Studies of inositol phospholipid-specific phospholipase C. *Science*, **244**, 546–50.

Rossier, M. F., Capponi, A. M. and Vallotton, M. B. (1989). The inositol 1,4,5-trisphosphate-binding site in adrenal cortical cells is distinct from the endoplasmic reticulum. *J. Biol. Chem.*, **264**, 14078–84.

Ryu, S. H., Suh, P. G., Cho, K. S., Lee, K. Y. and Rhee, S. G. (1987). Bovine brain cytosol contains three immunologically distinct forms of inositolphospholipid-specific phospholipase C. *Proc. Natl. Acad. Sci. USA*, **84**, 6649–53.

Saito, H., Okajima, F., Molski, T. F. P., Sha'afi, R. I., Ui, M. and Ishizaka, T. (1988). Effect of cholera toxin on histamine release from bone marrow-derived mouse mast cells. *Proc. Natl. Acad. Sci. USA*, **85**, 2504–8.

Saito, H., Ishizaka, K. and Ishizaka, T. (1989). Effect of nonhydrolyzable guanosine phosphate on IgE-mediated activation of phospholipase C and histamine release from rodent mast cells. *J. Immunol.*, **143**, 250–8.

Schwyzer, R. (1986). Estimated conformation, orientation and accumulation of dynorphin A-(1–13)-tridecapeptide on the surface of the neutral lipid membranes. *Biochemistry*, **25**, 4281–6.

Schwyzer, R. (1987). Membrane assisted molecular mechanism of neurokinin receptor subtype selection. *EMBO J.*, **6**, 2255–9.

Siraganian, R. P. (1983). Histamine secretion from mast cells and basophils. *Trends Pharmacol. Sci.*, **4**, 432–7.

Spiegel, A. M., Backlund, P. S., Butrynski, J. E., Jones, T. L. Z. and Simonds, W. F. (1991). The G protein connection: molecular basis of membrane association. *Trends Biochem. Sci.*, **16**, 339–41.

Strathmann, M. and Simon, M. I. (1990). G protein diversity: a distinct class of α subunits is present in vertebrates and invertebrates. *Proc. Natl. Acad. Sci. USA*, **87**, 9113–17.

Theocharides, T. C. (1990). Mast cells: the immune gate to the brain. *Life Sci.*, **46**, 607–17.

Tomita, U., Inanobe, A., Kobayashi, I., Takahashi, K., Ui, M. and Katada, T. (1991a). Direct interactions of mastoparan and compound 48/80 with GTP-binding proteins. *J. Biochem.*, **109**, 184–9.

Tomita, U., Takahashi, K., Ikenaka, K., Kondo, T., Fujimoto, I., Aimoto, S., Mikoshiba, K., Ui, M. and Katada, T. (1991b). Direct activation of GTP-binding proteins by venom peptides that contain cationic cluster within their alpha-helical structures. *Biochem. Biophys., Res. Commun.*, **178**, 400–6.

White, J. R., Pluznik, D. H., Ishizaka, K. and Ishizaka, T. (1985). Antigen-induced increase in protein kinase C activity in plasma membrane of mast cells. *Proc. Natl. Acad. Sci. USA*, **82**, 8193–7.

White, J. R., Zembryki, D., Hanna, N. and Mong, S. (1989). Differential inhibition of histamine release from mast cells by protein kinase C inhibitors: staurosporine and K-252a. *Biochem. Pharmacol.*, **40**, 447–56.

Wilson, B.S., Deanin, G. C. and Oliver, J. M. (1991). Regulation of IgE receptor-mediated secretion from RBL-2H3 mast cells by GTP binding-proteins and calcium. *Biochem. Biophys. Res. Commun.*, **174**, 1064–9.

Woldemussie, E., Ali, H., Takaishi, T., Siragagnian, R. P. and Beaven, M. A. (1987). Identification of variants of the basophilic leukemia (RBL-2H3) cells that have defective phosphoinositide responses to antigen and stimulants of guanosine 5′-triphosphate-regulatory proteins. *J. Immunol.*, **139**, 2431–8.

Yamada, K., Kanaho, Y., Miura, K. and Yoshinori, N. (1991). Antigen-induced phospholipase D activation in rat mast cells is independent of protein kinase C. *Biochem. Biophys. Res. Commun.*, **175**, 159–64.

9

Release of Granule Proteins by Eosinophils from Allergic Patients on Immunoglobulin-dependent Activation

M. Capron, M. Tomassini and A. Capron

Summary

Eosinophils possess receptors for IgG, IgE and IgA. These receptors are functional, since binding of insolubilized or cross-linked ligands can induce exocytosis of granule proteins. The comparison between eosinophil IgE receptor and CD23 recently revealed the low and variable expression of CD23 on eosinophils from patients, and the involvement of CD23 in IgE binding and IgE-mediated cytotoxicity. Cationic proteins present in eosinophil granules participate in the effector function of eosinophils in antiparasite defence as well as in hypersensitivity reactions. Whereas many studies have been related to functional and biochemical properties of these proteins, their mechanism of release is still poorly understood. The release of eosinophil peroxidase (EPO) and eosinophil cationic protein (ECP) was evaluated after incubation of eosinophils from allergic subjects with the specific allergen or with anti-IgE monoclonal antibodies (mAbs). High levels of EPO could be released after addition of the specific allergen (and not unrelated ones) or anti-IgE mAb. Moreover, EPO release with the two stimuli was significantly correlated both in allergic and in non-allergic patients. In the same supernatants, another granule protein, ECP, could not be detected, suggesting a lack of correlation between EPO and ECP release after IgE-dependent stimulation. However, when eosinophils with surface IgA antibodies were incubated with anti-IgA mAb, both EPO and

ECP were released. In contrast, incubation of eosinophils with anti-IgG mAb induced mainly the release of ECP and not EPO. These results indicate that pharmacologically active mediators can be released by eosinophils from allergic and non-allergic patients upon immunoglobulin-dependent activation. They also confirm the hypothesis of a selective release of the various granule proteins and raise the question of transduction signals delivered by the three Fc receptors (FcεR, FcαR and FcγR) present on human eosinophils. Such findings might be of relevance to the pathogenesis of asthma but also of other diseases characterized by eosinophilia involving mucosal surfaces.

9.1 Introduction

Over the past twenty years, several lines of evidence have raised growing interest in the effector functions of eosinophils, regarding a variety of clinical states associated with hypereosinophilia, including parasitic and allergic diseases (Gleich and Adolphson, 1986; Spry, 1988). Human eosinophils possess specific receptors and adhesion molecules which might be linked to their selective functions in allergy. Among those, distinct receptors for IgG, IgE and IgA immunoglobulins have been described.

Effector functions of eosinophils against parasites as well as against host cells appear to be mainly mediated by the release of cationic proteins, such as major basic protein (MBP), eosinophil cationic protein (ECP), eosinophil-derived neurotoxin (EDN) and eosinophil peroxidase (EPO). All these preformed mediators display a strong cytotoxic potential (Gleich and Adolphson, 1986). The precise mechanisms leading to eosinophil degranulation, however, are still poorly understood. It is not yet clear, in particular, whether eosinophils isolated from allergic patients could degranulate on exposure to allergens. Moreover, studies on parasite-infected patients have shown that not all the granule proteins were simultaneously released after the same stimulus of activation, suggesting a differential release of EPO and ECP (Khalife et al., 1986; Capron et al., 1989b).

In the present review, we summarize the characteristics of eosinophil receptors for IgG, IgE and IgA. These receptors are functional, as shown both by the inhibitory effects of anti-receptor monoclonal antibodies on eosinophil-mediated cytotoxicity and by the receptor-induced release of eosinophil granule proteins. In order to evaluate the functions of these receptors in allergic diseases, we have monitored the release of EPO, and ECP after incubation of eosinophils from allergic subjects with the specific allergen, with anti-IgE, anti-IgA or anti-IgG monoclonal antibodies (mAbs). Our results indicate that pharmacologically active mediators can be released by eosinophils from allergic and non-allergic patients upon immunoglobulin-dependent activation.

9.2 Receptors for the Fc Fragment of Immunoglobulins

The receptor for IgG (FcγR) was the first to be identified on eosinophil membrane, mainly by rosetting techniques. The possible use of monoclonal antibodies specifically directed against each type of FcγR has recently allowed the demonstration that unstimulated eosinophils expressed only FcγRII (CD32) (Hartnell et al., 1990). A panel of five different anti-FcγRII mAbs reacted similarly with eosinophils, monocytes and neutrophils, suggesting that this receptor is similar on the three cell types. However, eosinophils express about one-third as many as FcγRII (CD32) as neutrophils, and they do not have detectable expression of FcγRIII (CD16), which is detected at a very high density on neutrophils.

The existence of a low affinity receptor for IgE has been demonstrated on eosinophils by binding assays and more recently by immunosorbent chromatography (Capron et al., 1989a). The identification of structural similarities between eosinophil, macrophage, platelet and B cell IgE receptor (Jouault et al., 1988; Grangette et al., 1989) led to the concept of a second class of IgE receptors, called FcεRII (A. Capron et al., 1986). More recently, eosinophil IgE receptor has been compared with the B cell differentiation antigen CD23 (Capron et al., 1989a; Capron et al., 1991b). By flow cytometry, a significant correlation was found between the binding of myeloma IgE protein and the binding of one anti-CD23 mAb (135), which is directed against the IgE binding site of CD23, on a series of 16 hypereosinophilic patients. The binding of BB10, mAb 135 and two other anti-CD23 antibodies, directed (mAb 8–30), or not directed (mAb 3–5), against the IgE-binding site of CD23, was compared by flow cytometry. A low and variable expression of these CD23 epitopes was observed on eosinophils from different eosinophilic patients. Northern blot analysis of eosinophil RNA with the cDNA probe of CD23 revealed a weak message in three out of the six patients expressing membrane CD23. Finally, all the anti-CD23 under study inhibited in a dose-dependent manner the binding of radiolabelled IgE to eosinophils, even mAb 3–5, which did not inhibit IgE binding to B cells. Taken all together, these results are consistent with the expression, on eosinophil membrane, of molecules recognized by three non-cross-reactive anti-CD23 mAb. However, the low level of the corresponding mRNA, together with the inhibitory effect of mAb 3–5, suggests some differences between the molecules expressed by eosinophils and by B cells (Capron and Joseph, 1991). Another hypothesis, currently tested is that eosinophils might express a different type of IgE binding proteins, belonging to the family of carbohydrate-binding proteins. The cloning of the molecules involved in IgE binding to eosinophils will definitively clarify all these problems.

The first evidence of IgA binding to eosinophils was reported in 1988 by flow cytometry (Capron et al., 1988). Between 5% and 60% eosinophils from eosinophilic patients are able to bind serum IgA, as revealed by staining with fluorescein-labelled anti-human IgA. The large variations in the expression of IgA R in individual patients suggest a modulation of this receptor, as already shown for IgE R. Moreover, cytophilic IgA could be detected by this assay in some patients, mainly with parasitic infections or allergic diseases. Similarities in the molecular weight of IgA R on eosinophils, neutrophils and monocytes as well as recognition by the same mAb suggest that eosinophil FcαR is similar to the myeloid-cell-specific IgA R recently cloned (Maliszewski *et al.*, 1990). Besides FcαR, it has been recently reported that secretory IgA could bind to a lectin-type receptor on eosinophil membrane (Capron *et al.*, 1991a).

9.3 Release of Eosinophil Peroxidase (EPO) After Stimulation With Allergen or Anti-IgE Antibodies

Eosinophils isolated from seven allergic patients were incubated with the specific allergen (*Dactylis glomerata* or *Dermatophagoides pteronyssinus*). Eosinophils from 13 non-allergic patients with hypereosinophilia were tested in the same conditions and the release of EPO was evaluated. Only eosinophils isolated from allergic patients released significant amounts of EPO after stimulation with the specific allergen. To investigate the specificity of allergen-induced EPO release, eosinophils from allergic patients were incubated with unrelated allergen in five cases, no EPO release was observed in such experiments. In the same groups of patients, EPO release was measured after the addition of anti-human IgE antibodies. Similarly to stimulation with allergen, eosinophils from allergic patients released higher levels of EPO than eosinophils from non-allergic patients. Moreover, there was a significant correlation between EPO release induced by allergen and by anti-human IgE mAb ($r = 0.93$; $P < 0.001$) suggesting the participation of surface IgE in this mechanism of release.

9.4 Absence of Release of Eosinophil Cationic Protein (ECP) After IgE-dependent Stimulation

ECP was measured by a radioimmunoassay in aliquots of the same samples assayed for EPO. In none of the six allergic patients did the addition of the specific allergen or anti-human IgE induce a significant release of ECP. A similar comparison between EPO and ECP release after stimulation with anti-IgE antibodies in a total of 16 patients revealed the absence of correlation between EPO and ECP release.

9.5 Release of EPO and ECP After IgA-dependent Stimulation

In order to investigate the IgA-dependent eosinophil activation, the release of EPO and ECP was evaluated after incubation of eosinophils with anti-human IgA mAb. The release of EPO and ECP was compared in 14 patients. Six out of the 14 patients released significant levels of EPO after stimulation with anti-human IgA, whereas nine patients released significant amounts of ECP. Very interestingly, the individual results of EPO and ECP release were significantly correlated ($r = 0.6$; $p < 0.02$).

9.6 ECP but Low EPO Release After IgG-dependent Stimulation

Similarly, the release of EPO and ECP was compared on different aliquots of the same supernatants of eosinophils purified from 11 patients after incubation with anti-human IgG mAb. All the patient eosinophils released significantly high levels of ECP but did not release significant amounts of EPO, except for one patient, giving high levels of both EPO and ECP.

9.7 Discussion

Cross-linking of membrane receptors can induce cell activation and in some occasions release of mediators. This mechanism has been extensively studied in the case of FcεRI-mediated activation of mast cells. Theoretically, cross-linking can be achieved by addition of 'stimulator' anti-receptor antibodies, or by addition, after the binding of the ligand to its receptor, of a second stimulus, which might link the cell-bound ligands and induce cell activation. This second approach has been successfully used for eosinophils, taking advantage of the presence of cytophilic Ab bound *in vivo* to eosinophils from some eosinophilic patients (Capron *et al.*, 1985). Purified eosinophils were incubated with the specific antigen, which binds to the antigen binding site of cytophilic Ab, or with isotype-specific antibodies directed against the Fc portion of surface Ig.

In the present study, we show that surface IgE-bearing eosinophils purified from patients with allergic diseases release EPO after incubation with the specific antigen and not with unrelated ones (Tomassini *et al.*, 1991). The participation of IgE antibodies in this mechanism is suggested by the significant correlation between EPO release after incubation with allergen or with anti-IgE mAb. In contrast, no EPO can be detected after addition of anti-IgG antibodies, neither with allergic nor with non-allergic patients. Very surprisingly, ECP is not detected after incubation of eosinophils with anti-IgE whereas significant levels are measured after incubation with anti-IgG antibodies. It has also been shown that both EPO and ECP can be released by surface IgA-bearing eosinophils incubated with anti-IgA mAb. These results, associated with recently published ones (Abu-Ghazaleh et al., 1989), suggest that IgA and IgG antibodies are potent stimuli for the release of ECP and EDN but not IgE antibodies. The difference in eosinophil response to IgE, IgA and IgG antibodies might be linked to different signal transduction pathways delivered by the three Fc receptors (FcεR, FcαR, FcγR). In fact, other studies have shown a variability in eosinophil response to different activators.

The main factor could be related to human eosinophil heterogeneity (Winqvist et al., 1982; Khalife et al., 1986). Eosinophils with the 'hypodense' phenotype are thought to be more activated than normodense eosinophils. In addition, they express IgE Fc receptors with higher affinity as well as increased IgE-dependent cytotoxicity (M. Capron et al., 1986). It is therefore not surprising that hypodense eosinophils showed enhanced mediator release in response to IgE-dependent stimulation. It must be noticed that hypodense eosinophils represent the majority of tissue eosinophils as well as the highest proportion of blood eosinophils from hypereosinophilic patients, indicating therefore their potential role as effector inflammatory cells in IgE-dependent mechanisms (Capron et al., 1989a).

Taken all together, these results suggest that EPO is not released from human eosinophils in the same conditions of activation as ECP and raises the very interesting question of the mechanism of exocytosis of these granule proteins. We have no definitive arguments to answer this question but recent electron microscopy studies performed on tissue eosinophils by immunogold labelling suggest that the granule proteins might leave the granule through the cytoplasm, by a vesicular transport mechanism similar to that described for delayed type cutaneous basophil hypersensitivity (Capron et al., 1989a). These results suggest that eosinophil activation is a complex phenomenon depending upon the stimulus used but also on the state of activation or differentiation of cells.

Perhaps the most novel and interesting data are those concerning IgA-mediated eosinophil activation. Surface-bound IgA antibodies seemed to represent a potent stimulus, since both EPO and ECP could be released. These results confirm our previous findings on the interactions between IgA and eosinophils (Capron et al., 1988) and are in total agreement with recent reports on IgA-mediated release of EDN (Abu-Ghazaleh et al., 1989; Fujisawa et al., 1990). These findings might be of relevance to the pathogenesis of a variety of human diseases characterized by eosinophilia involving mucosal surfaces. It should be noted that eosinophils are increased in the nasal mucosa of allergic patients during natural pollen exposure, and there is a relationship between eosinophil activation and allergen-induced local inflammation (Pipkorn *et al.*, 1988). However, there is a lack of correlation between the variable ECP levels in nasal lavages and the local hyperresponsiveness observed after nasal allergen challenge (Andersson *et al.*, 1989). In contrast, elevated blood levels of MBP, ECP and EDN have been detected in patients with allergic asthma after bronchial challenge, whereas EPO levels were reduced (Durham *et al.*, 1989). All these data point to the selective release of eosinophil mediators *in vivo*. However, it cannot be excluded that *in vivo* pathways of eosinophil secretion might differ from the *in vitro* situation, depending for instance on exposure to a particular local microenvironment. In this respect, the influence of cell–cell interactions, mediated by intercellular adhesion molecules (Wegner *et al.*, 1990) or the role of soluble factors such as cytokines (Silberstein and David, 1987) have been recently suggested.

References

Abu-Ghazaleh, R. I., Fujisawa, T., Mestecky, J., Kyle, R. A. and Gleich, G. J. (1989). IgA-induced eosinophil degranulation. *J. Immunol.*, **142**, 2393–400.

Andersson, M., Andersson, P., Venge, P. and Pipkorn, U. (1989). Eosinophils and eosinophil cationic protein in nasal lavages in allergen-induced hyper-responsiveness: effect of topical glucocorticosteroid treatment. *Allergy*, **44**, 342–8.

Capron, A., Dessaint, J. P., Capron, M., Joseph, M., Ameisen, J. C. and Tonnel, A. B. (1986). From parasites to allergy: the second receptor for IgE (FcεR2). *Immunol. Today*, **7**, 15–18.

Capron, M. and Joseph, M. (1991). The low affinity receptor for IgE on eosinophils and platelets. In Karger, A. G. (ed.), *Monographs in Allergy*, Gordon, Basel, 63–75.

Capron, M., Kusnierz, J. P., Prin, L., Spiegelberg, H. L., Ovlaque, G., Gosset, P., Tonnel, A. B. and Capron, A. (1985). Cytophilic IgE on human blood and tissue eosinophils: detection by flow microfluorometry. *J. Immunol.*, **134**, 3013–18.

Capron, M., Spiegelberg, H. L., Prin, L., Bennich, H., Butterworth, A. E., Pierce, R. J., Ouaissi, M. A. and Capron, A. (1986). Role of IgE receptors in effector function of human eosinophils. *J. Immunol.*, **132**, 462–8.

Capron, M., Tomassini, M., Van der Vorst, E., Kusnierz, J. P., Papin, J. P. and Capron, A. (1988). Existence et fonctions d'un récepteur pour l'immunoglobuline A sur les éosinophiles humains. *C.R. Acad. Sci. Paris*, **307**, 397–402.

Capron, M., Grangette, C., Torpier, G. and Capron, A. (1989a). The second receptor for IgE in eosinophil effector function. *Chem. Immunol.*, **47**, 128–78.

Capron, M., Tomassini, M., Torpier, G., Kusnierz, J. P., McDonald, S. and Capron, A. (1989b). Selectivity of mediators released by eosinophils. *Int. Arch. Allergy Appl. Immunol.*, **88**, 54–8.

Capron, M., Gruart, V., Broussolle, A. and Capron, A. (1991a). Binding-site for secretory component on human eosinophils. *FASEB J.*, **5**, A640.

Capron, M., Truong, M. J., Aldebert, D., Gruart, V., Suemura, M., Delespesse, G., Tourvieille, B. and Capron, A. (1991b). Heterogeneous expression of CD23 epitopes by eosinophils from patients. Relationships with IgE-mediated functions. *Eur. J. Immunol.*, **21**, 2423–9.

Durham, S. R., Loegering, D. A., Dunnette, S. L., Gleich, G. J. and Kay, A. B. (1989). Blood eosinophils and eosinophil-derived proteins in allergic asthma. *J. Allergy Clin. Immunol.*, **84**, 931–6.

Fujisawa, T., Abu-Ghazaleh, R., Kita, H., Sanderson, C. J. and Gleich, G. J. (1990). Regulatory effect of cytokines on eosinophil degranulation. *J. Immunol.*, **144**, 642–6.

Gleich, G. J. and Adolphson, C. R. (1986). The eosinophilic leukocyte: structure and function. *Adv. Immunol.*, **39**, 177–253.

Grangette, G., Gruart, V., Ouaissi, M. A., Rizvi, F., Delespesse, G., Capron, A. and Capron, M. (1989). IgE receptor on human eosinophils: FcεRII: comparison with B cell CD23 and association with an adhesion molecule. *J. Immunol.*, **143**, 3580–8.

Hartnell, A., Moqbel, R., Walsh, G. M., Bradley, B. and Kay, A. B. (1990). Fcγ and CD11/CD18 receptor expression on normal density and low density human eosinophils. *Immunology*, **69**, 264.

Jouault, T., Capron, M., Balloul, J. M., Ameisen, J. C. and Capron, A. (1988). Quantitative analysis of the Fc receptor for IgE (FcεRII) on human eosinophils. *Eur. J. Immunol.*, **18**, 237–41.

Khalife, J., Capron, M., Cesbron, J. Y., Tai, P. C., Taelman, H., Prin, L. and Capron, A. (1986). Role of specific IgE antibodies in peroxidase (EPO) release from human eosinophils. *J. Immunol.*, **137**, 1659–64.

Maliszewski, R., March, C. J., Schoenborn, M. A., Gimpel, S. and Shen, L. (1990). Expression cloning of a human Fc receptor for IgA. *J. Exp. Med.*, **172**, 1665–72.

Pipkorn, U., Karlsson, G. and Enerback, L. (1989). The cellular response of the human allergic mucosa to natural allergen exposure. *J. Allergy Clin. Immunol.*, **82**, 1046–54.

Silberstein, D. S. and David, J. R. (1987). The regulation of human eosinophil function by cytokines. *Immunol. Today*, **8**, 380–5.

Spry, C. J. F. (1988). A comprehensive review and a guide to the literature. In *Eosinophils*, Oxford University Press, New York, 131.

Tomassini, M., Tsicopoulos, A., Tai, P. C., Gruart, V., Tonnel, A. B., Prin, L., Capron, A. and Capron, M. (1991). Release of granule proteins by eosinophils from allergic and non allergic patients with eosinophilia upon immunoglobulin-dependent activation. *J. Allergy Clin. Immunol.*, **88**, 365–75.

Wegner, C. D., Gundel, R. H., Reilly, P., Haynes, N., Letts, L. G. and Rothlein, R. (1990). Intercellular adhesion molecule-1 (ICAM1) in the pathogenesis of asthma. *Science*, **247**, 456–9.

Winqvist, I., Olofsson, T., Olsson, I., Persson, A. M. and Hallberg, T. (1982). Altered density, metabolism and surface receptors of eosinophils in eosinophilia. *Immunology*, **47**, 531–9.

10

Priming of the Eosinophil Granulocyte in Asthma

Per Venge, Marie Carlson and Lena Håkansson

10.1 Introduction

Previous studies have demonstrated the selective accumulation and activation of eosinophil granulocytes in the lungs of asthmatic subjects and concluded that these events are necessary ingredients in the complex process giving rise to the symptoms of asthma (Jeffery *et al.*, 1989; Frew and Kay, 1990; Diaz *et al.*, 1989; Azzawi *et al.*, 1990; Kay, 1991; Venge and Håkansson, 1991a; Venge, 1990; Ädelroth *et al.*, 1990; Bousquet *et al.*, 1990; Venge and Håkansson, 1991b; Laitinen *et al.*, 1991; Dahl *et al.*, 1988). The accumulation is seen in spite of the fact that the signals produced in the lung, and which may be operative in the attraction of the eosinophil, do not discriminate between eosinophils or neutrophils (Rak *et al.*, 1991; Venge and Håkansson, 1991a). That is, *in vitro*, both cells are attracted by these putative chemotactic signals. In order to explain this seeming paradox, therefore, we have to look for other more specific mechanisms. One such mechanism could be the selective adherence of eosinophils to the lung endothelial cells and indeed some data from animal experiments may support this possibility, since antibodies to the adherence molecule ICAM-1 (intercellular adhesion molecule-1) inhibited influx of eosinophils to the lung in parallel with the abrogation of lung hyper-reactivity (Wegner *et al.*, 1990). Another possibility would be that the response of the circulating eosinophils is altered in asthma, giving rise to an eosinophil population of increased responsiveness to the chemotactic signals. In the first part of this chapter, we will describe some clinical data which may be supportive of the latter possibility and also give a clue as to what mechanisms may be involved in the priming of the eosinophil to an enhanced responsiveness to chemotactic signals.

In the second part of the chapter we will discuss another phenomenon of great potential importance for the development of bronchial asthma and that is the mechanism of release of the cytotoxic granule proteins from the eosinophil granulocyte. Thus, it has been clearly shown that several of the eosinophil granule proteins such as ECP (eosinophil cationic protein), EPO (eosinophil peroxidase) and MBP (major basic protein) have profound effects on lung tissues in asthmatics. These effects include both the injury of lung epithelial cells (Dahl *et al.*, 1988; Venge *et al.*, 1988a; Filley *et al.*, 1982; Ayars *et al.*, 1985; Ayars *et al.*, 1989; Gleich, 1990; Gundel *et al.*, 1990; Gundel *et al.*, 1991) and the induction of hypersecretion by these cells (Lundgren *et al.*, 1991). Since the normal eosinophil *in vitro* is not a very efficient secretory cell, we speculated that the eosinophils of asthmatics may be altered and have an increased propensity to release their granule proteins in the tissue. The clinical studies described below indeed support this notion and we have therefore extended our studies in this direction in an attempt to understand the mechanisms underlying this phenomenon.

10.2 Priming of the Migratory Response of Eosinophils

Already in 1977 it had been shown (Atkins *et al.*, 1977), and later confirmed by several groups (Lee *et al.*, 1982; Venge *et al.*, 1982), that allergic asthmatic individuals have increased amounts of neutrophil chemotactic activity in their sera after allergen challenge. This was an interesting but curious finding, since it might suggest that neutrophil accumulation is an important and frequent finding in the asthmatic lung. Subsequent studies, however, have convincingly shown that neutrophil accumulation in the allergic asthmatic lung is rare (DeMonchy *et al.*, 1985; Bousquet *et al.*, 1990; Ädelroth *et al.*, 1990; Jeffery *et al.*, 1989; Diaz *et al.*, 1989; Laitinen *et al.*, 1991; Ferguson and Wong, 1989; Wardlaw *et al.*, 1988; Metzger *et al.*, 1987; Rossi *et al.*, 1991). On the contrary, these studies consistently demonstrated the presence of increased numbers of eosinophils. The problem of explaining this apparent paradox, though, was partially solved when we were able to show that these chemotactic signals also had the capacity to attract eosinophils (Håkansson *et al.*, 1989). The relevance of these chemotactic activities was suggested in several clinical studies and indicated to us that they are important signals in the process of accumulation of eosinophil granulocytes in the asthmatic lung and not just an epiphenomenon. In order, however, to be able to explain the selective attraction in spite of the production of unselective signals we had to postulate that asthmatic eosinophils had an altered and increased responsiveness to these signals.

Two studies have been finished so far, which address the above question. In one cross-sectional study on 57 asthmatics of varying severity, the chemotactic response of eosinophils was shown to be significantly raised as compared with a non-asthmatic reference group (Håkansson *et al.*, 1990). These raised eosinophil activities were contrasted by completely unaltered responses of the neutrophils. The raised activities were mainly found in patients with blood eosinophilia. Also, the chemokinetic response of eosinophils was increased, but only in patients with blood eosinophilia. These findings suggest that a common mechanism is operative in the priming of the migratory responses of eosinophils and in the mechanisms that are involved in eosinophilopoiesis. A common denominator is also suggested by the significant and linear correlation between the chemokinetic activity and the serum-ECP levels in these patients. The nature of this common denominator in activating the eosinophil will be discussed more below but may be such species as interleukin-5 (IL-5). In the second study on patients with asthma and eosinophilia we had very similar findings (Griffin *et al.*, 1991b). Thus, both the chemotactic and the chemokinetic responses of eosinophils were significantly raised as compared with non-asthmatics in contrast to the activities of the neutrophils, which were virtually unaltered. This group of patients was followed during a 5-week treatment period after which the activities were reinvestigated. On average the activities were unaltered after the treatment period. However, when the patients were separated in two groups, one of which had no clinical improvement and another in which lung function and other clinical tests of asthma had normalized, it appeared that the normalization of the migratory responses of the eosinophils parallelled the clinical improvement of the patients, and the reduction in blood eosinophil counts and serum-ECP levels. Both of these patient groups consisted of a mixture of asthmatics with different severities and with few patients actually untreated. The increased migratory responses of the eosinophils, therefore, may be grossly underestimated although we in these studies could not discern any effects of corticosteroid medication. It is therefore of interest that we in our further studies on very mild, asymptomatic and untreated asthmatic patient have found significantly increased migratory responses as well (unpublished).

In an attempt to explain the mechanisms underlying the selectively increased migratory response of asthmatic eosinophils we have recently performed a number of *in vitro* experiments investigating the effect of selected cytokines on eosinophil and neutrophil migration (to be published). Briefly, these experiments showed that IL-5 and to a lesser extent IL-3 enhance the chemotactic and chemokinetic response to a variety of chemotactic and chemokinetic stimuli. The effect, however, was not restricted to eosinophils, since the response of neutrophils was enhanced as well. Both IL-5 and IL-3, therefore, seem to be somewhat unselective in their actions. The results, however, also suggest that the effects of IL-5 on eosinophils occur at a somewhat lower concentration, which may give rise to some selectivity in its action towards eosinophils and neutrophils. Our conclusions from these studies, though, are that they do not satisfactorily explain the very selective increase in eosinophil response seen in asthmatic patients. A search for other principles is therefore needed. Finally, we have not yet ruled out the possibility that part of the explanation of this enhanced responsiveness is related to an inherent activity of asthma eosinophils. Thus, it might be a phenomenon directly related to the maturation process of eosinophils or a constitutional abnormality of asthmatics.

10.3 Priming of Eosinophil Degranulation

The estimation of the activity *in vivo* of the eosinophil granulocyte may be accomplished by means of the measurements of eosinophil products such as ECP in serum. This approach has been used extensively and been reviewed in several recent publications to which the interested reader is referred (Venge and Håkansson, 1991a; Rak *et al.*, 1988; Venge, 1990; Venge *et al.*, 1988b; Venge and Dahl, 1989a, b; Venge *et al.*, 1990; Venge, 1989; Venge and Carlson, 1990; Griffin *et al.*, 1991a; Venge and Håkansson, 1991b). Suffice it to be said in this chapter that the levels in serum of ECP probably to some extent reflect priming of the circulating eosinophil population (see also further below).

The more direct measurement of priming of eosinophils in asthma has been made by harvesting eosinophils from asthmatic patients and measuring their propensity *in vitro* to release their granule proteins, ECP and EPX (eosinophil protein X), after stimulation with a particulate stimulus coated with serum opsonins primarily complement factor 3b. In one study a group of 30 asthmatic patients with varying severity of the disease was studied (Carlson *et al.*, 1991). The results showed that the group of asthmatics released on average 50–100% more ECP or EPX as compared with the non-asthmatic reference group. There was, however, no discernible relationship between the activity of the eosinophils in this respect and the clinical findings in these patients. The release of MPO (myeloperoxidase) from the neutrophils was also measured in this group. These results showed a slightly, but significantly, elevated release of MPO from the neutrophils, which means that whatever primes the eosinophils to an enhanced release also primes the neutrophils.

In a second study we followed a group of seasonal asthmatic patients before, during and after the birch pollen season (Carlson *et al.*, 1992). The

eosinophils of these patients showed normal responses to the secretagogue
before and after season. During season the release of ECP and EPX was
increased on average 100% and the release activity peaked at the pollen
peak. In keeping with the cross-sectional study cited above the release of
MPO from the neutrophils was increased, although not to the same extent,
i.e. on average 50%, in this group as well. The peak of MPO release
coincided with the pollen peak. The serum-ECP levels were also measured
and were shown to be significantly raised even before the season but
increased further during the season. In contrast, the blood eosinophil
count, which was raised before the season, remained unaltered during the
season. Our interpretation of these findings was that the ECP-levels before
the season reflected the size of the population of the eosinophils whereas
the increment during the season was due to the priming of the eosinophils
to release their granule proteins. Thus, a given serum-ECP value is the sum
of the ECP derived from two or possibly three sources. One is related to
the size of the eosinophil pool in the body and the other to the state of
activity of the circulating population of eosinophils. A third source may be
the diffusion of ECP from a local process into the circulation.

In order to investigate the possible mechanisms of the enhancement of
eosinophil release further, we have investigated the effects of some cytokines, such as IL-5, on eosinophil and neutrophil release *in vitro* (to be
published). These studies showed that IL-5 had the capacity to enhance the
release of ECP from normal eosinophils, whereas there was no discernible
effect on neutrophil release activity. The effect of IL-5, therefore, seems to
be specifically directed towards the eosinophil and would therefore not
explain the fact that our clinical studies also suggest priming of the
neutrophil. As for the enhanced migratory response we have to extend our
search for additional mechanisms. The fact that eosinophil release activity
is normal out of season in contrast to the migratory activity, however,
definitely tells us that this phenomenon is an acquired quality of the
eosinophil.

References

Atkins, P. C., Norman, M., Weiner, H. and Zweiman, B. (1977). Release of
  neutrophil chemotactic activity during immediate hypersensitivity reactions in
  humans. *Ann. Intern. Med.*, **86**, 415–18.
Ayars, G. H., Altman, L. C., Gleich, G. J., Loegering, D. A. and Baker, C. B.
  (1985). Eosinophil- and eosinophil granule-mediated pneumocyte injury.
  J. Allergy Clin. Immunol., **76**, 595–604.
Ayars, G. H., Altman, L. C., McManus, M. M., Agosti, J. M., Baker, C., Luchtel,
  D. L., *et al.* (1989). Injurious effect of the eosinophil peroxide–hydrogen per-
  oxide–halide system and major basic protein on human nasal epithelium *in vitro*.
  Am. Rev. Respir. Dis., **140**, 125–31.

Azzawi, M., Bradley, B., Jeffery, P. K., Frew, A. J., Wardlaw, A. J., Knowles, G., et al. (1990). Identification of activated T lymphocytes and eosinophils in bronchial biopsies in stable atopic asthma. Am. Rev. Respir. Dis., 142, 1407–13.

Ädelroth, E., Rosenhall, L., Johansson, S.-Å., Linden, M. and Venge, P. (1990). Inflammatory cells and eosinophilic activity in asthmatics investigated by bronchoalveolar lavage: the effects of antiasthmatic treatment with Budesonide or Terbutaline. Am. Rev. Respir. Dis., 142, 91–9.

Bousquet, J., Chanez, P., Lacoste, J. Y., Barnéon, G., Ghavanian, N., Enander, L., et al. (1990). Eosinophilic inflammation in asthma. New Engl. J. Med., 323, 1033–9.

Carlson, M., Håkansson, L, Kämpe, M., Stålenheim, G., Peterson, C. and Venge, P. (1992). Degranulation of eosinophils from pollen atopic patients with asthma is increased during pollen season. J. Allergy Clin. Immunol., 89, 131–9.

Carlson, M., Håkansson, L., Peterson, C., Stålenheim, G. and Venge, P. (1991). Secretion of granule proteins from eosinophils and neutrophils is increased in asthma. J. Allergy Clin. Immunol., 87, 27–33.

Dahl, R., Venge, P. and Fredens, K. (1988). The eosinophil. In Barnes, P. J., Rodger, I. and Thomson, N. (eds.), Asthma: Basic Mechanisms and Clinical Management, Academic Press, London, 115–30.

DeMonchy, J. G. R., Kauffman, H. F., Venge, P., Koeter, G. H., Jansen, H. M., Sluiter, H. J., et al. (1985). Bronchoalveolar eosinophilia during allergen-induced late asthmatic reactions. Am. Rev. Respir. Dis., 131, 373–6.

Diaz, P., Gonzalez, M. C., Galleguillos, F. R., Ancic, P., Cromwell, O., Shepherd, D., et al. (1989). Leukocytes and mediators in bronchoalveolar lavage during allergen-induced late-phase asthmatic reactions. Am. Rev. Respir. Dis., 139, 1383–9.

Ferguson, A. C. and Wong, F. W. M. (1989). Bronchial hyperresponsiveness in asthmatic children: correlation with macrophages and eosinophils in broncholavage fluid. Chest, 96, 988–91.

Filley, W. V., Kephart, G. M., Holley, K. E. and Gleich, G. J. (1982). Identification by immunofluorescence of eosinophil granule major basic protein in lung tissues of patients with bronchial asthma. Lancet, 3, 11–16.

Frew, A. J. and Kay, A. B. (1990). Postgraduate course eosinophils and T-lymphocytes in late-phase allergic reactions. J. Allergy Clin. Immunol., 85, 533–9.

Gleich, G. J. (1990). The eosinophil and bronchial asthma: current understanding. J. Allergy Clin. Immunol., 85, 422–36.

Griffin, E., Håkansson, L., Formgren, H., Jörgensen, K., Peterson, C. and Venge, P. (1991a). Blood eosinophil number and activity in relation to lung function in asthmatic patients with eosinophilia. J. Allergy Clin. Immunol., 87, 548–57.

Griffin, E., Håkansson, L., Formgren, H., Jörgensen, K. and Venge, P. (1991b). Increased chemokinetic and chemotactic responses of eosinophils in asthmatic patients. Allergy, 46, 955–65.

Gundel, R. H., Gerritsen, M. E., Gleich, G. J. and Wegner, C. D. (1990). Repeated antigen inhalation results in a prolonged airway eosinophilia and airway hyperresponsiveness in primates. J. Appl. Physiol., 68, 779–86.

Gundel, R. H., Letts, L. G. and Gleich, G. J. (1991). Human eosinophil major basic protein induces airway constriction and airway hyperresponsiveness in primates. J. Clin. Invest., 87, 1470–3.

Håkansson, L., Rak, S., Dahl, R. and Venge, P. (1989). The formation of eosinophil and neutrophil chemotactic activity during a pollen season and after allergen challenge. J. Allergy Clin. Immunol., 83, 933–9.

Håkansson, L., Carlson, M., Stålenheim, G. and Venge, P. (1990). Migratory responses of eosinophil and neutrophil granulocytes from patients with asthma. *J. Allergy Clin. Immunol.*, **85**, 743–50.

Jeffery, P. K., Wardlaw, A. J., Nelson, F. C., Collins, J. V. and Kay, A. B. (1989). Bronchial biopsies in asthma: an ultrastructural, quantitative study and correlation with hyperreactivity. *Am. Rev. Respir. Dis.*, **140**, 1745–53.

Kay, A. B. (1991). Asthma and inflammation. *J. Allergy Clin. Immunol.*, **87**, 893–911.

Laitinen, L. A., Laitinen, A., Heino, M. and Haahtela, T. (1991). Eosinophilic airway inflammation during exacerbation of asthma and its treatment with inhaled corticosteroid. *Am. Rev. Respir. Dis.*, **143**, 423–7.

Lee, T. H., Nagy, L., Nagakura, T., Walport, M. J. and Kay, A. B. (1982). Identification and partial characterization of an exercise-induced neutrophil chemotactic factor in bronchial asthma. *J. Clin. Invest.*, **69**, 889–99.

Lundgren, J. D., Davey, R. T., Jr, Lundgren, B., Mullol, J., Marom, Z., Logun, C., *et al.* (1991). Eosinophil cationic protein stimulates and major basic protein inhibits airway mucus secretion. *J. Allergy Clin. Immunol.*, **87**, 689–98.

Metzger, W. J., Zavala, D., Richerson, H. B., Moseley, P., Iwamota, P., Monick, M., *et al.* (1987). Local allergen challenge and bronchoalveolar lavage of allergic asthmatic lungs. Description of the model of local airway inflammation. *Am. Rev. Respir. Dis.*, **135**, 433–40.

Rak, S., Löwhagen, O. and Venge, P. (1988). The effect of immunotherapy on bronchial hyperresponsiveness and eosinophil cationic protein in pollen-allergic patients. *J. Allergy Clin. Immunol.*, **82**, 470–80.

Rak, S., Björnson, A., Håkansson, L., Sörenson, S. and Venge, P. (1991). The effect of immunotherapy on eosinophil accumulation and production of eosinophil chemotactic activity in the lung of subjects with asthma during natural pollen exposure. *J. Allergy Clin. Immunol.*, **88**, 878–8.

Rossi, G. A., Crimi, E., Lantero, S., Gianiorio, P., Oddera, S., Crimi, P., *et al.* (1991). Late-phase asthmatic reaction to inhaled allergen is associated with early recruitment of eosinophils in the airways. *Am. Rev. Respir. Dis.*, **144**, 379–83.

Venge, P. (1989). Mediators from granulocytic blood cells. In Debelic, M. and Kunkel, G. (eds.), *Allergologie, Proceedings of the XIVth Congress of the European Academy of Allergology and Clinical Immunology, Berlin, September 17–22, 1989*, Dustri, Munich, 231–5.

Venge, P. (1990). What is the role of the eosinophil? *Thorax*, **45**, 161–3.

Venge, P. and Carlson, M. (1990). Eosinophil granule proteins in bronchial asthma. In Kay, A. B. (ed.), *Eosinophils, Allergy and Asthma*, Blackwell, Oxford, 96–105.

Venge, P., Dahl, R., Håkansson, L. and Peterson, C. (1982). Generation of heat-labile chemotactic activity in blood after inhalation challenge and its relationship to neutrophil and monocyte/macrophage turnover and activity. *Allergy*, **37**, 55–62.

Venge, P., Dahl, R. and Fredens, K. (1988a). Epithelial injury by human eosinophils. *Am. Rev. Respir. Dis.*, **138**, s54–s57.

Venge, P., Dahl, R. and Peterson, C. G. B. (1988b). Eosinophil granule proteins in serum after allergen challenge of asthmatic patients and the effects of anti-asthmatic medication. *Int. Arch. Allergy Appl. Immunol.*, **87**, 306–12.

Venge, P. and Dahl, R. (1989a). Are blood eosinophil number and activity important for the development of the late asthmatic reaction after allergen challenge? *Eur. J. Respir. Dis.*, **2** (Suppl. 6), 430s–434s.

Venge, P. and Dahl, R. (1989b). The eosinophil and intrinsic asthma. In Schmitz-

Schumann, M., Menz, G., Costabel, U. and Page, C. P. (eds.), *AAS 28: Intrinsic Asthma*, Birkhauser, Basel, 67–74.

Venge, P., Rak, S. and Håkansson, L. (1990). Study of inflammatory mediators in asthma by bronchoalveolar lavage. In Melillo, G., Norman, P. S. and Marone, G. (eds.), *Respiratory Allergy*, Decker, Toronto, 105–10.

Venge, P. and Håkansson, L. (1991a). The eosinophil and asthma. In Kaliner, M., Barnes, P. J. and Persson, C. G. A. (eds.), *Asthma. Its Pathology and Treatment*, Dekker, New York, 477–502.

Venge, P. and Håkansson, L. (1991b). Current understanding of the role of the eosinophil granulocyte in asthma. *Clin. Exp. Allergy*, **21** (Suppl. 3), 31–7.

Wardlaw, A. J., Dunnette, S., Gleich, G. J., Collins, J. V. and Kay, A. B. (1988). Eosinophils and mast cells in bronchoalveolar lavage in subjects with mild asthma. *Am. Rev. Respir. Dis.*, **137**, 62–9.

Wegner, C. D., Gundel, R. H., Reilly, P., Haynes, N., Letts, L. G. and Rothlein, R. (1990). Intercellular adhesion molecule-1 (ICAM-1) in the pathogenesis of asthma. *Science*, **247**, 456–9.

11

Lipoxygenase Derivatives in Asthma

J. P. Arm

11.1 Introduction

Leukotrienes are lipid mediators formed from the oxidative metabolism of arachidonic acid by the lipoxygenase enzyme cascade (Samuelsson, 1983). In contrast to mediators such as histamine, which are preformed and stored in granules, leukotrienes are lipid mediators and are newly synthesized upon cell activation. Leukotrienes have potent proinflammatory and spasmogenic properties and are present in asthmatic airways at rest and during an acute attack of asthma. The results of recent studies of potent and selective receptor antagonists and 5-lipoxygenase inhibitors provide compelling evidence that leukotrienes play an important role in the pathophysiology of bronchial asthma.

11.2 Synthesis and Metabolism

Synthesis

Arachidonic acid is released from membrane phospholipids by the action of phospholipase A_2. Metabolism by the 5-lipoxygenase generates the unstable intermediate 5-hydroperoxyeicosatetraenoic acid (5-HPETE) (Borgeat and Samuelsson, 1979c) which is reduced to 5-hydroxyeicosatetraenoic acid (5-HETE) or is converted to an epoxide, leukotriene (LT) A_4 (Borgeat and Samuelsson, 1979a; Rådmark *et al.*, 1980; Hammarström

114

and Samuelsson, 1980). LTA_4 is processed by an epoxide hydrolase to LTB_4 (Borgeat and Samuelsson, 1979b) or, by a glutathione-S-transferase, to LTC_4 (Murphy *et al.*, 1979; Bach *et al.*, 1980, 1984). LTC_4 is cleaved by τ-glutamyl-transpeptidase to LTD_4 which is cleaved by a dipeptidase to LTE_4 (Murphy *et al.*, 1979; Bach *et al.*, 1980; Lewis *et al.*, 1980a, b; Morris *et al.*, 1980; Örning *et al.*, 1980). LTA_4 also undergoes non-enzymatic hydrolysis to $5S,12R$- and $5S,12S$-dihydroxy-6-*trans*-LTB_4 diastereoisomers and to minor products, 5,6-dihydroxyeicosatetraenoic acid diastereoisomers (Borgeat and Samuelsson, 1979d).

With the molecular cloning of 5-lipoxygenase (5-LO) it became apparent that cellular 5-LO activity was dependent upon an additional factor. Osteosarcoma cells transfected with the cDNA for 5-LO were unable to generate leukotrienes upon stimulation with the calcium ionophore A23187 although cell lysates expressed active enzyme (Rouzer *et al.*, 1988). Furthermore, a class of compounds, of which MK-886 is an example, has been described, which inhibit the generation of cellular leukotrienes but have no inhibitory effect on soluble 5-LO (Gillard *et al.*, 1989). The target of MK-886 was identified as a membrane protein of molecular weight 18 000, termed 5-LO activating protein (FLAP) (Miller *et al.*, 1990). *N*-terminal and internal amino acid sequence were used to design oligonucleotide probes, with which cDNA clones were isolated from both rat and human cell lines (Dixon *et al.*, 1990). The cDNA encodes a protein of 161 amino acids with three transmembrane domains. Osteosarcoma cells transfected with 5-LO or FLAP alone did not generate leukotrienes upon activation with A23187. Transfection with cDNAs for both 5-LO and FLAP was required for significant generation of leukotrienes.

The distribution and action of 5-lipoxygenase is limited. Peripheral blood neutrophils generate about 50 ng $LTB_4/10^6$ cells and only one-tenth as much LTC_4 in response to activation with A23187 (Weller *et al.*, 1983; Lee *et al.*, 1983), the quantities and ratio being reversed for eosinophils (Weller *et al.*, 1983). Peripheral blood monocytes produce about 70 ng LTB_4 and 30 ng $LTC_4/10^6$ cells (Williams *et al.*, 1984), whereas adherent alveolar macrophages generate 100–400 ng $LTB_4/10^6$ cells, in an average 20-fold excess relative to LTC_4 (Fels *et al.*, 1982; Martin *et al.*, 1984). The quantities of leukotriene generated by each of these cells in response to physiological stimuli, for example unopsonized (Mahauthaman *et al.*, 1988; Williams *et al.*, 1985) or opsonized (Walsh *et al.*, 1981) zymosan and immunoglobulin G (IgG) coated sepharose beads (Shaw *et al.*, 1985) are generally less than those obtained with ionophore activation. The stimulation of neutrophils and eosinophils with unopsonized zymosan results in a significant cellular retention of 5-lipoxygenase products, suggesting that release of these metabolites may be an event that is regulated separately from their generation. Lam and colleagues have shown that the export of LTC_4 by cultured human eosinophils and of LTB_4 from human neutrophils is a specific biochemical step distinct from their biosynthesis (Lam *et al.*, 1989, 1990).

Human mast cells isolated from both skin and lung generate LTC_4 in response to IgE-mediated stimulation (Benyon *et al.*, 1987; MacGlashan *et al.*, 1982); PGD_2 is the major eicosanoid released from human mast cells in an approximate 10-fold molar excess compared with LTC_4 (Leung *et al.*, 1987). The LTA_4 hydrolase that converts LTA_4 to LTB_4 is widely distributed. Thus LTA_4 may be released from one cell for transcellular metabolism by another, leading to the generation of LTB_4 by erythrocytes (McGee and Fitzpatrick, 1986), or LTC_4 by platelets (Edenius *et al.*, 1988; Maclouf and Murphy, 1988) endothelial cells (Feinmark and Cannon, 1986), and mast cells (Dahinden *et al.*, 1985).

Metabolism

LTB_4 is converted intracellularly by a hydroxylase to 20-hydroxy LTB_4, and by further oxidation to a biologically inactive molecule, 20-aldehyde LTB_4 (Soberman *et al.*, 1985; Shak and Goldstein, 1984; Soberman *et al.*, 1988). LTB_4-20 hydroxylase is a member of the P450 cytochrome family and is located in neutrophils. 20-aldehyde LTB_4 is converted irreversibly to 20-carboxy-LTB_4 which is converted back to 20-OH LTB_4 by a microsomal aldehyde reductase.

In addition to their generation by inflammatory cells, leukotrienes may be synthesized and metabolized by lung tissue. Thus, the conversion of LTA_4 to LTB_4, LTC_4, LTD_4 and LTE_4 has been demonstrated in guinea-pig lung (Aharony *et al.*, 1985), and of LTC_4 to LTD_4 and LTE_4 in human lung parenchyma (Conroy *et al.*, 1989). In addition to the bioconversion of LTC_4 to LTD_4 and to LTE_4, the sulphidopeptide leukotrienes may be metabolized by granulocytes, upon the triggering of the respiratory burst (Lee *et al.*, 1983). Neutrophils metabolize LTC_4, LTD_4 and LTE_4 and eosinophils metabolize LTC_4 through an extracellular hydrogen peroxide–peroxidase chloride-dependent reaction. More than 70% of the metabolites are composed of the 6-*trans*-LTB_4-diastereoisomers and the subclass specific diastereoisomeric leukotriene sulphoxides.

11.3 Biological Activities

Leukotriene B₄

LTB_4 is a potent pro-inflammatory mediator. Its *in vitro* activities are apparent at concentrations as low as 10^{-9} M and include chemokinesis and chemotaxis of human neutrophils and eosinophils (Ford-Hutchinson *et al.*, 1980; Nagy *et al.*, 1982), chemokinesis of monocytes (Palmer *et al.*, 1980), aggregation of neutrophils (Ford-Hutchinson *et al.*, 1980), enhanced expression of complement receptors on granulocytes (Lee *et al.*, 1988), release of lysosomal enzymes from neutrophils (Showell *et al.*, 1982), and augmentation of neutrophil adherence to endothelial cell monolayers (Hoover *et al.*, 1984). *In vivo*, intradermal injection of LTB_4 promotes a prolonged neutrophil infiltration into human skin, with induration and tenderness 4–6 h after injection (Soter *et al.*, 1983). LTB_4 also contracts smooth muscle through the biosynthesis of cyclooxygenase products (Sirois *et al.*, 1981).

Radioligand binding studies suggest the existence of a heterogeneous population of LTB_4 binding sites. The dissociation constant (K_d) of the high affinity receptor was approximately 0.5 nM and the K_d of the low affinity receptor was approximately 300 nM (Goldman and Goetzl, 1982). The high affinity receptor is believed to mediate chemotaxis, and the low affinity receptor lysosomal enzyme release (Lin *et al.*, 1984).

Sulphidopeptide Leukotrienes

Sulphidopeptide leukotrienes constrict non-vascular smooth muscle, enhance mucus secretion, constrict arterioles, and enhance venopermeability. Bronchial mucosal explants respond in tissue culture by enhanced mucus secretion to as little as 10^{-9} M LTC_4 (Marom *et al.*, 1982; Coles *et al.*, 1983). The capacity of LTC_4 and, to a lesser extent, LTD_4 to constrict arterioles was initially demonstrated in guinea-pig skin at the site of intradermal administration, requiring less than 10^{-7} M of either compound (Lewis *et al.*, 1980a; Drazen *et al.*, 1980), and was confirmed by the response to topical administration to the hamster cheek pouch (Dahlén *et al.*, 1981) and by blanching at the injection site in normal human skin (Soter *et al.*, 1983; Camp *et al.*, 1983). In addition the intradermal administration of LTC_4, LTD_4 and LTE_4 in normal human subjects produces a local wheal and flare response, in which the wheal representing enhanced venopermeability, is sustained for 2–4 h (Soter *et al.*, 1983; Camp *et al.*, 1983). The sulphidopeptide leukotrienes are potent contractile agonists for bronchial smooth muscle both *in vitro* and *in vivo*.

The activity and binding of the sulphidopeptide leukotrienes in various tissues and cells have been characterized. With regard to the lung, there are limited data on human tissues and most attention has focused on the guinea-pig, in which stereospecific, reversible and saturable binding of LTC_4, LTD_4, and LTE_4 have been demonstrated. The existence of receptor heterogeneity for these agonists in guinea-pig lung is suggested by differences in the contractile properties and kinetics of action of the separate leukotrienes, the effects of leukotriene receptor antagonists, and radioligand binding studies (Lee *et al.*, 1984; Lewis *et al.*, 1980a; Drazen *et al.*, 1980, 1983; Krilis *et al.*, 1983; Snyder and Krell, 1984; Weichman and Tucker, 1985; Cheng and Townley, 1984; Krell *et al.*, 1983; Hay *et al.*, 1988; Aharony *et al.*, 1989).

In contrast to the results in guinea-pig tissues, a study conducted in the presence of bioconversion inhibitors on intralobar airways isolated from human subjects undergoing surgery for carcinoma of the bronchus did not reveal evidence for multiple leukotriene receptors. FPL 55712 and SK&F 104353 are selective LTD_4–LTE_4 antagonists in guinea-pig lung, but antagonize the actions of LTC_4, LTD_4 and LTE_4 in isolated human bronchi (Buckner *et al.*, 1986; Hay *et al.*, 1987), with similar PA_2 values for each agonist. However, it should be emphasized that data from human tissue are very limited. Furthermore, the effects of underlying disease on the expression of the different leukotriene receptors have not been studied and data are not available for asthmatic lung.

11.4 Leukotrienes in Bronchial Asthma

Potency

LTC_4 and LTD_4 are potent constrictors of human airways both *in vitro* and *in vivo* (Lee *et al.*, 1984; Roberts *et al.*, 1987; Dahlén *et al.*, 1980). LTC_4 and LTD_4 are approximately 1000-fold more potent than histamine on a molar basis in contracting isolated human bronchi *in vitro* (Dahlén *et al.*, 1980). In normal subjects the concentrations of LTC_4 and histamine required to produce a 30% fall in V_{30} (flow at 30% of vital capacity) were 2–20 µg/ml and 2–10 mg/ml respectively (Weiss *et al.*, 1982a). LTC_4 was 600- to 9500-fold more potent than histamine and LTD_4 was 6000-fold more potent than histamine on a molar basis (Weiss *et al.*, 1983). While LTC_4 and LTD_4 have similar potencies in human airways *in vivo* they have a different time course of contraction, maximal bronchoconstriction occurring 10 to 15 min after inhalation of LTC_4 and 2 min after inhalation of LTD_4 (Weiss *et al.*, 1983).

In asthmatic subjects, Griffin *et al.* (1983) reported that LTD_4 was 140-fold more potent than histamine in eliciting a 30% fall in $V_{30}P$. This contrasts with the data in normal subjects in whom LTD_4 was 6000-fold more potent than histamine (Weiss *et al.*, 1983). A comparison between these two groups of subjects revealed that the asthmatic subjects were only 1/3 more responsive to LTD_4 than the normal subjects, despite an approximate 100-fold hyperresponsiveness to inhaled histamine. The relative lack of hyperresponsiveness to LTC_4 and LTD_4 in asthmatic subjects was confirmed by other studies (Barnes *et al.*, 1984a; Adelroth *et al.*, 1986). A correlation was also observed between airways responsiveness to methacholine and the relative responsiveness to LTC_4 and LTD_4; subjects with the most responsive airways demonstrated the lowest relative responsiveness to LTC_4 and LTD_4 as compared with methacholine (Adelroth *et al.*, 1986). The study by Smith *et al.* (1985) contrasts with these results, reporting that a group of asthmatic subjects who were 35-fold more responsive to methacholine than normal controls were 100-fold more responsive to LTD_4.

There are limited data on the bronchoconstrictor properties of LTE_4 *in vivo*. Using V_{30} as an index of bronchoconstriction, Davidson found LTE_4 to be 39-fold more potent than histamine in normal subjects and 14-fold more potent than histamine in asthmatic subjects (Davidson *et al.*, 1987). Using airways specific conductance (SGaw) as an index of bronchoconstriction, the relative potency of LTE_4 compared with histamine and methacholine was 2 to 3 times greater in asthmatic than in normal subjects (O'Hickey *et al.*, 1988). This contrasts with the relative hyporesponsiveness of asthmatic subjects to LTC_4 and LTD_4. Because of the inherent difficulties in comparing studies performed in different subjects using different methodologies, we compared the potencies of LTC_4, LTD_4 and LTE_4 with one another and with both histamine and methacholine in normal and asthmatic subjects (Arm *et al.*, 1990). The airways of asthmatic subjects were 14-fold, 15-fold, 6-fold, 9-fold and 219-fold more responsive than the airways of normal subjects to histamine, methacholine, LTC_4, LTD_4 and LTE_4 respectively. Furthermore, while LTC_4 and LTD_4 were 100- to 150-fold more potent than LTE_4 in constricting the airways of normal subjects they were only 4- to 5-fold more potent than LTE_4 in asthmatic subjects. The cumulative data therefore suggest that the airways of asthmatic subjects are relatively unresponsive to LTC_4 and LTD_4, but have a marked hyperresponsiveness to LTE_4.

Differences between asthmatic and normal individuals in the predominant site of response to leukotrienes within the tracheobronchial tree have been described. Initial studies found that the inhalation of LTC_4 and LTD_4 elicited a fall in V_{30} with little change in forced expired volume in 1 s (FEV_1), suggesting a predominantly peripheral site of action in normal subjects (Holroyde *et al.*, 1981). Weiss established that in normal subjects a 50-fold greater concentration of LTC_4 was required to achieve a 20% fall in FEV_1 compared with the concentration needed to achieve a 30% fall in V_{30} (Weiss *et al.*, 1982b). However, in other studies inhalation of leukotriene was noted to have a similar effect on both SGaw and V_{30} (Barnes *et al.*, 1984b; Kern *et al.*, 1986; Smith *et al.*, 1985). Studies in asthmatic subjects suggest that leukotrienes may elicit a response which is more marked in the central than the peripheral airways. Bisgaard and co-workers reported that the airways of asthmatic subjects were more responsive to LTD_4 than non-asthmatic subjects (Bisgaard *et al.*, 1985). The relative difference in potency between asthmatic and normal subjects was 100- to 1000-fold when measured in terms of FEV_1 but only 15-fold in terms of V_{30}. Smith *et al.* (1985) found that a 30% fall in V_{30} in response to LTD_4 was accompanied by a 60% fall in SGaw in asthmatic subjects, but only a 30% fall in SGaw in normal controls. The study by Davidson also suggested a predominantly central effect of LTE_4 in asthmatic subjects compared with normal controls (Davidson *et al.*, 1987). A 30% fall in $V_{30}P$ in response to LTE_4 was accompanied by a 2.6% fall in FEV_1 in normal subjects, but a 15% fall in FEV_1 in asthmatic subjects. In contrast a 30% fall in $V_{30}P$ induced by histamine was accompanied by comparable falls in FEV_1 in both groups of subjects (Davidson *et al.*, 1987). Using both density dependence of velocity maximum (V_{max}) and the effects of a deep breath on expiratory flow rates as indices of the predominant site of response to LTC_4 or histamine, Pichurko *et al.* (1989) found that there was predominantly central airway response to inhaled LTC_4 in asthmatic subjects which was not seen with histamine inhalation.

The mechanism whereby leukotrienes produce a contractile response is unknown. The fact that prior administration of aspirin (Weiss *et al.*, 1983) or indomethacin (Smith *et al.*, 1987) does not change leukotriene responsiveness suggests that secondary generation of cyclooxygenase products is not important. The calcium channel blocker verapamil has been shown to inhibit LTD_4-induced bronchoconstriction in normal humans suggesting that extracellular calcium entry is required for LTD_4-induced bronchoconstriction (Roberts *et al.*, 1986b). In contrast, verapamil did not inhibit the response of asthmatic subjects to inhaled LTD_4 suggesting that there may be a different mechanism of action of LTD_4 in asthmatic subjects compared with normal subjects (Roberts *et al.*, 1986a).

Leukotrienes and Airway Hyperresponsiveness

Brocklehurst demonstrated that slow reacting substance of anaphylaxis enhanced the contractile response of guinea-pig ileum to histamine *in vitro* (Brocklehurst, 1962). Lee subsequently demonstrated that pretreatment of guinea-pig tracheal spirals with 10 to 23 nM LTE_4, but not LTC_4 or LTD_4, enhanced the subsequent contractile response to histamine (Lee *et al.*, 1984). This effect was not observed when parenchymal strips were contracted with LTE_4. Further studies have shown that LTE_4-induced hyperresponsiveness of guinea-pig tracheal spirals is selective for histamine and is not seen for carbachol or substance P (Jacques *et al.*, 1991). LTE_4-induced hyperresponsiveness is blocked by indomethacin and by the thromboxane B_2 receptor (TBX_2 receptor) antagonist GR32191, atropine, and tetrodotoxin. Preincubation of tracheal spirals with LTE_4 also potentiated the contractile response to electrical field stimulation (Jacques *et al.*, 1991). These results suggest that LTE_4 augments the contractile response of guinea-pig tracheal spirals to histamine by facilitating cholinergic neurotransmission, and is mediated via the secondary generation of cyclooxygenase products acting at the TBX_2 receptor. Treatment of human bronchus with 4.8 nM LTE_4 produced a 4-fold leftwards displacement of the histamine dose–response curve. This effect was blocked by atropine and by GR32191, suggesting a similar mechanism to that defined for guinea-pig trachea (Jacques *et al.*, 1991).

In vivo studies support a role for the sulphidopeptide leukotrienes in enhancing airways hyperresponsiveness in asthma. Inhalation of a bronchoconstricting dose of LTD_4 in normal subjects produced an approximate 2-fold increase in airway methacholine responsiveness (Kern *et al.*, 1986). The maximal effect on methacholine responsiveness was observed at day 7, and persisted for up to 2 to 3 weeks (Kaye and Smith, 1990). The degree and duration of changes in the airways responsiveness to methacholine were comparable with those observed following inhalation of platelet activating factor (PAF) in the same individuals (Kaye and Smith, 1990). In normal subjects inhalation of LTD_4 did not significantly enhance the airway response to exercise (Bisgaard and Groth, 1987) or histamine (Barnes *et al.*, 1984a), although it increased the sensitivity of the airways to inhaled $PGF_{2\alpha}$ by approximately 7-fold (Barnes *et al.*, 1984a).

Normal and asthmatic airway responses *in vivo* differ not only in their sensitivity to a wide range of pharmacological and non-pharmacological stimuli (Holgate *et al.*, 1987), but also by the presence of maximal airway narrowing to histamine and methacholine in non-asthmatic subjects. Asthmatic subjects show a leftward shift of the dose–response curve and progressive airway narrowing with increasing dose of agonist, whereas the airway response in normal subjects reaches a plateau at mild degrees of airway narrowing (Woolcock *et al.*, 1984; Sterk *et al.*, 1986). Bel and colleagues investigated the effect of LTD_4 on both the position and the plateau of the dose–response curve to methacholine (Bel *et al.*, 1987). The degree of maximal airway narrowing was consistently greater in response to LTD_4 than to methacholine. Administration of LTD_4 did not change the position of the dose–response curve to methacholine, although the maximal airway response to methacholine increased. The authors suggested that the effects of LTD_4 were due to changes in vascular permeability leading to oedema of the mucosa, and possibly increased mucus production. Consistent with this suggestion, the maximal airway narrowing to LTD_4 was diminished and the LTD_4-induced augmentation of maximal airway narrowing to methacholine was prevented by pretreatment with inhaled budesonide for 1 week (Bel *et al.*, 1989).

Studies in asthmatic subjects have been more limited. The inhalation of bronchoconstricting doses of LTC_4 did not enhance the airway response to ultrasonically nebulized distilled water (Bianco *et al.*, 1985). In contrast, preinhalation of a bronchoconstricting dose of LTE_4 in asthmatic subjects increased histamine responsiveness by approximately 3-fold (Arm *et al.*, 1988). Changes in airways histamine responsiveness were maximal at 4 to 7 h after inhalation of LTE_4 and had returned to baseline values by 1 week. Subsequent work has shown that bronchoconstricting doses of LTC_4 and LTD_4 elicit a comparable increase in airways responsiveness to histamine in asthmatic individuals (O'Hickey *et al.*, 1991). None of LTC_4, LTD_4 or LTE_4 elicited any change in airways responses to histamine in normal subjects, although each mediator was administered in a dose which elicited a mean 35% fall in SGaw (Arm *et al.*, 1988; O'Hickey *et al.*, 1991). The lack of effect in normal individuals is in contrast to the studies of Kaye *et al.* (1990) and Kern *et al.* (1986) (above), and may be due to a selective effect of LTD_4 on normal airways responses to methacholine (as opposed to histamine), to the timing of measurements of airways responsiveness, or to individual variability.

In addition to the capacity of inhaled leukotrienes to enhance subsequent airways responses to histamine in subjects with asthma, LTC_4 may interact synergistically with histamine and PGD_2 in the acute bronchoconstrictor response (Phillips and Holgate, 1989). This is in contrast to the additive effects of PGD_2 with histamine in asthmatic subjects (Hardy *et al.*, 1986).

Release of Leukotrienes in Asthma

Leukotrienes have been detected in bronchoalveolar lavage (BAL) fluid of asthmatic subjects, both at rest and following bronchial challenge. Lam *et al.* (1988) used fast atom bombardment mass spectroscopy to demonstrate LTE_4 in the BAL fluid of 15 out of 17 asthmatic subjects. LTD_4 was detected in two subjects, and 20-hydroxy LTB_4 in 12 subjects with asthma. Leukotrienes were not detected in the BAL fluid of healthy subjects. Other studies have confirmed the presence of significant quantities of LTC_4 and LTB_4 in BAL fluid of asthmatic subjects compared with normal controls (Wardlaw *et al.*, 1989). Leukotrienes have been detected in BAL fluid following local endobronchial challenge with allergen (Wenzel *et al.*, 1990) and following isocapnic hyperventilation (Pliss *et al.*, 1990). As assessed by HPLC the predominant sulphidopeptide leukotriene in lavage fluid of atopic asthmatics prior to allergen challenge was LTC_4, with lesser amounts of LTD_4 and LTE_4. Following allergen challenge mean LTC_4 levels rose from 64 pg/ml of lavage fluid to 616 pg/ml (Wenzel *et al.*, 1990). LTC_4 was detected in lavage fluid in 1 out of 7 atopic non-asthmatic subjects prior to challenge and was undetectable in non-atopic controls before and after allergen challenge. Following asthma provoked by isocapnic hyperventilation, BAL concentrations of LTB_4 and immunoreactive sulphidopeptide leukotrienes rose from baseline levels of 10 pg/ml and 46 pg/ml respectively, to 121 pg/ml and 251 pg/ml respectively (Pliss et al., 1990).

Measurement of urinary LTE_4 concentration has been used as a marker of systemic release of sulphidopeptide leukotrienes (Örning et al., 1985; Tagari et al., 1989; Maltby et al., 1990). Taylor et al. (1989) demonstrated that urinary LTE_4 levels increase during acute severe asthma and at 3 h following antigen challenge of asthmatic subjects. Manning also demonstrated a rise in urinary LTE_4 in the first 3 h following the early asthmatic response to allergen, which correlated with the severity of bronchoconstriction. No increases in urinary LTE_4 were observed during the development of the late asthmatic response, 3 to 7 h after challenge (Manning et al., 1990a). Smith et al. (1991) also demonstrated release of urinary leukotrienes following allergen challenge, but not following exercise-induced asthma despite a similar fall in FEV_1.

Leukotriene Antagonists and Inhibitors

If leukotrienes play a significant role in the pathogenesis of asthma, then attempts to inhibit their generation or to antagonize their action at specific receptors should be of some benefit in asthma. Studies have now been reported of the effects of 5-lipoxygenase (5-LO) inhibitors and sulphidopeptide leukotriene antagonists on asthma induced by exercise, inhalation of antigen, and by cold, dry air. In addition there are preliminary data on the effects of leukotriene receptor antagonists on the clinical severity of day-to-day asthma.

One of the earliest leukotriene antagonists was FPL 55712, which is an antagonist of LTD_4 and LTE_4 in guinea-pig trachea (Snyder et al., 1984; Weichman and Tucker, 1985), and of all three sulphidopeptide leukotrienes in isolated human bronchi (Buckner et al., 1986). It is a weak antagonist with a short half-life, and is not bio-available via the oral route. LY 171,883 is very similar in structure to FPL 55712, has a similar low potency and can be given orally (Fleisch et al., 1985). LY 171,883 is only a weak antagonist of inhaled LTD_4 in non-asthmatic subjects, shifting the dose–response curve to LTD_4 to the right by approximately 5-fold (Phillips et al., 1988). Nevertheless, oral administration of LY 171,883 led to a significant attenuation of the early response to inhaled antigen (Fuller et al., 1989), and to isocapnic hyperventilation (Israel et al., 1989). The effect of LY 171,883 in chronic asthma was evaluated in a multicentre trial of 138 subjects (Cloud et al., 1989). Following active treatment with 600 mg of active drug for 6 weeks, mean FEV_1 rose from 78.8% of predicted to 83.3%, and was significantly different from the change in placebo-treated subjects. This was associated with a decrease in severity of both day time and night time wheezing and breathlessness. In those patients who took >23 mg/week of metaproterenol prior to entry into the study there was a significant decrease in its use compared with placebo-treated subjects. Recently, highly potent and selective leukotriene antagonists have become available, allowing a more critical evaluation of the role of leukotrienes in asthma.

MK-571 has high affinity for the LTD_4 receptor and is a potent antagonist of the spasmogenic activity of LTD_4 *in vitro* (Ford-Hutchinson, 1990). Although it is orally active, early trials have been carried out with intravenous infusions. It is well tolerated in normal human volunteers up to blood levels of 300 µg/ml (Ford-Hutchinson, 1990). Administration of the drug in asthmatic subjects, but not normal subjects, produced bronchodilatation, suggesting that LTD_4 may contribute to resting airway tone in asthma (Kips *et al.*, 1989, 1990; Gaddy *et al.*, 1990). This effect was additive to that of inhaled albuterol (Gaddy *et al.*, 1990). Complete antagonism of the bronchoconstrictor response to LTD_4 was achieved in normal subjects with blood levels as low as 1 µg/ml (Kips *et al.*, 1989). In asthmatic subjects as >40-fold and >80-fold shift in the dose–response curve to inhaled LTD_4 was achieved with intravenous infusions of 28 mg and 277 mg respectively (Kips *et al.*, 1990). The effect of MK-571 upon exercise-induced asthma was evaluated in 12 asthmatic subjects (Manning *et al.*, 1990b). The mean fall in FEV_1 following exercise was 9.2% in subjects given 160 mg MK-571 compared with 25.2% in subjects given placebo, the extent of the protection afforded by MK-571 varying from 29% to 100%. MK-571 has also been evaluated in chronic asthma (Gaddy *et al.*, 1991). Subjects received either placebo or 75 mg of MK-571 three times daily (tds) for 2 weeks followed by 150 mg tds for 4 weeks. Compared with placebo, treatment with MK-571 led to a mean 8% to 14% improvement in FEV_1, a 30% decrease in morning and evening symptom scores, and an approximate 30% decrease in usage of albuterol.

Following inhalation of 800 µg of SKF-104353 in asthmatic subjects there was a modest but significant 23% increase in baseline SGaw, and 5% increase in baseline FEV_1, accompanied by a mean shift in the dose–response curve to LTD_4 of approximately 8-fold (PC_{35} SGaw) and 12-fold (PC_{20} FEV_1) (Joos *et al.*, 1991). In a separate study, prior inhalation of 900 µg aerosolized SK&F 104353, 30 min prior to challenge, led to at least a 10-fold shift in the dose–response curve to LTC_4 and LTE_4 (Christie *et al.*, 1991c). Interestingly, a significant inhibition of PAF-induced bronchoconstriction was noted (Torphy *et al.*, 1991), consistent with the suggestion that PAF may stimulate leukotriene generation (Voelkel *et al.*, 1982; Taylor *et al.*, 1990). Preliminary data also indicate that this compound inhibits the bronchoconstriction induced by allergen (Eiser *et al.*, 1989) and exercise (Torphy *et al.*, 1991) in asthmatic subjects.

ICI 204,219 is a structural analogue of ICI 198,615 with an improved profile of bio-availability when given orally (Krell *et al.*, 1990). In normal subjects a single oral dose of 40 mg given 2 h, 12 h and 24 h prior to LTD_4 inhalation challenge increased the PD_{35} SGaw by 117-fold, 9-fold and 5-fold respectively (Smith *et al.*, 1990). Administration of 40 mg of ICI 204,219, 2 h prior to allergen challenge, led to a significant attenuation of both early and late asthmatic responses, and inhibited the increase in airways responses to histamine 6 h after allergen challenge (Taylor *et al.*, 1991).

There are relatively few data on the effects of 5-LO inhibitors in asthma. A-64077 has been evaluated in asthma induced by cold, dry air (Israel *et al.*, 1990) and by allergen (Hui *et al.*, 1991). 800 mg of A-64077 or placebo were administered 3 h prior to challenge with cold dry air. The *ex vivo* ionophore-induced production of LTB_4 was inhibited by 74% following treatment with A-64077, with no inhibition of the generation of thromboxane B_2. This was accompanied by a significant 47% increase in the respiratory heat exchange required to produce a 10% fall in FEV_1. There was no significant difference in baseline lung function between placebo and active treatment. In a separate study, 800 mg of oral A-64077, administered 3 h prior to allergen challenge, led to a mean 93% inhibition in the *ex vivo* generation of LTB_4 in response to ionophore (Hui *et al.*, 1991), and a 48% reduction in the urinary excretion of LTE_4 production following allergen challenge. The small attenuation of the early asthmatic response to allergen was not statistically significant. Nevertheless, there was a correlation between the inhibition of urinary leukotriene excretion and the attenuation in the early asthmatic response, suggesting that the lack of clinical effect may have been related to insufficient inhibition of 5-LO.

The overall impression from these studies is that leukotrienes contribute to the resting airways tone in asthma, the early asthmatic response to a range of stimuli including exercise, allergen and cold–dry air, the late asthmatic response to allergen and the airways hyperresponsiveness induced by allergen challenge of sensitized subjects. Studies of the effects of these drugs in day-to-day asthma suggest a role for leukotrienes in the pathophysiology of asthma. However, further studies are needed to evaluate the possible place of leukotriene antagonists and inhibitors in the management of asthma.

11.5 Aspirin-induced Asthma

A proportion of subjects with asthma are intolerant of aspirin. In these subjects ingestion of aspirin is followed within 1–2 h by the onset of bronchospasm that may be accompanied by rhinitis and/or urticaria (Samter and

Beers, 1968). Inhibition of cyclooxygenase appears to be central to the mechanism of aspirin-induced asthma (AIA). This is suggested by the observation that aspirin-sensitive subjects also react to other inhibitors of this enzyme (Szczeklik *et al.*, 1975, 1977) and by the observation of cross-desensitization between these drugs (Pleskow *et al.*, 1982). Several hypotheses have been advanced proposing a loss of protective prostaglandins or a shunting of arachidonate metabolism leading to increased generation of leukotrienes in susceptible individuals. Several groups have therefore explored the contribution of the peptidoleukotrienes to AIA. Ferreri demonstrated release of LTC_4 into nasal secretions in AIA associated with naso-ocular symptoms (Ferreri *et al.*, 1988). In two subjects in whom the asthmatic response occurred without naso-ocular symptoms there was no increase in LTC_4. Histamine release was also noted in three of four aspirin-sensitive subjects, but no increase in immunoreactive LTB_4 was detected. There were no changes in LTC_4 levels in nasal washings of subjects with AIA who had been desensitized, in aspirin-tolerant asthmatics, and in normal controls following ingestion of 650 mg aspirin. Ortolani *et al.* (1987) detected significant increases in histamine, immunoreactive LTC_4 and bioactive SRS-A, 60 min after intranasal aspirin challenge of aspirin-sensitive subjects. No significant increases in histamine, LTC_4 or SRS-A were found in aspirin-tolerant individuals. Christie *et al.* (1991a) reported a mean four-fold increase in urinary LTE_4 following aspirin-induced asthma which was not observed following placebo challenge or methacholine challenge in the same individuals, or following either aspirin or placebo challenge in aspirin-tolerant asthmatics. Increased urinary LTE_4 concentrations were noted in subjects with AIA compared with aspirin-tolerant asthmatics prior to challenge, suggesting an upregulation of arachidonate metabolism in aspirin-sensitive subjects.

An additional mechanism of AIA might be an increased sensitivity of the airways to leukotrienes released following aspirin challenge. We therefore measured airways responses to LTE_4 and histamine in asthmatic subjects with and without AIA (Arm *et al.*, 1989). Whilst airway responses to histamine were comparable between the 2 groups of subjects, subjects with AIA were on average 16-fold more responsive to LTE_4 than asthmatics without AIA. Following oral desensitization to aspirin there was a mean 20-fold decrease in the sensitivity of the airways to LTE_4 but not to histamine. The role of leukotrienes in the pathogenesis of AIA is supported by the inhibition of AIA following inhalation of the leukotriene antagonist SK&F 104353 (Christie *et al.*, 1991b).

In conclusion, inhibition of cyclooxygenase appears to be central to the mechanism of AIA. There is evidence that this is accompanied by release of leukotrienes. An increased sensitivity of the airways to leukotrienes may contribute to the mechanism of AIA. Desensitization may result from a decrease in airways responsiveness to leukotrienes, combined with an attenuation of leukotriene release in response to aspirin. The role of leukotriene antagonists in the management of AIA requires further evaluation.

References

Adelroth, E., Morris, M. M., Hargreave, F. E. and O'Byrne, P. M. (1986). Airway responsiveness to leukotrienes C_4 and D_4 and to methacholine in patients with asthma and normal controls. *N. Engl. J. Med.*, **315**, 480–4.

Aharony, D., Dobson, P. T. and Krell, R. D. (1985). *In vitro* metabolism of [^{3}H]-peptide leukotrienes in human and ferret lung: a comparison with the guinea pig. *Biochem. Biophys. Res. Commun.*, **131**, 892–8.

Aharony, D., Catanese, C. A. and Falcone, R. C. (1989). Kinetic and pharmacological analysis of [^{3}H]-leukotriene E_4 binding to receptors on guinea pig lung membranes: evidence of selective binding to a subset of leukotriene D_4 receptors. *J. Pharm. Exp. Ther.*, **248**, 581–8.

Arm, J. P., Spur, B. W. and Lee, T. H. (1988). The effects of inhaled leukotriene E_4 on the airway responsiveness to histamine in subjects with asthma and normal subjects. *J. Allergy Clin. Immunol.*, **82**, 654–60.

Arm, J. P., O'Hickey, S. P., Spur, B. W. and Lee, T. H. (1989). Airway responsiveness to histamine and leukotriene E_4 in subjects with aspirin-induced asthma. *Am. Rev. Respir. Dis.*, **140**, 148–53.

Arm, J. P., O'Hickey, S. P., Hawksworth, R. J., Fong, C. Y., Crea, A. E. G., Spur, B. W. and Lee, T. H. (1990). Asthmatic airways have a disproportionate hyperresponsiveness to LTE_4, as compared with normal airways, but not to LTC_4, LTD_4, methacholine, and histamine. *Am. Rev. Respir. Dis.*, **142**, 1112–18.

Bach, M. K., Brashler, J. R., Hammarström, S. and Samuelsson, B. (1980). Identification of leukotriene C-1 as a major component of slow-reacting substance from rat mononuclear cells. *J. Immunol.*, **125**, 115–17.

Bach, M. K., Brashler, J. R. and Morton, D. R. (1984). Solubilization and characterization of the leukotriene C_4 synthetase of rat basophilic leukaemia cells: a novel particulate glutathione-*S*-tranferase. *Arch. Biochem. Biophys.*, **230**, 455–65.

Barnes, N. C., Piper, P. J. and Costello, J. F. (1984a). Actions of inhaled leukotrienes and their interactions with other allergic mediators. *Prostaglandins*, **28**, 629–30.

Barnes, N. C., Watson, A., Piper, P. J. and Costello, J. F. (1984b). Action of inhaled leukotriene C and D on large and small airways. Effect of pre-inhalation of leukotriene D on histamine dose–response curve. *Am. Rev. Respir. Dis.*, **129**, A1.

Bel, E. H., van der Veen, H., Kramps, J. A., Dijkman, J. H. and Sterk, P. J. (1987). Maximal airway narrowing to inhaled leukotriene D_4 in normal subjects. Comparison and interaction with methacholine. *Am. Rev. Respir. Dis.*, **136**, 979–84.

Bel, E. H., van der Veen, H., Dijkman, J. H. and Sterk, P. J. (1989). The effect of inhaled budesonide on the maximal degree of airway narrowing to leukotriene D_4 and methacholine in normal subjects *in vivo*. *Am. Rev. Respir. Dis.*, **139**, 427–31.

Benyon, R. C., Lowman, M. A. and Church, M. K. (1987). Human skin mast cells: their dispersion, purification, and secretory characterization. *J. Immunol.*, **138**, 861–7.

Bianco, S., Robuschi, M., Vaghi, A., Simone, P., Folco, G., Berti, F. and Pasargiklian, M. (1985). Effects of leukotriene C_4 on the bronchial response to an ultrasonic mist of water. In Herzog, H. and Perruchoud, A. P. (eds.), *Progress in Respiratory Research*, Volume 19, *Asthma and Bronchial Hyperreactivity*, Karger, Basel, 82–6.

Bisgaard, H., and Groth, S. (1987). Bronchial effects of leukotriene D_4 inhalation in normal human lung. *Clin. Sci.*, **72**, 585–92.

Bisgaard, H., Groth, S. and Madsen, F. (1985). Bronchial hyperreactivity to leukotriene D_4 and histamine in exogenous asthma. *Br. Med. J.*, **290**, 1468–71.

Borgeat, P. and Samuelsson, B. (1979a). Arachidonic acid metabolism in polymorphonuclear leukocytes: unstable intermediate in the formation of dihydroxy acids. *Proc. Natl. Acad. Sci. USA*, **76**, 3213–17.

Borgeat, P. and Samuelsson, B. (1979b). Arachidonic acid metabolism in polymorphonuclear leukocytes: effects of ionophore A23187. *Proc. Natl. Acad. Sci. USA*, **76**, 2148–52.

Borgeat, P. and Samuelsson, B. (1979c). Metabolism of arachidonic acid by polymorphonuclear leukocytes: structural analysis of novel hydroxylated compounds. *J. Biol. Chem.*, **254**, 7865–9.

Borgeat, P. and Samuelsson, B. (1979d). Transformation of arachidonic acid by rabbit polymorphonuclear leukocytes. Formation of a novel dihydroxyeicosatetraenoic acid. *J. Biol. Chem.*, **254**, 2643–6.

Brocklehurst, W. E. (1962). Slow reacting substance and related compounds. *Prog. Allergy*, **6**, 539–58.

Buckner, C. K., Krell, R. D., Lavaruso, R. B., Coursin, D. B., Bernstein, P. R. and Will, J. A. (1986). Pharmacological evidence that human intralobar airways do not contain different receptors that mediate contractions to leukotriene C_4 and leukotriene D_4. *J. Pharm. Exp. Ther.*, **237**, 558–62.

Camp, R. D. R., Coutts, A. A., Greaves, M. W., Kay, A. B. and Walport, M. J. (1983). Response of human skin to intraadermal injection of leukotrienes C_4, D_{4s} and B_4. *Br. J. Pharmacol.*, **80**, 497–502.

Cheng, J. B. and Townley, R. G. (1984). Identification of leukotriene D_4 receptor binding sites in guinea pig lung homogenates using $[^3H]$-leukotriene D_4. *Biochem. Biophys. Res. Commun.*, **118**, 20–6.

Christie, P. E., Tagari, P., Ford-Hutchinson, A. W., Charleson, P., Chee, P., Arm, J. P. and Lee, T. H. (1991a). Urinary leukotriene E_4 concentrations increase after aspirin challenge in aspirin-sensitive asthmatic subjects. *Am. Rev. Respir. Dis.*, **143**, 1025–9.

Christie, P. E., Smith, C. M. and Lee, T. H. (1991b). The potent and selective sulfidopeptide leukotriene antagonist, SK&F 104353, inhibits aspirin-induced asthma. *Am. Rev. Respir. Dis.*, **144**, 957–8.

Christie, P. E., Spur, B. W. and Lee, T. H. (1991c). The effect of inhalation of the leukotriene receptor antagonist SKF 104353 on LTC_4 and LTE_4-induced bronchoconstriction in asthmatic subjects. *J. Allergy Clin. Immunol.*, **88**, 193–8.

Cloud, M. L., Enas, G. G., Kemp, J., Platts-Mills, T., Altman, L. C., Townley, R., Tinkelman, D., King, T., Jr, Middleton, E., Sheller, A. L., *et al.* (1989). A specific LTD_4/LTE_4-receptor antagonist improves pulmonary function in patients with mild, chronic asthma. *Am. Rev. Respir. Dis.*, **140**, 1336–9.

Coles, S. J., Neill, K. H., Reid, L. M., Austen, K. F., Nii, Y., Corey, E. J. and Lewis, R. A. (1983). Effects of leukotrienes C_4 and D on glycoprotein and lysozyme secretion by human bronchial mucosa. *Prostaglandins*, **25**, 155–70.

Conroy, D. M., Piper, P. J., Samhoun, M. N. and Yacoub, M. (1989). Metabolism and generation of cysteinyl containing leukotrienes by human airways *in vitro*. *Br. J. Pharmacol.*, **96**, 72P.

Dahinden, C. A., Clancy, R. M., Gross, M., Chiller, J. M. and Hugli, T. E. (1985). Leukotriene C_4 production by murine mastocytoma cells: evidence for a role for extracellular leukotriene A_4. *Proc. Natl. Acad. Sci. USA*, **82**, 6632–6.

Dahlén, S.-E., Hedqvist, P., Hammarström, S. and Samuelsson, B. (1980). Leukotrienes are potent constrictors of human bronchi. *Nature (London)*, **288**, 484–6.

Dahlén, S.-E., Björk, J., Hedqvist, P., Arfors, K. E., Hammarström, S., Lindgren, J. A. and Samuelsson, B. (1981). Leukotrienes promote plasma leakage and leukocyte adhesion in postcapillary venules: *in vivo* effects with relevance to the acute inflammatory response. *Proc. Natl. Acad. Sci. USA*, **78**, 3887–91.

Davidson, A. B., Lee, T. H., Scanlon, P. D., Solway, J., McFadden, E. R., Jr, Ingram, R. H., Jr, Corey, E. H., Austen, K. F. and Drazen, J. M. (1987). Bronchoconstrictor effects of leukotriene E_4 in normal and asthmatic subjects. *Am. Rev. Respir. Dis.*, **135**, 333–7.

Dixon, R. A. F., Diehl, R. E., Opas, E., Rands, E., Vickers, P. J., Evans, J. F., Gillard, J. W. and Miller, D. K. (1990). Requirement of a 5-lipoxygenase-activating protein for leukotriene synthesis. *Nature (London)*, **343**, 282–4.

Drazen, J. M., Austen, K. F., Lewis, R. A., Clark, O. A., Goto, G., Marfat, A. and Corey, E. J. (1980). Comparative airway and vascular activities of leukotrienes C-1 and D *in vivo* and *in vitro*. *Proc. Natl. Acad. Sci. USA*, **77**, 4354–8.

Drazen, J. M., Lewis, R. A., Austen, K. F. and Corey, E. J. (1983). Pulmonary pharmacology of the SRS-A leukotrienes. In Berti, F., Folco, G. and Velo, G. P. (eds.), *Leukotrienes and Prostacyclin*, Plenum, New York, 125–34.

Edenius, C., Heidvall, K. and Lindgren, J. A. (1988). Novel transcellular interaction: conversion of granulocyte-derived leukotriene A_4 to cysteinyl-containing leukotrienes by human platelets. *Eur. J. Biochem.*, **178**, 81–6.

Eiser, N. M., Hayhurst, M. and Denman, W. (1989). The contribution of histamine and leukotriene release to the production of early and late asthmatic responses to antigen. *Am. Rev. Respir. Dis.*, **139**, A462.

Feinmark, S. J. and Cannon, P. J. (1986). Endothelial cell leukotriene C_4 synthesis results from intercellular transfer of leukotriene A_4 synthesized by polymorphonuclear leukocytes. *J. Biol. Chem.*, **261**, 16466–72.

Fels, A. O., Pawlowski, N. A., Cramer, E. B., King, T. K. C., Cohn, Z. A. and Scott, W. A. (1982). Human alveolar macrophages produce leukotriene B_4. *Proc. Natl. Acad. Sci. USA*, **79**, 7866–70.

Ferreri, N. R., Howland, W. C., Stevenson, D. D. and Spiegelberg, H. L. (1988). Release of leukotrienes, prostaglandins, and histamine into nasal secretions of aspirin-sensitive asthmatics during reaction to aspirin. *Am. Rev. Respir. Dis.*, **137**, 847–54.

Fleisch, J. H., Rinkema, L. E., Haisch, K. D., Swanson-Bean, D., Goodson, T., Ho, P. P. and Marshall, W. S. (1985). LY171883, 1-[2-hydroxy-3-propyl-4-[4-(tetrazol-5-yl)butoxy]phenyl]ethanone, an orally active leukotriene D_4 antagonist. *J. Pharm. Exp. Ther.*, **233**, 148–57.

Ford-Hutchinson, A. W., (1990). Regulation of the production and action of leukotrienes by MK-571 and MK-886. In Samuelsson, B., Ramwell, P. W., Paoletti, R., Folco, G. and Granström, E. (eds.), *Advances in Prostaglandin, Thromboxane, and Leukotriene Research*, Vol. 21, Raven Press, New York, 9–16.

Ford-Hutchinson, A. W., Bray, M. A., Doig, M. V., Shipley, M. E. and Smith, M. J. H. (1980). Leukotriene B, a potent chemokinetic and aggregating substance released from polymorphonuclear leukocytes. *Nature (London)*, **286**, 264–5.

Fuller, R. W., Black, P. N. and Dollery, C. T. (1989). Effect of the oral leukotriene D₄ antagonist LY171,883 on inhaled and intradermal challenge with allergen and leukotriene D₄ in atopic subjects. *J. Allergy Clin. Immunol.*, **83**, 939–44.

Gaddy, J., Bush, R. K., Margolskee, D., Williams, V. C. and Busse, W. (1990). The effects of a leukotriene D₄ (LTD₄) antagonist (MK-571) in mild to moderate asthma. *J. Allergy Clin. Immunol.*, **85**, 197 (Abstract).

Gaddy, J., McCreedy, W., Margolskee, D., Williams, V. and Busse, W. (1991). A potent leukotriene D₄ antagonist (MK-571) significantly reduces airway obstruction in mild to moderate asthma. *J. Allergy Clin. Immunol.*, **87**, 306 (Abstract).

Gillard, J., Ford-Hutchinson, A. W., Chan, C., Charleson, S., Denis, D., Foster, A., Fortun, R., Leger, S., McFarlane, C. S., Morton, H., *et al.* (1989). L-663,536 (MK-886) (3-[1-(4-chlorobenzyl)-3-t-butyl-thio-5-isopropylindol-2-yl]-2,2-dimethylpropanoic acid), a novel, orally active leukotriene biosynthesis inhibitor. *Can. J. Physiol. Pharmacol.*, **67**, 456–64.

Goldman, D. W. and Goetzl, E. J. (1982). Specific binding of leukotriene B₄ to receptors on human polymorphonuclear leukocytes. *J. Immunol.*, **129**, 1600–4.

Griffin, M., Weiss, J. W., Leitch, A. G., McFadden, E. R., Jr, Corey, E. J., Austen, K. F. and Drazen, J. M. (1983). Effects of leukotriene D on the airways in asthma. *N. Engl. J. Med.*, **308**, 436–9.

Hammarström, S. and Samuelsson, B. (1980). Detection of leukotriene A₄ as an intermediate in the biosynthesis of leukotrienes C₄ and D₄. *FEBS. Lett.*, **122**, 83–6.

Hardy, C. C., Bradding, P., Robinson, C. and Holgate, S. T. (1986). The combined effects of two pairs of mediators, adenosine with methacholine and prostaglandin D₂ with histamine, on airway calibre in asthma. *Clin. Sci.*, **71**, 385–92.

Hay, D. W. P., Muccitelli, R. M., Tucker, S. S., Vickery-Clark, L. M., Wilson, K. A., Gleason, J. G., Hall, R. F., Wasserman, M. A. and Torphy, T. J. (1987). Pharmacological profile of SK&F 104353: a novel, potent and selective peptidoleukotriene receptor antagonist in guinea-pig and human airways. *J. Pharm. Exp. Ther.*, **243**, 474–81.

Hay, D. W. P., Muccitelli, R. M., Wilson, K. A., Wasserman, M. A. and Torphy, T. J. (1988). Functional antagonism by salbutamol suggests differences in the relative efficacies and dissociation constants of the peptidoleukotrienes in guinea pig trachea. *J. Pharm. Exp. Ther.*, **244**, 71–8.

Holgate, S. T., Beasley, C. R. W. and Twentyman, O. P. (1987). The pathogenesis and significance of bronchial hyperresponsiveness in airways disease. *Clin. Sci.*, **73**, 561–72.

Holroyde, M. C., Altounyan, R. E. C., Cole, M., Dixon, M. and Elliott, E. V. (1981). Bronchoconstriction produced in man by leukotrienes C and D. *Lancet*, **2**, 17–18.

Hoover, R. L., Karnovsky, M. J., Austen, K. F., Corey, E. J. and Lewis, R. A. (1984). Leukotriene B₄ action of endothelium mediates augmented neutrophil/endothelial adhesion. *Proc. Natl. Acad. Sci. USA*, **81**, 2191–3.

Hui, K. P., Taylor, I. K., Taylor, G. W., Rubin, P., Kesterson, J., Barnes, N. C. and Barnes, P. J. (1991). Effect of a 5-lipoxygenase inhibitor on leukotriene generation and airway responses after allergen challenge in asthmatic patients. *Thorax*, **46**, 184–9.

Israel, E., Juniper, E. F., Callaghan, J. T., Mathur, P. N., Morris, M. M., Dowell,

A. R., Enas, G. G., Hargreave, F. E. and Drazen, J. M. (1989). Effect of a leukotriene antagonist, LY171883, on cold air-induced bronchoconstriction in asthmatics. *Am. Rev. Respir. Dis.*, **140**, 1348–53.

Israel, E., Dermarkarian, R., Rosenberg, M., Sperling, R., Taylor, G., Rubin, P. and Drazen, J. M. (1990). The effects of a 5-lipoxygenase inhibitor on asthma induced by cold, dry air. *N. Engl. J. Med.*, **323**, 1740–4.

Jacques, C. A., Spur, B. W., Johnson, M. and Lee, T. H. (1991). Mechanism of LTE_4-induced histamine hyperresponsiveness in guinea-pig tracheal and human bronchial smooth muscle, *in vitro*. *Br. J. Pharmacol.*, **104**, 859–66.

Joos, G. F., Kips, J. C., Pauwels, R. A. and Van Der Staeten, M. E. (1991). The effect of aerosolized SK&F 104353-Z_2 on the bronchoconstrictor effect of leukotriene D_4 in asthmatics. *Pulm. Pharmacol.*, **4**, 37–42.

Kaye, M. G. and Smith, L. J. (1990). Effects of inhaled leukotriene D_4 and platelet-activating factor on airway reactivity in normal subjects. *Am. Rev. Respir. Dis.*, **141**, 993–7.

Kern, R., Smith, L. J., Patterson, R., Krell, R. D. and Bernstein, P. R. (1986). Characterization of the airway response to inhaled leukotriene D_4 in normal subjects. *Am. Rev. Respir. Dis.*, **133**, 1127–32.

Kips, J. C., Joos, G., Margolskee, D., De Lepelevie, I., Rogers, J. D., Pauwels, R. and Van Der Straeten, M. (1989). L-660.711: a potent antagonist of LTD_4-induced bronchoconstriction in man. *Am. Rev. Respir. Dis.*, **139**, A63 (Abstract).

Kips, J., Joos, G., Pauwels, R., Van Der Straeten, M., De Lepelevie, I., Williams, V. and Margolskee, D. (1990). MK-571 (L-660.771): a potent LTD_4 antagonist in asthmatic men. *Am. Rev. Respir. Dis.*, **141**, A117 (Abstract).

Krell, R. D., Tsai, B. S., Berdoulay, A., Barone, M. and Giles, R. E. (1983). Heterogeneity of leukotriene receptors in guinea pig trachea. *Prostaglandins*, **25**, 171–8.

Krell, R. D., Aharony, D., Buckner, C. K., Keith, R. A., Kusner, E. J., Snyder, D. W., Bernstein, P. R., Matassa, V. G., Yee, Y. K., Brown, F. J. *et al.* (1990). The preclinical pharmacology of ICI 204,219. *Am. Rev. Respir. Dis.*, **141**, 978–87.

Krilis, S., Lewis, R. A., Corey, E. J. and Austen, K. F. (1983). Bioconversion of C-6 sulfidopeptide leukotrienes by the responding guinea pig ileum determines the time course of its contraction. *J. Clin. Invest.*, **71**, 909–15.

Lam, B. K., Owen, W. F., Jr., Austen, K. F. and Soberman, R. J. (1989). The identification of a distinct export step following the biosynthesis of leukotriene C_4 by human eosinophils. *J. Biol. Chem.*, **264**, 12885–9.

Lam, B. K., Gagnon, L., Austen, K. F. and Soberman, R. J. (1990). The mechanism of leukotriene B_4 export from human polymorphonuclear leukocytes. *J. Biol. Chem.*, **265**, 13438–41.

Lam, S., Chan, H., LeRiche, J. C., Chan-Yeung, M. and Salari, H. (1988). Release of leukotrienes in patients with bronchial asthma. *J. Allergy Clin. Immunol.*, **81**, 711–17.

Lee, C. W., Lewis, R. A., Tauber, A. I., Mehrotra, M., Corey, E. J. and Austen, K. F. (1983). The myeloperoxidase-dependant metabolism of leukotrienes C_4, D_4 and E_4 to 6-*trans*-leukotriene B_4 diastereoisomers and the subclass specific S-diastereoisomeric sulfoxides. *J. Biol. Chem.*, **258**, 15004–10.

Lee, T. H., Austen, K. F., Corey, E. J. and Drazen, J. M. (1984). Leukotriene E_4-induced airway hyperresponsiveness of guinea pig tracheal smooth muscle to histamine and evidence for three separate sulfidopeptide leukotriene receptors. *Proc. Natl. Acad. Sci. USA*, **81**, 4922–5.

Lee, T. H., Sethi, T., Crea, A. E. G., Peters, W., Arm, J. P., Horton, C. E., Walport, M. J. and Spur, B. W. (1988). Characterization of leukotriene B_3: comparison of its biological activities with leukotriene B_4 and leukotriene B_5 in complement receptor enhancement, lysozyme release and chemotaxis of human neutrophils. *Clin. Sci.*, **74**, 467–75.

Leung, K. B. P., Flint, K. C., Hudspith, B. N., Brostoll, J., Johnson, M. M., Seager, K., Hammond, M. and Pearce, F. L. (1987). Mast cells and basophils. Some further properties of human pulmonary mast cells recovered by bronchoalveolar lavage and enzymic dispersion of lung tissue. *Agents Actions*, **20**, 213–15.

Lewis, R. A., Drazen, J. M., Austen, K. F., Clark, D. A., and Corey, E. J. (1980a). Identification of the C(6)–S-conjugate of leukotriene A with cysteine as a naturally occurring slow reacting substance of anaphylaxis (SRS-A). Importance of the 11-*cis*-geometry for biological activity. *Biochem. Biophys. Res. Commun.*, **96**, 271–7.

Lewis, R. A., Austen, K. F., Drazen, J. M., Clark, D. A., Marfat, A. and Corey, E. J. (1980b). Slow reacting substance of anaphylaxis: identification of leukotriene C-1 and D from human and rat sources. *Proc. Natl. Acad. Sci. USA*, **77**, 3710–14.

Lin, A. H., Ruppel, P. L. and Gorman, R. R. (1984). Leukotriene B_4 binding to human neutrophils. *Prostaglandins*, **28**, 837–49.

MacGlashan, D. W., Schleimer, R. P., Peters, S. P., Schulman, E. S., Adams, K., Newball, H. H. and Lichtenstein, L. M. (1982). Generation of leukotrienes by purified human lung mast cells. *J. Clin. Invest.*, **70**, 747–51.

Maclouf, J. A. and Murphy, R. C. (1988). Transcellular metabolism of neutrophil-derived leukotriene A_4 by human platelets. *J. Biol. Chem.*, **263**, 174–181.

Mahauthaman, R., Howell, C. J., Spur, B. W., Youlten, L. J., Clark, T. J., Lessof, M. H. and Lee, T. H. (1988). The generation and cellular distribution of leukotriene C_4 in human eosinophils stimulated by unopsonized zymosan and glucan particles. *J. Allergy Clin. Immunol.*, **81**, 696–705.

Maltby, N. H., Taylor, G. W., Ritter, J. M., Moore, K., Fuller, R. W. and Dollery, C. T. (1990). Leukotriene C_4 elimination and metabolism in man. *J. Allergy Clin. Immunol.*, **85**, 3–9.

Manning, P. J., Rokach, J., Malo, J.-L., Ethier, D., Cartier, A., Girard, Y., Charleson, S. and O'Byrne, P. M. (1990a). Urinary leukotriene E_4 levels during early and late asthmatic responses. *J. Allergy Clin. Immunol.*, **86**, 211–20.

Manning, P. J., Watson, R. M., Margolskee, D. J., Williams, V. C., Schwartz, J. I. and O'Byrne, P. M. (1990b). Inhibition of exercise-induced bronchoconstriction by MK-571, a potent leukotriene D_4 antagonist. *N. Engl. J. Med.*, **323**, 1736–9.

Marom, Z., Shelhamer, J. H., Bach, M. K., Morton, D. R. and Kaliner, M. (1982). Slow-reacting substances, leukotrienes C_4 and D_4, increase the release of mucus from human airways *in vitro*. *Am. Rev. Respir. Dis.*, **126**, 449–51.

Martin, T.R., Altman, L. C., Albert, R. K. and Henderson, W. R. (1984). Leukotriene B_4 production by the human alveolar macrophage: a potential mechanism for amplifying inflammation in the lung. *Am. Rev. Respir. Dis.*, **129** 106–11.

McGee, J. E. and Fitzpatrick, F. A. (1986). Erythrocyte–neutrophil interactions: formation of leukotriene B_4 by transcellular biosynthesis. *Proc. Natl. Acad. Sci. USA*, **83**, 1349–53.

Miller, D. K., Gillard, J. W., Vickers, P. J., Sadowski, S., Léveillé, C., Mancini, J. A., Charleson, P., Dixon, R. A., Ford-Hutchinson, A. W., Fortin, R., *et al.* (1990). Identification and isolation of a membrane protein necessary for leukotriene production. *Nature (London)*, **343**, 278–81.

Morris, H. R., Taylor, G. W., Piper, P. J. and Tippins, J. R. (1980). Structure of slow reacting substance of anaphylaxis from guinea-pig lung. *Nature (London)*, **285**, 104–6.

Murphy, R. C., Hammarström, S. and Samuelsson, B. (1979). Leukotriene C: a slow reacting substance from murine mastocytoma cells. *Proc. Natl. Acad. Sci. USA*, **76**, 4275–9.

Nagy, L., Lee, T. H., Goetzl, E. J., Pickett, W. C. and Kay, A. B. (1982). Complement receptor enhancement and chemotaxis of human neutrophils and eosinophils by leukotrienes and other lipoxygenase products. *Clin. Exp. Immunol.*, **47**, 541–7.

O'Hickey, S. P., Arm, J. P., Rees, P. J., Spur, B. W. and Lee, T. H. (1988). The relative responsiveness to inhaled leukotriene E_4, methacholine and histamine in normal and asthmatic subjects. *Eur. Respir. J.*, **1**, 913–17.

O'Hickey, S. P., Hawksworth, R. J., Fong, C. Y., Arm, J. P., Spur, B. W. and Lee, T. H. (1991). Leukotrienes C_4, D_4, and E_4 enhance histamine responsiveness in asthmatic airways. *Am. Rev. Respir. Dis.*, **144**, 1053–7.

Örning, L., Hammarström, S. and Samuelsson, B. (1980). Leukotriene D: a slow reacting substance from rat basophilic leukaemia cells. *Proc. Natl. Acad. Sci. USA*, **77**, 2014–17.

Örning, L., Kaijser, L. and Hammarström, S. (1985). *In vivo* metabolism of leukotriene C_4 in man. *Biochem. Biophys. Res. Commun.*, **130**, 214–20.

Ortolani, C., Mirone, C., Fontana, A., Folco, G. C., Miadomma, A., Montalbetti, N., Rinaldi, M., Sala, A., Tedeschi, A. and Valente, D. (1987). Study of mediators of anaphylaxis in nasal fluids after aspirin and sodium metabisulfite nasal provocation in intolerant rhinitic patients. *Ann. Allergy*, **59**, 106–12.

Palmer, R. M. J., Stepney, R. J., Higgs, G. A. and Eakins, K. E. (1980). Chemokinetic activity of arachidonic acid lipoxygenase products on leukocytes of different species. *Prostaglandins*, **20**, 411–18.

Phillips, G. D. and Holgate, S. T. (1989). Interaction of inhaled LTC_4 with histamine and PGD_2 on airway calibre in asthma. *J. Appl. Physiol.*, **66**, 304–12.

Phillips, G. D., Rafferty, P., Robinson, C. and Holgate, S. T. (1988). Dose-related antagonism of leukotriene D_4-induced bronchoconstriction by p.o. administration of LY-171883 in nonasthmatic subjects. *J. Pharm. Exp. Ther.*, **246**, 732–8.

Pichurko, B. M., Ingram, R. H., Jr, Sperling, R., Lafleur, J. E., Corey, E. J., Austen, K. F. and Drazen, J. M. (1989). Localization of the site of the broncho-constrictor effects of leukotriene C_4 compared with that of histamine in asthmatic subjects. *Am. Rev. Respir. Dis.*, **140**, 334–9.

Pleskow, W. W., Stevenson, D. D., Mathison, D. A., Simon, R. A., Schatz, M. and Zeiger, R. S. (1982). Aspirin desensitization in aspirin-sensitive asthmatic patients: clinical manifestations and characterization of the refractory period. *J. Allergy Clin. Immunol.*, **69**, 11–19.

Pliss, L. B., Ingenito, E. P., Ingram, R. H. and Pichurko, B. (1990). Assessment of bronchoalveolar cell and mediator response to isocapnic hyperpnea in asthma. *Am. Rev. Respir. Dis.*, **142**, 73–8.

Rådmark, O., Malmsten, C., Samuelsson, B., Goto, G., Marfat, A. and Corey, E. J. (1980). Leukotriene A: isolation from human polymorphonuclear leukocytes. *J. Biol. Chem.*, **255**, 11828–31.

Roberts, J. A., Rodger, I. W. and Thomson, N. C. (1986a). Effect of verapamil and sodium cromoglycate on leukotriene D_4 induced bronchoconstriction in patients with asthma. *Thorax*, **41**, 753–8.

Roberts, J. A., Giembycz, M. A., Raeburn, D., Rodger, I. W. and Thomson, N. C. (1986b). *In vitro* and *in vivo* effect of verapamil on human airway responsiveness to leukotriene D_4. *Thorax*, **41**, 12–16.

Roberts, J. A., Rodger, I. W. and Thomson, N. C. (1987). *In vivo* and *in vitro* human airway responsiveness to leukotriene D_4 in patients without asthma. *J. Allergy Clin. Immunol.*, **80**, 688–94.

Rouzer, C. A., Rands, E., Kargman, S., Jones, R. E., Register, R. B. and Dixon, R. A. (1988). Characterization of cloned human leukocyte 5-lipoxygenase expressed in mammalian cells. *J. Biol. Chem.*, **263**, 10135–40.

Samter, M. and Beers, R. F. (1968). Intolerance to aspirin: clinical studies and consideration of its pathogenesis. *Ann. Intern. Med.*, **68**, 975–83.

Samuelsson, B. (1983). Leukotrienes: mediators of hypersensitivity reactions and inflammation. *Science*, **220**, 568–75.

Shak, S. and Goldstein, I. M. (1984). Omega-oxidation is the major pathway for the catabolism of leukotriene B_4 in human polymorphonuclear leukocytes. *J. Biol. Chem.*, **259**, 10181–7.

Shaw, R. J., Walsh, G. M., Cromwell, O., Moqbel, R., Spry, C. J. F. and Kay, A. B. (1985). Activated human eosinophils generate SRS-A leukotrienes following IgG-dependent stimulation. *Nature (London)*, **316**, 150–2.

Showell, H. J., Naccache, P. H., Borgeat, P., Picard, S., Vallerand, P., Becker, E. L. and Sha'afi, R. I. (1982). Characterization of the secretory activity of leukotriene B_4 toward rabbit neutrophils. *J. Immunol.*, **128**, 811–16.

Sirois, P., Roy, S. and Borgeat, P. (1981). The lung parenchymal strip as a sensitive assay for leukotriene B_4. *Prostaglandins*, **6**, 153–9.

Smith, C. M., Christie, P. E., Hawksworth, R. J., Thien, F. and Lee, T. H. (1991). Urinary leukotriene E_4 levels following allergen and exercise challenge in bronchial asthma. *Am. Rev. Respir. Dis.*, **144**, 1411–3.

Smith, L. J., Greenberger, P. A., Patterson, R., Krell, R. D. and Bernstein, P. R. (1985). The effect of inhaled leukotriene D_4 in humans. *Am. Rev. Respir. Dis.*, **131**, 368–72.

Smith, L. J., Kern, R., Patterson, R., Krell, R. D. and Bernstein, P. R. (1987). Mechanism of leukotriene D_4-induced bronchoconstriction in normal subjects. *J. Allergy Clin. Immunol.*, **80**, 338–45.

Smith, L. J., Geller, S., Ebright, L., Glass, M. and Thyrum, P. T. (1990). Inhibition of leukotriene D_4-induced bronchoconstriction in normal subjects by the oral LTD_4 receptor antagonist ICI 204,219. *Am. Rev. Respir. Dis.*, **141**, 988–92.

Snyder, D. W. and Krell, R. D. (1984). Pharmacological evidence for a distinct leukotriene C_4 receptor in guinea-pig trachea. *J. Pharm. Exp. Ther.*, **231**, 616–22.

Soberman, R. J., Harper, T. W., Murphy, R. C. and Austen, K. F. (1985). Identification and functional characterization of leukotriene B_4 20-hydroxylase of human polymorphonuclear leukocytes. *Proc. Natl. Acad. Sci. USA*, **82**, 2292–5.

Soberman, R. J., Sutyak, J. P., Okita, R. T., Wendelborn, D. F., Roberts, L. J. and Austen, K. F. (1988). The identification and formation of 20-aldehyde leukotriene B_4. *J. Biol. Chem.*, **263**, 7996–8002.

Soter, N. A., Lewis, R. A., Corey, E. J. and Austen, K. F. (1983). Local effects of synthetic leukotrienes (LTC_4, LTD_4, LTE_4 and LTB_4) in human skin. *J. Invest. Dermatol.*, **80**, 115–19.

Sterk, P. J., Timmers, M. C. and Dijkman, J. H. (1986). Maximal airway narrowing in humans *in vivo*: histamine compared with methacholine. *Am. Rev. Respir. Dis.*, **34**, 714–18.

Szczeklik, A., Gryglewski, R. J. and Czerniawska-Mysik, G. (1975). Relationship of inhibition of prostaglandin biosynthesis by analgesics to asthma attacks in aspirin-sensitive patients. *Br. Med. J.*, **1**, 67–9.

Szczeklik, A., Gryglewski, R. J. and Czerniawska-Mysik, G. (1977). Clinical patterns of hypersensitivity to nonsteroidal anti-inflammatory drugs and their pathogenesis. *J. Allergy Clin. Immunol.*, **60**, 276–84.

Tagari, P., Ethier, D., Carry, M., Korley, V., Charleson, S., Girard, Y. and Zambani, R. (1989). Measurement of urinary leukotrienes by reversed-phase liquid chromatography and radioimmunoassay. *Clin. Chem.*, **35**, 388–91.

Taylor, G. W., Taylor, I., Black, P., Maltby, N. H., Turner, N., Fuller, R. W. and Dollery, C. T. (1989). Urinary leukotriene E_4 after antigen challenge and in acute asthma and allergic rhinitis. *Lancet*, **1**, 584–8.

Taylor, I. K., Taylor, G. W. and Fuller, R. W. (1990). Platelet activating factor (PAF) induced bronchoconstriction in asthmatics: role of cysteinyl leukotrienes. *Thorax*, **45**, 790 (Abstract).

Taylor, I. K., O'Shaughnessy, K. M., Fuller, R. W. and Dollery, C. T. (1991). Effect of cysteinyl-leukotriene receptor antagonist ICI 204.219 on allergen-induced bronchoconstriction and airway hyperreactivity in atopic subjects. *Lancet*, **337**, 690–4.

Torphy, T. J., Faiferman, I., Gleason, J. G., *et al.* (1991). The clinical and preclinical pharmacology of SK&F 104353, a potent and selective peptidoleukotriene receptor antagonist. *Ann. NY Acad. Sci.*, **629**, 157–67.

Voelkel, N. F., Worthen, S., Reeves, J. T., Henson, P. M. and Murphy, R. C. (1982). Nonimmunological production of leukotrienes induced by platelet-activating factor. *Science*, **218**, 286–8.

Walsh, C. E., Waite, B. M., Thomas, M. J. and DeChatelet, L. R. (1981). Release and metabolism of arachidonic acid in human neutrophils. *J. Biol. Chem.*, **256**, 7228–34.

Wardlaw, A. J., Hay, H., Cromwell, O., Collins, J. V. and Kay, A. B. (1989). Leukotrienes, LTC_4 and LTB_4, in bronchoalveolar lavage in bronchial asthma and other respiratory diseases. *J. Allergy Clin. Immunol.*, **84**, 19–26.

Weichman, B. M. and Tucker, S. S. (1985). Differentiation of the mechanisms by which leukotrienes C_4 and D_4 elicit contraction of the guinea pig trachea. *Prostaglandins*, **29**, 547–60.

Weiss, J. W., Drazen, J. M., Coles, N., McFadden, E. R., Jr, Weller, P. F., Corey, E. J., Lewis, R. A. and Austen, K. F. (1982a). Bronchoconstrictor effects of leukotriene C in humans. *Science*, **216**, 196–8.

Weiss, J. W., Drazen, J. M., McFadden, E. R., Jr, Weller, P. F., Corey, E. J., Lewis, R. A. and Austen, K. F. (1982b). Comparative bronchoconstrictor effects of histamine, leukotriene C, and leukotriene D in normal human volunteers. *Trans. Assoc. Am. Physicians*, **95**, 30–5.

Weiss, J. W., Drazen, J. M., McFadden, E. R., Jr, Weller, P. F., Corey, E. J., Lewis, R. A. and Austen, K. F. (1983). Airway constriction in normal humans produced by inhalation of leukotriene D. Potency, time course, and effect of aspirin theraphy. *J. Am. Med. Assoc.*, **249**, 2814–17.

Weller, P. F., Lee, C. W., Foster, D. W., Corey, E. J., Austen, K. F. and Lewis, R. A. (1983). Generation and metabolism of 5-lipoxygenase pathway leukotrienes by human eosinophils: predominant production of leukotriene C_4. *Proc. Natl. Acad. Sci. USA*, **80**, 7626–30.

Wenzel, S. E., Larsen, G. L., Johnston, K., Voelkel, N. F. and Westcott, J. Y. (1990). Elevated levels of leukotriene C_4 in bronchoalveolar lavage fluid from atopic asthmatics after endobronchial allergen challenge. *Am. Rev. Respir. Dis.*, **142**, 112–19.

Williams, J. D., Czop, J. K. and Austen, K. F. (1984). Release of leukotrienes by

human monocytes on stimulation of their phagocytic receptor for particulate
activators. *J. Immunol.*, **132**, 3034–40.

Williams, J. D., Lee, T. H., Lewis, R. A. and Austen, K. F. (1985). Intracellular
retention of the 5-lipoxygenase pathway product, leukotriene B_4, by human
neutrophils activated with unopsonised zymosan. *J. Immunol.*, **134**, 2624–30.

Woolcock, A. J., Salome, C. M. and Yan, K. (1984). The shape of the dose–
response curve to histamine in asthmatic and normal subjects. *Am. Rev. Respir.
Dis.*, **130**, 71–5.

12

Prostanoid and Leukotriene Biosynthesis in Peritoneal and Airway Macrophages of Various Animal Species and Man

B. Pipy, M. F. Forgue, C. M'Rini-Puel, Ph. Carre, M. Beraud,
C. Cambon and A. Didier

12.1 Introduction

Among the biologically active mediators generated under normal physiological conditions and during injury and inflammation, few compounds have received more interest than those derived from the oxygenation of arachidonic acid (AA). This fatty acid can be released from membrane phospholipids via the activity of phospholipase A2 or the combined activities of phospholipase C and diglycerol lipase. The intracellularly released arachidonic acid can then be metabolized via the cyclooxygenase pathway to generate prostaglandins E_2, D_2, $F_{2\alpha}$ (PGE$_2$, PGD$_2$, PGF$_{2\alpha}$), thromboxane A_2 (TXA$_2$), prostacyclin (PGI$_2$), and hydroxyheptadecatrienoic acid (HHT) and, via the lipoxygenase pathways, to produce monohydroxyeicosatetraenoic acids (5-, 11-, 12-, 15-HETEs). The 5-lipoxygenase pathway results in the formation of leukotriene B$_4$ (LTB$_4$) and the sulphidopeptide leukotrienes LTC$_4$, LTD$_4$, LTE$_4$, formerly called the slow reacting substance of anaphylaxis (SRS-A). These eicosanoids have been demonstrated to modulate a lot of biological functions and are thought to play a key role in the pathogenesis of chronic inflammatory disorders (Davies *et al.*, 1980), fibrosis and the immune response (Goldyne and Strobo, 1981; Henderson, 1987). These arachidonic acid metabolites have powerful actions on airway smooth muscle and airway mucociliary clearance. PGD$_2$, PGF$_{2\alpha}$ and TXA$_2$

cause contraction in mammalian airways (Beasly *et al.*, 1987; Hardy *et al.*, 1984) and PGE_2 and PGI_2 most often cause relaxation in both normal and asthmatic subjects, although sometimes bronchoconstriction was observed (Walters and Davies, 1982; Roberts *et al.*, 1985). A functional antagonism or a synergistic action between the secreted prostanoids and leukotrienes can often be observed; LTC_4–D_4–E_4 are potent bronchoconstrictors both *in vivo* and *in vitro*.

Leukotrienes and prostaglandins are synthesized in various cells, in particular in macrophages. In addition to their direct cytotoxic and phagocytic effects, tissue macrophages are involved in the regulation of the local homeostasis by the secretion of extracellular signalling molecules. Of the growing array of cellular signalling molecules, only the eicosanoids will be considered in this study.

Several soluble and particulate stimuli induce the release of AA from plasma membrane phospholipids and the synthesis of prostaglandins and leukotrienes by these cells (Humes *et al.*, 1982). In this review, we will summarize the available information on the conditions under which arachidonic acid is mobilized and the nature of its oxygenation products in macrophage populations derived from various sources in different species, particularly mouse, rat, guinea-pig and man. It is established that there are marked qualitative and quantitative differences in these arachidonic acid metabolites, according to the source of the cells, the environment from which they are obtained, as well as the stimuli to which the cells are exposed.

The various AA oxygenation products released by cells in culture can be measured in one of several ways: bioassays, gas–liquid chromatography mass spectrometry, release of radiolabelled products and radioimmunoassay. The results presented in this report were obtained from the release of radiolabelled products from radiolabelled cells as used in our laboratory (Forgue *et al.*, 1991). The metabolites from AA were extracted, separated by thin layer chromatography (TLC) and HPLC and identified by measurement of the radioactivity and by radioimmunoassay.

The capacity of cells to synthesize arachidonic oxygenation products is dependent on the release of this fatty acid substrate from phospholipids. The highest proportion of arachidonic acid is contained in phosphatidylcholine. [^{3}H]AA is efficiently incorporated into cellular phospholipids of a variety of cells. Resident or activated peritoneal macrophages and alveolar macrophages used in these studies incorporate into cellular phospholipids considerable amounts of [^{3}H]AA over 4 h incubation periods in cell cultures. The primary advantage of this method is that it measures *de novo* synthesis of an AA oxygenation product. In addition, this method evaluates the synthesis from endogenous, and thus relevant, substrate pools. This radiorelease method allows the evaluation of the products derived from both the cyclooxygenase and the lipoxygenase pathways separated one from the other by TLC and HPLC (Forgue *et al.*, 1991).

12.2 Arachidonic Acid Incorporation in Various Mononuclear Phagocyte Populations

Studies in our laboratory indicated that 40–45% of exogenous labelled AA was incorporated by mouse resident peritoneal macrophages within 4 h. The highest proportion of labelled AA was found in phospholipids (PLs). The major phospholipids labelled by AA were phosphatidylcholine (PC), 38.4±0.9% of the radioactivity, and phosphatidylethanolamine (PE), 22.7±1.1% (de Maroussem et al., 1985). A small amount of radioactivity was also found in phosphatidylserine–phosphatidylinositol (8.5%). The diacylglycerols, triacylglycerols and cholesterol esters contained 16% of the radioactivity. Activated mouse peritoneal macrophages incorporated 60% of labelled AA within 4 h (Fig. 12.1). Approximately 90% of the [^{3}H]AA was incorporated into the phospholipids of activated mouse peritoneal macrophages; 38.5±0.8% of the radioactivity was found in PC, 29.5±1.2% in PE and 21.1±0.9% in PS–PI; the diacylglycerols, triacylglycerols and cholesterol esters contained 6.5±0.4% of the radioactivity. Resident rat peritoneal macrophages incorporated 60% of added AA into cellular lipid within 4 h. Approximately 60.2±1.2% of the labelled AA was incorporated into the PC of resident rat peritoneal macrophages during this period, and 17.4±0.7% into PE and 11.8±0.9% into PS–PI; the diacylglycerols, triacylglycerols and cholesterol esters contained 6.3±0.6% of the radioactivity. Guinea-pig alveolar macrophages incorporated 62.6±0.9% of added AA into cellular lipids within 4 h. Approximately

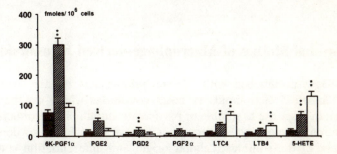

Fig. 12.1 Release of ^{3}H-labelled arachidonic acid metabolites from resident mouse peritoneal macrophages in response to opsonized zymosan. Resident macrophages were collected from male Swiss mice by intraperitoneal lavage. The cells (10^6 per 24 multiwell plate Falcon) were labelled by incubation in culture medium containing 1 μCi [^{3}H]arachidonic acid for 4 h. They were then washed and incubated for 30 min without zymosan (control group) (■), with opsonized zymosan (200 μg/ml) (▨) or with opsonized zymosan (200 mg/ml) plus indomethacin (0.1 mM) (□). The [^{3}H]arachidonic acid metabolites released in the culture medium were extracted and separated by TLC. The results are means for three experiments. The bar represents the standard error.
*indicates, for each metabolite, values significantly different from control: $^*P < 0.05$; $^{**}P < 0.01$.

63.2±1.4% of the labelled AA was incorporated into the PC during this period, 10.7±0.9% into PE, 16.5±0.8% into PS-PI, and the diacylglycerols, triacylglycerols and cholesterol esters contained 6.3±0.6%. Exogenous AA incorporated by human alveolar macrophages within 4 h was found in PL, distributed principally between PC and PE.

12.3 Synthesis of Arachidonic Acid Metabolites in Mononuclear Phagocytes

Macrophages represent a group of cells that widely differ in their functional capacities. Macrophages are capable of secreting a variety of eicosanoids. Certain arachidonic acid metabolites are produced in greatest amounts by resident macrophages. Other eicosanoids are produced by activated macrophages. Furthermore, the state of differentiation, harvesting technique and other aspects of experimental methods all influence the proportion of the different eicosanoids released by these cells (Nathan, 1987; Scott *et al.*, 1982). It is apparent that different macrophage populations from different tissue beds produce different combinations of eicosanoids. The studies in our laboratory have been concerned with the difference in the nature of products of the cyclooxygenase and lipoxygenase pathways synthesized by peritoneal macrophages and by macrophages from other sources (liver, lungs) and species, particularly by human peripheral blood monocytes and alveolar macrophages.

12.4 Animal Studies of Macrophage-derived Eicosanoids

Macrophages prelabelled with [³H]arachidonic acid release small quantities of labelled eicosanoids in basal conditions which can be greatly increased in response to soluble or particulate stimuli. The products of AA oxygenation by monocytes–macrophages have been found to depend on the nature of the stimulus, cellular origin and differentiation state. The metabolic profile also depends on the *in vitro* culture conditions, on the duration of culture and on the species studied.

Dependence on Nature of the Stimulus

The synthesis of PGs and LTs is dependent on the stimulus that triggers the macrophages. Zymosan (a particulate inflammatory stimulus) added to cultures of resident mouse peritoneal macrophages causes the synthesis

and release of large amounts of ^{3}H-labelled prostaglandins and leukotrienes in a time- and concentration-dependent manner (Forgue *et al.*,
1990). Radioactive AA metabolites were quantified in culture medium
after stimulation with opsonized zymosan for 30 min. As shown in Fig. 12.1
significant increases in the synthesis and release of AA products are
observed after the addition of zymosan. Chromatographic separation of
arachidonic acid metabolites shows that the most abundant radioactive
oxygenation products were 6K-PGF$_{1\alpha}$ (stable product of PGI$_2$), PGE$_2$, and
HETE$_s$, followed by both PGD$_2$ and PGF$_{2\alpha}$. The production of this
metabolite was inhibited completely by the cyclooxygenase inhibitor indomethacin. Zymosan also induced the formation of leukotriene (LT) C$_4$
and B$_4$; these lipoxygenase metabolites were increased by indomethacin at
0.1 μM. Analysis of the phospholipid content of cell cultures exposed to
zymosan for 1 h showed that the majority of net depletion of [^{3}H]AA was
from phosphatidylcholine with little net depletion of label from phosphatidylethanolamine. The decrease in the amount of [^{3}H]AA in phosphatidylcholine in these cells was accompanied by an increase in the amount of
labelled fatty acid in triacylglycerol, suggesting that some of the fatty acids
released by zymosan were reacylated while another part of this radioactive
pool was utilized for eicosanoid synthesis.

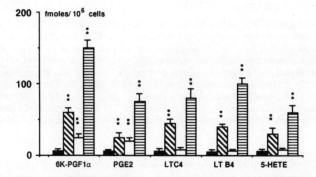

Fig. 12.2 Release of ^{3}H-labelled arachidonic acid metabolites from resident mouse peritoneal microphages in response to TPA and A23187. Resident macrophages were collected,
cultured and prelabelled as described in Figure. 12.1. The cells were incubated for 30 min
without stimulator (■) (control group), with TPA alone (100 nM) (□), with A23187 alone
(2.5 μM) (◨), or with TPA (100 nM) + A23187 (2.5 μM) (▤). The results are means for three
experiments. The bar represents the standard error.
* indicates, for each metabolite, values significantly different from control: * $P < 0.05$; ** $P <$
0.01.

In a similar manner, calcium ionophore A23187, which increases the
intracellular calcium, induced the formation of 6K-PGF$_{1\alpha}$, LTC$_4$ and
leukotriene B$_4$ (Fig. 12.2). In contrast, we have shown that in resident
mouse peritoneal macrophages the direct protein kinase C (PKC) activator

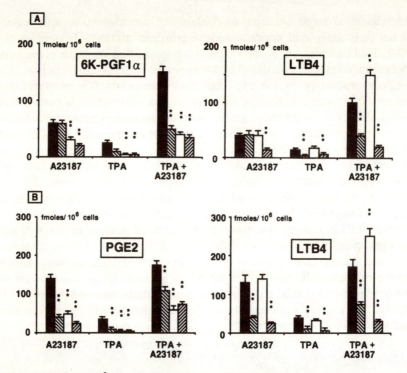

Fig. 12.3 Release of ^{3}H-labelled arachidonic acid metabolites from (A) resident and (B) activated mouse peritoneal macrophages in response to TPA and A23187. Activated macrophages were isolated from trehalose dimycolate-treated mice after 7 days. Resident and activated macrophages were collected, cultured and prelabelled as described in Fig. 12.1. The cells were incubated for 15 min in the absence of metabolic inhibitors (■) or in the presence of 100 μM H7 (▨), 0.1 μM indomethacin (□) or 0.1 μM BW755C (▨). The cells were stimulated for 30 min by TPA alone (100 nM), A23187 alone (2.5 μM), or with TPA (100 nM) + A23187 (2.5 μM). The results are means for three experiments. The bar represents the standard error. * indicates, for each metabolite, values significantly different from control: * $P<0.05$; **$P < 0.01$.

12-O-tetradecanoylphorbol 13-acetate at 100 nM (TPA) exclusively stimulated the formation of cyclooxygenase metabolites in particular 6K-PGF$_{1\alpha}$ with no effect on the production of leukotrienes (Fig. 12.2).

The synthesis of PGs and LTs by resident and peritoneal macrophages responding to particulate and soluble inflammatory stimuli depends on PKC and also Ca^{2+}. Studies in this laboratory have shown that preincubation of resident peritoneal macrophages with PKC inhibitors (100 μM H7 or 70 μM staurosporine) caused a concentration-dependent inhibition of both AA release and eicosanoid synthesis stimulated by either TPA or zymosan. These PKC inhibitors have no effect on CO and LO metabolite productions triggered by A23187 (Fig. 12.3(A)). The synthesis of cyclooxygenase products was found to be inhibited by the cyclooxygenase inhibitor indomethacin; inversely this inhibitor increased lipoxygenase metabolite production. The synthesis of arachidonic acid metabolites of the cyclooxygenase and lipoxygenase pathways was inhibited in the presence of BW755C (dual inhibitor of cyclooxygenase and lipoxygenase). Besides adenosine triphosphate (ATP) and several additional components, calcium is an absolute requirement for 5-lipoxygenase translocation to the membrane and activation (Rouzer and Kargman, 1988; Wong et al., 1988). We have also demonstrated that arachidonic acid metabolite synthesis by mouse resident peritoneal macrophages could be synergistically enhanced, by the simultaneous addition of TPA and A23187. At high intracellular calcium levels PKC activation preferentially produced LTs and fewer cyclooxygenase metabolites were formed (Fig. 12.2). Measurement of intracellular calcium by fluo-3 revealed that the observed synergism induced by low concentrations of TPA plus calcium ionophore was not a result of an additional intracellular calcium increase as a consequence of the phorbol ester addition. When resident cells were preincubated with PKC inhibitors, the potentiation of TPA by A23187 disappeared and metabolite release decreased (Fig. 12.3(A)). The results of Kaever et al. (1990) suggest that drugs specifically lowering the intracellular calcium level could result in a shift from leukotriene to prostanoid synthesis. Thus, in macrophages the ratio of cyclooxygenase and lipoxygenase products caused by mediators, acting via phospholipase C or D, and the breakdown of inositol lipids could be regulated by the extent of intracellular calcium increase.

Differentiation State

Nature and extent of the cyclooxygenase and lipoxygenase product formation by macrophages are dependent on the differentiation state of the cells. Humes et al. (1980) have shown that thioglycolate-elicited macrophages synthesize much less PGE_2 and $6K-PGF_{1\alpha}$ than resident macrophages responding to the same stimulus (zymosan). Macrophages harvested from inflammatory sites have been demonstrated to have a dramatically reduced capacity to release AA metabolites (Humes et al., 1980; Scott et al., 1982), and the magnitude of this reduction correlates closely with the cells' state of activation as measured by their microbicidal capacity. Based on this model, it has been hypothesized that down-regulation of AA metabolism may serve to limit the local inflammatory response. Contrary to these findings, Kunkel and Chensue (1983) demonstrated that macrophages harvested 2 weeks after the inflammatory stimulus had an increased production of AA metabolites. In the murine model we have established that the resident and activated peritoneal macrophages differ in their capacity to secrete prostaglandins and leukotrienes (Fig. 12.4). So, for resident peritoneal macrophages $6K-PGF_{1\alpha}$ was the major AA metabolite; for trehalose dimycolate-activated mouse peritoneal macrophages, PGE_2 and

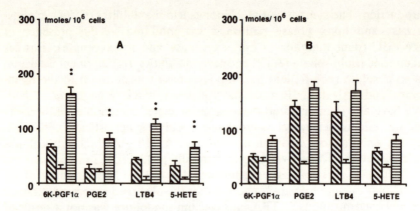

Fig. 12.4   Release of ^{3}H-labelled arachidonic acid metabolites from (A) resident and (B) activated mouse peritoneal macrophages in response to TPA and A23187. Activated macrophages were isolated from trehalose dimycolate-treated mice after 7 days. Resident and activated macrophages were collected, cultured and prelabelled as described in Fig. 12.1. The cells were stimulated for 30 min by TPA alone (100 nM) (□), A23187 alone (2.5 μM) (▨), or TPA (100 nM) + A23187 (2.5 μM) (▤). The results are means for three experiments. The bar represents the standard error.
** indicates, for each metabolite, significant potentiation with respect to the effects induced by TPA or A23187 alone: ** $P < 0.01$.

LTB$_4$ were the most abundant eicosanoids formed. The ratio as well as the absolute quantities of the AA metabolites released into the extracellular medium are undoubtedly important in determining the differentiation state of macrophages.

For activated cells TPA did not affect the amounts of lipoxygenase and cyclooxygenase products released in response to A23187; the potentiation of TPA by A23187 did not appear (Fig. 12.4). However, the TPA plus A23187-induced production was greater for activated macrophages than for resident macrophages, particularly for PGE$_2$ and LTB$_4$.

When activated peritoneal macrophages were preincubated with PKC inhibitors the metabolite production triggered by TPA plus A23187 decreased (Fig. 12.3(B)); in parallel, the synthesis of AA oxygenation products induced by A23187 alone was found to be inhibited by PKC inhibitors (Fig. 12.3(B)). These findings suggest that in activated peritoneal macrophages PKC was implicated in A23187-induced AA metabolite production. In activated peritoneal macrophages the activation of PKC by A23187 alone should influence synergetic AA release induced by TPA and A23187.

Species Origin

We established that the arachidonic acid metabolic profile was also a function of the species studied. In comparable studies of populations of

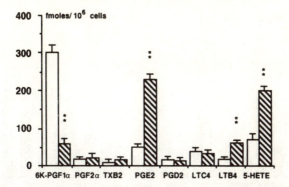

Fig. 12.5   Release of ^{3}H-labelled arachidonic acid metabolites from resident mouse and rat peritoneal mecrophages in response to zymosan. Resident macrophages were collected, cultured and prelabelled as described in Fig. 12.1. Resident mouse peritoneal macrophages (□) and resident rat peritoneal macrophages (▨) were stimulated for 1 h by zymosan. The results are means for three experiments. The bar represents the standard error.
** indicates, for each metabolite, values significantly different from control: **$P < 0.01$.

mouse and rat resident peritoneal macrophages, quantitative differences in AA oxygenation product formation were demonstrated. In contrast with mouse resident peritoneal macrophages (Fig. 12.5), rat resident peritoneal macrophages responding to the same stimulus (zymosan) produced large amounts of PGE_2 but much less $6K\text{-}PGF_{1\alpha}$.

In Vitro *Culture Conditions*

In studies of populations of rat resident peritoneal macrophages, quantitative differences in AA oxygenation product formation were shown according to the conditions under which they were maintained *ex vivo*, and to the nature of the stimuli to which the cells were exposed in culture. Recent studies in our laboratory have shown that normal rat serum (without LPS contamination) at a concentration higher than 30% is able to trigger the release and catabolism of AA from prelabelled resident rat peritoneal macrophages (Fig. 12.6).

Macrophages contain low affinity receptors for IgE (Capron *et al.*, 1986) which induce cellular activation when exposed to IgE and allergen (or anti-IgE). Thus, the IgE-dependent activation of macrophages may play an important role in allergic diseases. In order to determine the allergenic effects on the generation of pro-inflammatory products by macrophages, a large number of studies have used a passively sensitized model with IgE-rich serum. However, an effect of serum used for passive sensitization of macrophage functions has not been reported. Compared with culture conditions without serum, normal rat serum and IgE-rich rat serum induced a significant increase of both lipoxygenase and cyclooxygenase

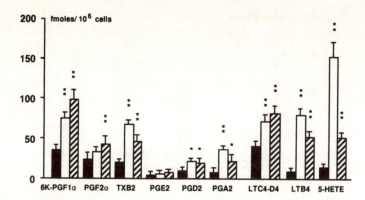

Fig. 12.6   Effect of serum on the release of ^{3}H-labelled arachidonic acid metabolites from resident rat peritoneal macrophages. Resident macrophages were collected, cultured and prelabelled as described in Fig. 12.1. Cells were incubated for 1 h without serum (■) or in the presence of 30% normal rat serum (□) or 30% IgE-rich rat serum (▨). The results are means for three experiments. The bar represents the standard error.
*indicates, for each metabolite, values significantly different from control: * $P < 0.05$; **$P < 0.01$.

products. Normal rat serum induced a significantly greater increase in LTB$_4$ and 5-HETE than IgE-rich rat serum. For both sera, the lipoxygenase pathway was stimulated more than the cyclooxygenase pathway (Fig. 12.6). Serum did not fully stimulate macrophage functions. Thus, cells were still able to respond to further stimuli, zymosan or allergen (if the serum was an IgE-rich serum). Furthermore, after allergenic challenge of sensitized macrophages, we demonstrated that allergen (ovalbumin) increases the AA metabolism by both lipoxygenase and cyclooxygenase pathways. In particular, the allergen stimulates the secretion of LTC$_4$–D$_4$ and TXB$_2$ (Fig. 12.7). TXA$_2$ and LTC$_4$ are the most important arachidonic acid metabolites in the induction of bronchoconstriction of the lung. Additionally, our findings suggested that, when serum was rich in specific IgE, it prepares the macrophage for allergen challenge and that the sulphidopeptide leukotriene pathway may be activated by IgE-dependent stimuli.

Cellular Origin

Alveolar macrophages were found to release greater amounts of AA metabolites than peritoneal macrophages. Down-regulation of AA metabolism in alveolar populations may be due to chronic macrophage exposure to the inflammatory stimuli from the airways. Alveolar macrophages can metabolize AA by cyclooxygenase and lipoxygenase pathways in order to form various PGs and LTs (Bertram *et al.*, 1988; Kouzan *et al.*, 1985; Rouzer *et al.*, 1982). This metabolism by alveolar macrophages is induced

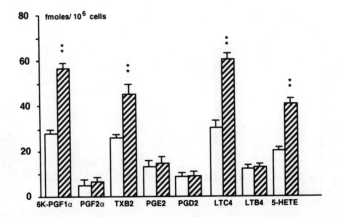

Fig. 12.7   Release of ^{3}H-labelled arachidonic acid metabolites from resident rat peritoneal macrophages in response to allergen. Resident macrophages were collected, cultured and prelabelled as described in Fig. 12.1. Cells were incubated for 4 h in the presence of 30% normal rat serum (control group without IgE) (□), or in the presence of 30% of IgE-rich rat serum (sensitized group) (▨). The cells were then washed and incubated for 1 h with allergen (ovalbumin). The results are means for three experiments. The bar represents the standard error.
* indicates, for each metabolite, values significantly different from control: * $P < 0.05$; ** $P < 0.01$.

by zymosan, TPA, A23187 and asbestos. The major cyclooxygenase metabolite produced by non-stimulated guinea-pig alveolar macrophages was TXB_2; these cells treated with A23187 exhibited an increased production of LTC_4. Alveolar macrophages challenged with TPA released large quantities of $PGF_{2\alpha}$, TXB_2, HHT and 5-HETE (Fig. 12.8). For guinea-pig alveolar macrophages TPA increases the amounts of TXB_2 and HHT released in response to A23187. Guinea-pig alveolar macrophages cultured from sensitized animals exhibited no difference in the quantities or profiles of basal eicosanoid synthesis. For sensitized cells TPA did not affect the amounts of lipoxygenase or cyclooxygenase products released in response to A23187; the potentiation between TPA and A23187 did not appear (Fig. 12.8). However, the A23187-induced production was greater for alveolar macrophages cultured from sensitized animals than for control animals, particularly for TXB_2, LTC_4 and 5-HETE (Fig. 12.9).

12.5 Clinical Studies of Macrophage-derived Eicosanoids

Studies of human macrophage subpopulations also suggested considerable heterogeneity in the release of oxidative products of arachidonic acid. Human peripheral blood monocytes from healthy individuals, prelabelled

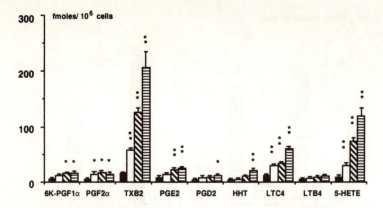

Fig. 12.8   Release of ^{3}H-labelled arachidonic acid metabolites from guinea-pig alveolar macrophages in response to TPA or A23187. Alveolar macrophages were collected from female Heartley guinea-pig by bronchoalveolar lavage. The cells (10^6 per 24 multiwell plate Falcon) were labelled by incubation in culture medium containing 1 μCi [3H]arachidonic acid for 4 h. At this time the cells were washed and incubated for 1 h without agonist (control group unstimulated) (■) or in the presence of TPA alone (100 nM) (▨), A23187 alone (2.5 μM) (□), or TPA (100 nM) + A23187 (2.5 μM) (▤). The results are means for three experiments. The bar represents the standard error.
* indicates, for each metabolite, values significantly different from control: * $P < 0.05$; ** $P <$ 0.01.

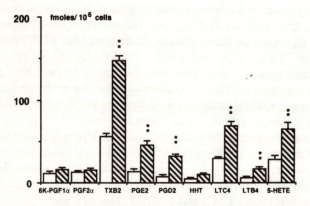

Fig. 12.9   Release of ^{3}H-labelled arachidonic acid metabolites from alveolar macrophages of guinea-pig sensitized with ovalbumin or not sensitized in response to A23187. Alveolar macrophages of guinea-pig sensitized with ovalbumin (▨) or not (□) were collected and prelabelled as described in Fig. 12.8. The cells were stimulated for 1 h by A23187 alone (2.5 μM). The results are means for three experiments. The bar represents the standard error.
* indicates, for each metabolite, values significantly different from control: * $P < 0.05$; ** $P <$ 0.01.

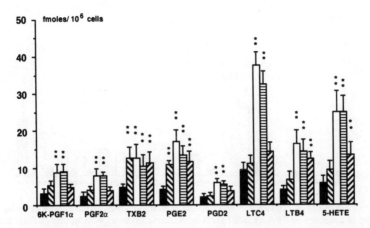

Fig. 12.10   Release of ^{3}H-labelled arachidonic acid metabolites from human monocytes in response to TPA, A23187 or zymosan. Blood monocytes were taken from healthy donors. The cells (10^6 per 24 multiwell plate Falcon) were labelled by incubation in culture medium containing 1 µCi [^{3}H]arachidonic acid for 4 h. They were then washed and incubated for 1 h without agonist (control group unstimulated) (■) or in the presence of TPA alone (100 nM) (▧), A23187 alone (2.5 µM) (□), TPA (100 nM) + A23187 (2.5 µM) (▤) or opsonized zymosan (200 µg per ml) (▨). The results are means for three experiments. The bar represents the standard error.
* indicates, for each metabolite, values significantly different from control: * $P < 0.05$; ** $P < 0.01$.

with [^{3}H]AA, released labelled cyclooxygenase metabolites in response to serum-treated zymosan (100 µg/ml), TPA (100 nM) and A23187 (2.5 µM). TXB$_2$ and PGE$_2$ were the major metabolites observed (Fig. 12.10). 6K-PGF$_{1\alpha}$, PGF$_{2\alpha}$, PGD$_2$ were also secreted but in lesser amounts. The metabolic profile obtained from zymosan- or A23187-stimulated cells differed by the presence of labelled 5-lipoxygenase products (LTC$_4$, LTB$_4$ and 5-HETE). Combined treatment with individually optimal doses of TPA and A23187 had no additional effect (Fig. 12.10). The calcium dependence of 5-lipoxygenase activation was confirmed by the inhibition of 5-lipoxygenase metabolites production in ionophore-stimulated cells incubated in calcium-free medium. The formation of metabolites of arachidonic acid was also determined in human alveolar macrophages obtained from bronchoalveolar lavage from healthy individuals. In this measurement the cells were stimulated with TPA, A23187 or zymosan. After zymosan challenge, TXB$_2$ was the cyclooxygenase product present in the highest amount followed by PGE$_2$, PGF$_{2\alpha}$ and PGD$_2$. The amounts of the lipoxygenase products are 5-HETE, LTB$_4$ and LTC$_4$-D$_4$-E$_4$. Kinetic studies of A23187-stimulated macrophages showed a rapid release of arachidonate followed by the 5-lipoxygenase products LTB$_4$ and 5-HETE. A23187 stimulates the cyclooxygenase and lipoxygenase pathways whereas TPA selectively stimulates the cyclooxygenase pathway (Fig. 12.11). The

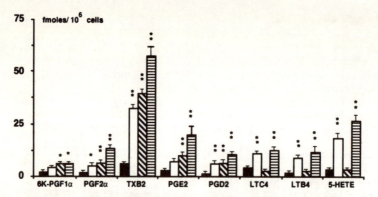

Fig. 12.11   Release of ³H-labelled arachidonic acid metabolites from human alveolar macrophages in response to TPA or A23187. Alveolar macrophages were collected from healthy man by bronchoalveolar lavage. The cells (10^6 per 24 multiwell plate Falcon) were labelled by incubation in culture medium containing 1 µCi [³H]arachidonic acid for 4 h. They were then washed and incubated for 1 h without agonist (unstimulated control group) (■) or in the presence of TPA alone (100 nM) (▧), A23187 alone (2.5 µM) (□), or TPA (100 nM) + A23187 (2.5 µM) (▤). The results are means for three experiments. The bar represents the standard error.
* indicates, for each metabolite, values significantly different from control: * $P < 0.05$; ** $P < 0.01$.

activity of 5-lipoxygenase increases markedly in blood monocytes relative to alveolar macrophages, suggesting substantial changes in regulation processes of this enzyme during cellular differentiation.

12.6 Conclusions

The various macrophage characteristics concerning arachidonic acid metabolism serve to emphasize the biological versatility of these cells. Macrophages are obviously multipotential cells that may develop a variety of characteristics depending on the nature of the precise signals that they receive. This functional heterogeneity is strictly controlled and could result from a change in the sequence of intracellular messenger which leads to the activation of AA metabolism. In particular this heterogeneity is, therefore, the final consequence of a series of down-regulations and up-regulations of some cellular processes. The role of PKC and the intracellular calcium level could be particularly important in the control of macrophage differentiation and in the ratio of prostanoid and leukotriene production. This process bears important clinical implications since drugs affecting the intracellular calcium level could alter the amount of macrophage eicosanoid synthesis and the ratio of prostanoid and leukotriene production.

References

Beasly, C. R. W., Robinson, C., Feathersstone, R. L., Varley, G. J., Hardy, C. C., Church, M. K. and Holgate, S. T. (1987). 9a,11b-Prostaglandin $F_{2\alpha}$, a novel metabolite of prostaglandin D_2 is a potent contractile agonist of human and guinea-pig airways. *J. Clin. Invest.*, **79**, 978–83.

Bertram, T. A., Overby, L. H., Danilowicz, R., Eling, T. E. and Brody, A. R. (1988). Pulmonary intravascular macrophages metabolize arachidonic acid *in vitro*. Comparison with alveolar macrophages. *Am. Rev. Respir. Dis.*, **138**, 936–44.

Capron, A., Dessaint, J. P., Capron, M., Joseph, M., Ameisen, J. C. and Tonnel, A. B. (1986). From parasites to allergy: the second receptor for IgE (FcERII). *Immunol. Today*, **7**, 15–18.

Davies, P., Bonney, R. J., Humes, J. L. and Kuehl, F. A. (1980). The role of macrophage secretory products in chronic inflammatory processes. *J. Invest. Dermatol.*, **74**, 292–6.

Forgue, M. F., Pipy, B., Beraud, M., Souqual, M. C. and Combis, J. M. (1990), 1-Naphthyl-*N*-methyl carbamate effect on intra and extracellular concentrations of arachidonic acid metabolites and on chemiluminescence generation by mouse peritoneal macrophages. *Int. J. Immunopharmacol.*, **12**, 155–63.

Forgue, M. F., Pipy, B., Beraud, M., Pinelli, E., Cambon-Gros, C., Didier, A., Souqual, M. C. and Vandaele, J. (1991). Possible implication of arachidonic acid metabolism in the decrease of chemiluminescence production after exposure of murine peritoneal macrophages to diethylnitrosamine and tumor promoter, 12-*O*-tetradecanoyl-phorbol-13 acetate. *Carcinogenesis*, **12**, 449–57.

Goldyne, M. E. and Stobo, J. D. (1981). Immunoregulation role of prostaglandins and related lipids. *CRC Crit. Rev. Immunol.*, **2**, 189–223.

Hardy, C. C., Robinson, C., Tattersfield, E. and Holgate, S. T. (1984). The bronchoconstrictor effect of inhaled prostaglandin D_2 in normal and asthmatic men. *N. Engl. J. Med.*, **311**, 209–13.

Henderson, W. R. (1987). Eicosanoids and lung inflammation. *Am. Rev. Respir. Dis.*, **135**, 1176–85.

Humes, J. H., Burgen, S., Galavage, M., Kuchl, F. A., Wightman, P. D., Dahlgren, M. E., Davies, P. and Bonney, R. J. (1980). The diminished production of arachidonic acid oxygenation products by elicited mouse peritoneal macrophages: possible mechanisms. *J. Immunol.*, **124**, 2110–16.

Humes, J. L., Sadowski, S., Galavage, M., Goldenberg, M., Subers, E., Bonney, R. J. and Kuehl, F. A. (1982). Evidence for two sources of arachidonic acid for oxidative metabolism by mouse peritoneal macrophages. *J. Biol. Chem.*, **257**, 1591–4.

Kaever, V., Pfannkuche, H.-J., Wessel, K. and Resch, K. (1990). The ratio of macrophage prostaglandin and leukotriene synthesis is determined by the intracellular free calcium level. *Biochem. Pharmacol.*, **39**, 1313–19.

Kouzan, S., Brodu, A. R., Nettesheim, P. and Eling, T. (1985). Production of arachidonic acid metabolites by macrophages exposed *in vitro* to asbestos, carbonyl iron particles, or calcium ionophore. *Am. Rev. Respir. Dis.*, **131**, 624–32.

Kunkel, S. L. and Chensue, S. (1983). Production of superoxide anion prostaglandins and hydroxyeicosatetraenoic acid by macrophages from hypersensitivity type (*Schistosoma mansoni* egg) and foreign body-type granulomas. *Infect. Immunol.*, **42**, 1116–25.

de Maroussem, D., Pipy, B., Beraud, M., Derache, P. and Mathieu, J. R. (1985).

[1-^{14}C]arachidonic acid incorporation into glycerolipids and prostaglandin synthesis in macrophages: effect of chloramphenicol. *Biochim. Biophys. Acta*, **834**, 8–23.

Nathan, C. F. (1987). Secretory products of macrophages. *J. Clin. Invest.*, **79**, 319–26.

Roberts, A. M., Schultz, H. D., Green, J. F., Armstrong, D. J., Kaufman, M. P., Coleridge, H. M. and Coleridge, J. C. G. (1985). Reflex tracheal contraction evoked in dogs by bronchodilatator prostaglandin E_2 and I_2. *J. Appl. Physiol.*, **58**, 1823–31.

Rouzer, C. A. and Kargman, S. (1988). Translocation of 5-lipoxygenase to the membrane in human leukocytes challenged with ionophore A23187. *J. Biol. Chem.*, **263**, 10980–8.

Rouzer, C. A., Scott, W. A., Hammill, A. L., Liu, F. T., Katz, H. and Cohn, Z. A. (1982). Secretion of leukotriene C and other arachidonic acid metabolites by macrophages challenged with immunoglobulin E immune complexes. *J. Exp. Med.*, **156**, 1077–86.

Scott, W. A., Pawlowski, N. A., Murray, H. W., Andreach, M., Zrike, J. and Cohn, Z. A. (1982). Regulation of arachidonic acid metabolism by macrophage activation. *J. Exp. Med.*, **155**, 1148–60.

Walters, E. H. and Davies, B. H. (1982). Dual effect of prostaglandin E_2 on normal airways smooth muscle *in vivo*. *Thorax*, **37**, 918–27.

Wong, A., Hwang, S. M., Cook, M. N., Hogaboom, G. K. and Crooke, S. T. (1988). Interaction of 5-lipoxygenase with membranes: studies on the association of soluble enzyme with membranes and alterations in enzyme activity. *Biochemistry*, **27**, 6763–9.

13

The Role of T-lymphocytes in Asthma

C. J. Corrigan, A. Bentley, D. S. Robinson, Q. Hamid, Sun Ying,
M. Azzawi, B. Bradley, S. R. Durham and A. B. Kay

13.1 Introduction

It is now widely accepted that bronchial mucosal inflammation plays an important role in the pathogenesis of asthma, despite the fact that the precise relationship of this inflammation to accepted measures of asthma severity, such as non-specific bronchial hyperresponsiveness, remains unclear. The bronchial mucosal inflammatory response observed in asthma is characteristic, with infiltration of the mucosa predominantly by eosinophils and lymphocytes.

There exists much circumstantial evidence that eosinophils may act as pro-inflammatory cells in asthma, being responsible at least in part for the associated mucosal damage, while lymphocytes, aided by antigen presenting cells, probably play a role in all inflammatory responses that are antigen driven, since they are the only cells that can recognize and respond directly to such antigens. It has long been recognized that activated T-lymphocytes have the propensity to orchestrate chronic inflammatory responses to foreign antigens, independently of the presence or absence of a specific antibody response ('cell-mediated' immunity). More recently, it has become clear that this control of inflammatory reactions is exerted through the release of lymphokines, protein mediators which influence the production, recruitment, life-span and activation of specific granulocytes as well as other cell types. For example, interleukin-5 (IL-5) selectively promotes the development of eosinophils from bone marrow precursor cells, causes specific adherence of eosinophils to vascular endothelium (whence they enter the tissues), and enhances the survival and degree of

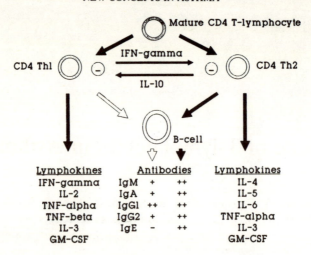

Lymphokines	Antibodies		Lymphokines
IFN-gamma	IgM +	++	IL-4
IL-2	IgA +	++	IL-5
TNF-alpha	IgG1 ++	++	IL-6
TNF-beta	IgG2 +	++	TNF-alpha
IL-3	IgE -	++	IL-3
GM-CSF			GM-CSF

Fig. 13.1 Two functional types of CD4 T-lymphocyte in the mouse. Little is known about the factors which influence the development of Th1 and Th2 cells from putative Th0 cells. Once formed, each can inhibit the proliferation of the other as shown. As a result of their differing lymphokine synthesis, Th1 cells are better equipped to elicit DTH reactions, whereas Th2 cells tend to promote allergic inflammation and antibody synthesis.

activation of eosinophils in the tissues. The actions of lymphokines such as IL-5 may at least partly explain the preferential accumulation and activation of eosinophils in the asthmatic bronchial mucosa, a phenomenon whose mechanism has until recently been poorly understood.

Of great interest has been the recent demonstration (Fig. 13.1) of two major functional subsets of CD4 T-lymphocytes, Th1 and Th2 (Mosmann and Coffman, 1989). Th1 cells, following activation, preferentially secrete IL-2 and interferon-Γ, and are implicated in the pathogenesis of delayed-type hypersensitivity reactions (Cher and Mosmann, 1987). Th2 cells preferentially secrete a number of lymphokines (including IL-4 and IL-5) which are particularly implicated in the pathogenesis of eosinophil-rich inflammatory responses such as those seen in the asthmatic bronchial mucosa and in allergic inflammatory responses. In addition, these lymphokines promote the preferential synthesis of IgE by antigen-specific B-lymphocytes, whereas interferon-Γ inhibits IgE synthesis (Pene et al., 1988). Furthermore, early evidence suggests that allergen-specific T-lymphocytes may be predominantly of the Th2 type and that atopic patients have regulatory abnormalities confined to these allergen-specific T-lymphocytes (Wierenga et al., 1990). If, therefore, bronchial mucosal inflammation is indeed of fundamental importance in clinical asthma, it would appear to follow that a full appreciation of the functional capacity (antigen specificity and profile of lymphokine secretion) of activated CD4 T-lymphocytes in the asthmatic bronchial mucosa will play a large part in our further understanding of the pathogenesis of this disease.

13.2 Activated T-lymphocytes in Asthma

We demonstrated (Corrigan et al., 1988), using immunostaining and flow cytometry, that activated CD4 T-lymphocytes could be detected in the peripheral blood of patients with acute severe asthma but not control groups (normals, mild asthma, chronic obstructive pulmonary disease). Activation was assessed by expression of well-characterized T-lymphocyte activation markers (IL-2 receptor, HLA-DR and VLA-1). In addition, the serum concentrations of two products of activated T-lymphocytes (interferon-Γ and the soluble form of the IL-2 receptor) were elevated in these patients but not the controls (Corrigan and Kay, 1990). The numbers of activated CD4 T-lymphocytes and the concentrations of soluble IL-2 receptor decreased after therapy of the patients for seven days to a degree which could be correlated with the degree of clinical improvement. These observations provide circumstantial evidence implicating activated CD4 T-lymphocytes in the pathogenesis of acute severe asthma.

We have examined the nature of the cells infiltrating the bronchial mucosa in bronchial biopsies obtained from patients with asthma of diverse aetiology. Cells were identified, and their activation status documented by immunostaining with monoclonal antibodies against cellular phenotypic and activation markers. In mild atopic asthmatics, infiltration of the mucosa with activated (IL-2 receptor bearing) CD4 T-lymphocytes and eosinophils was the most striking feature (Azzawi et al., 1990; Bradley et al., 1991). The numbers of neutrophils and macrophages in the mucosa were not significantly elevated as compared with normal controls. Although the total numbers of T-lymphocytes in these biopsies were similar to those in biopsies from normal controls, only the asthmatic biopsies showed evidence of T-lymphocyte activation. Very few eosinophils were seen in biopsies from normal controls. The numbers of activated T-lymphocytes in the biopsies from the asthmatics could be correlated with the severity of their disease, as assessed by measurement of the methacholine PC_{20}. Furthermore, in individual biopsies the numbers of activated CD4 T-lymphocytes also correlated with the numbers of activated eosinophils. These observations support the hypotheses that, in asthma,

(a) the degree of bronchial mucosal T-lymphocyte activation is at least one factor which influences disease severity, and
(b) products of activated T-lymphocytes regulate the numbers and activation status of eosinophils locally in the inflamed mucosa.

We have also examined the histopathology of the bronchial mucosa in patients with 'intrinsic' and occupational asthma (Bentley et al., 1992a, b). As in the case of atopic asthma, the mucosa was infiltrated with increased numbers of activated T-lymphocytes and eosinophils, although again the total numbers of lymphocytes were not increased as compared with normal controls. The numbers of neutrophils and tissue macrophages were not increased as compared with normal controls. In fact, in terms of relative cell numbers in the bronchial mucosa, all three forms of asthma were indistinguishable. These data suggest that the pathogenesis of asthma is uniform irrespective of any putative causative factor, and lend weight to the hypothesis that the atopic state alone is irrelevant to asthma pathogenesis. This is in accord with common clinical experience that not all atopic patients develop asthma, whereas not all asthmatics are apparently atopic. The atopic state is therefore neither necessary nor sufficient for the development of asthma.

13.3 Lymphokines in Asthma

Direct measurement of lymphokine production by T-lymphocytes in clinical situations such as asthma is extremely difficult, even though sensitive ELISA and radioimmunoassays are now available, owing to their low concentrations and rapid metabolism. Measurements of lymphokines in the peripheral blood and bronchoalveolar lavage (BAL) fluid of asthmatics are likely to reflect only dimly those concentrations released locally in the inflamed bronchial mucosa, and are subject to unquantifiable dilutional effects. Furthermore, access to the bronchial mucosa in patients with severe disease is at present neither practically nor ethically feasible.

One possible alternative approach to the direct measurement of lymphokine concentrations is the detection of the synthesis of their mRNA using the technique of *in situ* hybridization with lymphokine-specific cDNA probes or riboprobes. Although this is not a strictly quantitative technique, it does have the advantage that it can localize the secretion of lymphokines within cells and tissues. Using this technique we recently showed (Hamid *et al.*, 1991) that IL-5 mRNA was elaborated by cells in the bronchial mucosa of a majority of mild asthmatics but not normal controls. The amount of mRNA detected correlated broadly with the numbers of activated CD4 T-lymphocytes and eosinophils in biopsies from the same subjects, providing direct evidence supporting the hypothesis that activated CD4 T-lymphocytes secrete IL-5 in the asthmatic bronchial mucosa which regulates the numbers and activation status of eosinophils. The detection of mRNA does not necessarily equate with protein synthesis and it will need to be shown that translation and secretion of these lymphokines also occur. Furthermore, T-lymphocytes are not the sole potential source of lymphokines, since granulocytes including mast cells and eosinophils have been shown to elaborate certain lymphokines at least *in vitro*. Nevertheless, these observations provide direct evidence in support of the hypothesis that activated CD4 T-lymphocytes, through their patterns of lymphokine secretion, regulate the types of granulocytes which participate in inflammatory reactions. Furthermore, they demonstrate that Th1 and Th2 CD4 T-lymphocyte responses can be detected in humans under physiological conditions.

13.4 T-lymphocytes and Asthma Therapy

Glucocorticoids form the mainstay of treatment of asthma and are the only anti-asthma drugs which have been shown unequivocally to reduce the degree of bronchial hyperresponsiveness in asthma of wide ranging severity and aetiology. If bronchial mucosal inflammation is indeed important in the pathogenesis of bronchial hyperresponsiveness, the effects of glucocorticoids might be associated with a reduction in the amount of this inflammation. Although glucocorticoids are classified as 'anti-inflammatory', their precise mechanism of action is quite unknown. One possibility is that glucocorticoids act at least in part through a direct inhibitory effect on inflammatory leukocytes. There is now a large body of evidence suggesting that, whereas T-lymphocytes and antigen presenting cells are exquisitely sensitive to glucocorticoid inhibition in the majority of subjects, B-lymphocytes and granulocytes, particularly eosinophils and mast cells, are insensitive to inhibition by glucocorticoids at therapeutic concentrations (Schleimer et al., 1989). Taken together, these observations allow the hypothesis that the activated T-lymphocyte may be one primary target for glucocorticoid therapy in asthma (and other inflammatory diseases).

We have recently provided evidence in support of this hypothesis in a study of glucocorticoid-resistant asthma (Corrigan et al., 1991a, b). A group of chronic, severe (forced expiratory volume in 1 s (FEV_1) < 70% of the predicted value) asthmatic patients with documented reversible airways obstruction were classified as clinically sensitive or resistant to oral glucocorticoid therapy on the basis of their FEV_1 response to a two week course of oral prednisolone (20 mg daily for one week followed by 40 mg daily for a further week). Sensitive patients were defined as those showing a 15% or greater improvement in FEV_1. The resistant patients showed no significant improvement in FEV_1 or a number of other measurements of airways obstruction despite this therapy. Peripheral blood mononuclear cells from sensitive and resistant patients were cultured in vitro with the T-lymphocyte mitogen PHA and in the presence of various concentrations of dexamethasone. Mitogen-induced proliferation of T-lymphocytes from the sensitive, but not the resistant, patients was inhibited by therapeutic ($10^{-8}-10^{-7}$ mol/l) concentrations of dexamethasone in vitro. Similarly, release of IL-2 and interferon-Γ by the proliferating cells was significantly inhibited by these concentrations of dexamethasone only in T-lymphocytes derived from the clinically sensitive patients. Absorption and elimination of orally administered glucocorticoid did not differ between the sensitive and resistant patients, and the characteristics of their cellular glucocorticoid receptors were similar. These observations support the hypothesis that clinical glucocorticoid resistance in asthma reflects, at least in part, a relative resistance of T-lymphocytes to the inhibitory effects of glucocorticoid therapy, with the corollary that activated T-lymphocytes have an important role in the pathogenesis of the disease. It was similarly noted that monocytes isolated from glucocorticoid-resistant asthmatics were relatively resistant to the inhibitory effects of glucocorticoids *in vitro* (Wilkinson *et al.*, 1989).

13.5 Conclusions and Future Prospects

In summary, asthma is characterized by inflammation of the bronchial mucosa, and a question central to the understanding of asthma pathogenesis is how this inflammation is initiated and propagated. CD4 T-lymphocytes can respond directly to antigens encountered at mucosal surfaces and, by the secretion of lymphokines, bring about the accumulation and activation of particular granulocytes. The direct activation of T-lymphocytes by antigen and their subsequent direct effects on granulocytes form one possible mechanism for the genesis of bronchial inflammation, which is independent of the presence or absence of antibodies including IgE (Fig. 13.2). B-lymphocytes in atopic subjects may secrete IgE in response to airborne allergens and other antigens. The control of this process is evidently very complex, but is in part dependent upon T-lymphocyte products. In atopic subjects, allergen-specific IgE bound to granulocyte F_c receptors may activate these cells directly on exposure to allergens, with release of inflammatory mediators. This forms a second possible mechanism for the genesis of asthmatic inflammation which is obviously applicable only to atopic subjects (Fig. 13.2).

It will be important in future studies to delineate the relative contributions of these two parallel mechanisms to the pathogenesis of asthma. Whereas acute degranulation of mast cells and eosinophils on exposure to allergens may be important in producing acute exacerbations of disease in atopic subjects, inflammation orchestrated by activated CD4 T-lymphocytes may be more important in maintaining chronic ongoing disease. The studies from our department demonstrating that activated CD4 T-lymphocytes secreting lymphokines are present in the asthmatic bronchial mucosa, and a consideration of the possible mechanism of action of glucocorticoids in this disease, provide considerable support for this hypothesis.

If activated T-lymphocytes are indeed important in the pathogenesis of

Mechanisms in asthma

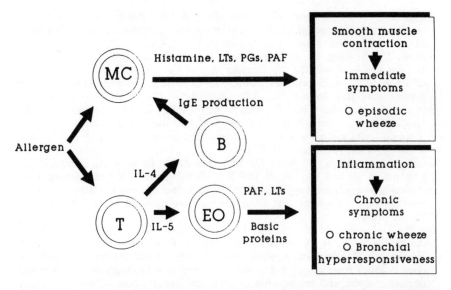

Fig. 13.2   Two pathways for antigen-induced bronchial mucosal inflammation in asthma. Antigens (including allergens) may activate T-lymphocytes directly, leading to release of lymphokines which subsequently activate granulocytes such as eosinophils. This mechanism need not involve Ig (lower pathway). Antigens may also activate granulocytes directly if the latter possess surface-bound IgE which is cross-linked after allergen exposure. This mechanism is not obviously applicable to non-atopic subjects. The first mechanism (which is inhibited by glucocorticoids) may be more important in chronic ongoing disease, whilst the second might be responsible for acute exacerbations following acute exposure of atopic subjects to allergens. MC, mediator cell; B, B-lymphocyte; T, T-lymphocyte; EO, eosinophil.

asthma, it follows that other anti-T-lymphocyte drugs might be efficacious in this disease. A recent double-blind cross-over study performed by our department on the effects of cyclosporin A (CsA) therapy in a group of chronic, severe corticosteroid-dependent asthmatics (Alexander *et al.*, 1991) showed that CsA did improve lung function in a proportion of these patients, in some cases to a spectacular degree. This is even more remarkable when it is remembered that these patients were taking maximal doses of inhaled therapy in addition to up to 20 mg oral prednisolone daily, and therefore had airways obstruction which would previously have been considered to be irreversible. Although CsA has its own range of unwanted effects, it is probable that newer anti-T-lymphocyte drugs with an improved efficacy–safety profile will appear in the near future, providing an exciting new approach to the therapy of asthmatics, particularly those patients who suffer from intractable disease despite debilitating doses of glucocorticoids.

References

Alexander, A. G., Barnes, N. C. and Kay, A. B. (1992). Cyclosporin A in corticosteroid-dependent chronic severe asthma. A randomized double-blind placebo-controlled crossover trial. *Lancet*, **339**, 324–8.

Azzawi, M., Bradley, B., Jeffery, P. K., Frew, A. J., Wardlaw, A. J., Knowles, G., Assoufi, B., Collins, J. V., Durham, S. and Kay, A. B. (1990). Identification of activated T-lymphocytes and eosinophils in bronchial biopsies in stable atopic asthma. *Am. Rev. Respir. Dis.*, **142**, 1407–13.

Bentley, A. M., Maestrelli, P., Saetta, M., Fabbri, L. M., Robinson, D. S., Bradley, B. L., Jeffery, P. K., Durham, S. R. and Kay, A. B. (1992a). Activated T-lymphocytes and eosinophils in the bronchial mucosa in occupational asthma. *J. Allergy Clin. Immunol.*, **89**, 821–9.

Bentley, A. M., Menz, G., Storz, C., Robinson, D. S., Bradley, B., Jeffery, P. K., Durham, S. R. and Kay, A. B. (1992b). Identification of T-lymphocytes, macrophages and activated eosinophils in the bronchial mucosa in intrinsic asthma: relationship to symptoms and bronchial responsiveness. *Am. Rev. Respir. Dis.* (in the press).

Bradley, B. L., Azzawi, M., Assoufi, B., Jacobson, M., Collins, J. V., Irani, A.-M. A., Schwartz, L. B., Durham, S. R., Jeffery, P. K. and Kay, A. B. (1991). Eosinophils, T-lymphocytes, mast cells, neutrophils and macrophages in bronchial biopsies from atopic asthmatics: comparison with atopic non-asthma and normal controls and relationship to bronchial hyperresponsiveness. *J. Allergy Clin. Immunol.*, **88**, 661–74.

Cher, D. J. and Mosmann, T. R. (1987). Two types of murine helper T-cell clone: 2. Delayed type hypersensitivity is mediated by Th1 clones. *J. Immunol.*, **138**, 3688–94.

Corrigan, C. J. and Kay, A. B. (1990). CD4 T-lymphocyte activation in acute severe asthma. Relationship to disease severity and atopic status. *Am. Rev. Respir. Dis.*, **141**, 970–7.

Corrigan, C. J., Hartnell, A. and Kay, A. B. (1988). T-lymphocyte activation in acute severe asthma. *Lancet*, **1**, 1129–31.

Corrigan, C. J., Brown, P. H., Barnes, N. C., Szefler, S. J., Tsai, J.-J., Frew, A. J. and Kay, A. B. (1991a). Glucocorticoid resistance in chronic asthma: glucocorticoid pharmacokinetics, glucocorticoid receptor characteristics and inhibition of peripheral blood T-lymphocytes by glucocorticoids *in vitro*. *Am. Rev. Respir. Dis.*, **144**, 1016–25.

Corrigan, C. J., Brown, P. H., Barnes, N. C., Tsai, J.-J., Frew, A. J. and Kay, A. B. (1991b). Glucocorticoid resistance in chronic asthma: peripheral blood T-lymphocyte activation and a comparison of the T-lymphocyte inhibitory effects of glucocorticoids and cyclosporin A. *Am. Rev. Respir. Dis.*, 1026–32.

Hamid, Q., Azzawi, M., Ying, S., Moqbel, R., Wardlaw, A. J., Corrigan, C. J., Bradley, B., Durham, S. R., Collins, J. V., Jeffery, P. K., Quint, D. J. and Kay, A. B. (1991). Expression of mRNA for interleukin-5 in mucosal bronchial biopsies from asthma. *J. Clin. Invest.*, **87**, 1541–6.

Mosmann, T. R. and Coffman, R. L. (1989). Th1 and Th2 cells: different patterns of lymphokine secretion lead to different functional properties. *Annu. Rev. Immunol.*, **7**, 145–73.

Pene, I., Rousset, F., Briere, F., Chretien, I., Bonnefoy, J. Y., Spits, H., Yokota, T., Arai, K., Banchereau, J. and de Vries, J. (1988). IgE production by normal human lymphocytes is induced by interleukin-4 and suppressed by interferons Γ and α and prostaglandin E_2. *Proc. Natl. Acad. Sci. USA*, **85**, 6880–4.

Schleimer, R. P., Claman, H. N. and Oronsky, A. (eds.) (1989). *Anti-inflammatory Steroid Action: Basic and Clinical Aspects*, Academic Press, London.

Wierenga, E. A., Snoek, M., de Groot, C., Chretien, L., Bos, J. D., Jansen, H. M. and Kapsenberg, M. I. (1990). Evidence for compartmentalization of functional subsets of CD4+ T-lymphocytes in atopic patients. *J. Immunol.*, **144**, 4651–6.

Wilkinson, J. R. W., Crea, A. E. G., Clark, T. J. H. and Lee T. H. (1989). Identification and characterization of a monocyte-derived neutrophil activating factor in corticosteroid-resistant bronchial asthma. *J. Clin. Invest.*, **84**, 1930–41.

14

T-lymphocyte–Eosinophil Interactions in Allergic Inflammation

P. L. B. Bruijnzeel, C. A. F. M. Bruijnzeel-Koomen, G. C. Mudde,
R. A. J. Warringa, L. Koenderman, R. Moser, T. T. Hansel and
C. Walker

14.1 Introduction

There is increasing evidence that eosinophils are important contributors to allergic inflammation (Gleich, 1990). This is mainly due to their capacity to release of a variety of mediators (Bruijnzeel, 1989). One distinguishes granule-derived mediators such as major basic protein (MBP), eosinophil cationic protein (ECP) and eosinophil peroxidase (EPO) and membrane-derived mediators such as leukotriene C4 (LTC4) and platelet-activating factor (PAF). The granule-derived mediators are present in a preformed state, whereas the membrane-derived mediators are generated upon stimulation. The above-mentioned mediators are considered important for the allergic inflammation, because they are able to act toxic on cells surrounding the eosinophil in the tissue. In addition, they may mobilize more eosinophils or other inflammatory cells and may cause physiological responses such as induced by histamine (Bruijnzeel, 1989). Based on this knowledge eosinophils are thought to participate actively in the pathogenesis of asthma, allergic rhinitis and even atopic dermatitis (AD) (Bousquet et al., 1990; Bruijnzeel-Koomen et al., 1988; Frew and Kay, 1990).

Currently, lymphocyte-derived factors, called cytokines, are thought to modulate role in eosinophil formation, eosinophil activation state and eosinophil tissue infiltration. The most important cytokines in this respect are granulocyte–macrophage colony stimulating factor (GM-CSF), inter-leukin 3 (IL-3) and interleukin 5 (IL-5) (Owen, 1991).

To illustrate possible lymphocyte–eosinophil interactions *in vivo*, the patch test reaction to aeroallergens in AD patients will be used. The observed cellular infiltration during the patch test reaction has demon-strated the simultaneous tissue infiltration of both lymphocytes (T-lymphocytes) and eosinophils. Although not yet shown this simultaneous infiltration strongly suggests cell–cell interaction. Based on this *in vivo* observation an attempt will be made to explain why in particular eosino-phils infiltrate the skin during this patch test reaction. This explanation is largely based on *in vitro* studies dealing with T-lymphocytes, the cyto-kines GM-CSF, IL-3 and IL-5 and their influence on eosinophil migration. Finally, a hypothetical model will be described which tries to explain the lymphocyte–eosinophil interaction within the tissue.

Here, the patch test reaction to aeroallergens in AD patients is taken as a model system. This model system may be representative for the allergic inflammatory reaction observed in asthma and in allergic rhinitis as well.

14.2 The Patch Test Reaction to Aeroallergens in Atopic Dermatitis

Atopic dermatitis (AD) patients may, upon patch testing with aeroal-lergens, develop an eczematous skin lesion after 24–48 h. Since positive patch test reactions to aeroallergens only occur in AD patients and not in patients suffering from other allergic diseases this reaction may be con-sidered characteristic for AD. Not only macroscopically but also micro-scopically this eczematous skin lesion resembles active eczematous skin. Biopsies taken after patch testing AD patients show a T-cell infiltrate which is similar to the one observed in active AD skin. Therefore, the patch test reaction to aeroallergens in AD patients may be considered an *in vivo* model to study AD (Bruijnzeel-Koomen *et al.*, 1988, 1990).

Based on the demonstration of IgE bound to epidermal Langerhans cells (Bruijnzeel-Koomen, 1986), Bruijnzeel-Koomen *et al.* (1986) have pro-posed the following model for the patch test reaction to aeroallergens in AD patients. Aeroallergens, applied onto the skin, can bind to epidermal Langerhans cells (Bruijnzeel-Koomen *et al.*, 1986; Mudde *et al.*, 1990), and consecutively be presented to dermal T-lymphocytes resulting in a lym-phoproliferative response (see Fig. 14.1).

To understand better the cellular reaction sequence after epicutaneous application of aeroallergens to the skin, the cellular infiltration has been examined in more detail by taking sequential biopsies, which were investi-gated immunohistologically. It was shown that 2 h after patch testing

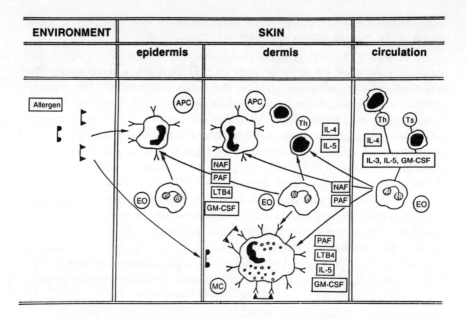

Fig. 14.1   Epicutaneously applied aeroallergens to the skin of AD patients can bind to IgE present on Langerhans cells (LC) in the epidermis. In the dermis these LC can present cell-bound allergens to T-lymphocytes, resulting in a lymphoproliferative response. These activated T-lymphocytes (Th) may by the release of cytokines (IL-4, IL-5, GM-CSF) on the one hand stimulate B cells to synthesize IgE (via IL-4) and on the other hand cause increased differentiation and maturation of eosinophils (via IL-5 and GM-CSF). Increased IgE levels and increased peripheral blood eosinophilia are present in the circulation. Diffusion of IgE in the tissue is facilitated by the release of vasoactive mediators. This IgE may bind to various cell types present in both the dermis and the epidermis. At the same time as T-lymphocytes infiltrate the dermis also eosinophils (EO) (but no neutrophils) penetrate the dermis and at a later stage the epidermis. This is probably not due to an increased vascular permeability but to the presence of lymphocyte-derived cytokines such as IL-3, IL-4, IL-5 and GM-CSF in the circulation which give the eosinophil the capacity to adhere to the endothelium and to transmigrate across it in a selective way. Once the eosinophil has passed the endothelium, chemotactic factors locally synthesized within the tissue may exert their mobilizing action. Because of the influence of the above-mentioned cytokines the eosinophil may show an increased chemotactic responsiveness to a great number of chemotactic factors such as NAF-1 or IL-8, PAF, and LTB4. On the other hand other locally synthesized factors may act on the eosinophil to induce the expression of surface receptor molecules such as IgE receptor, ICAM-1, HLA-DR and others. Because of the expression of these molecules the eosinophil is able to interact with the lymphocyte. The outcome of this interaction is, however, not yet fully clear. Abbreviations: APC, antigen presenting cell; MC, mast cell; LC, Langerhans cell; EO, eosinophil; Th, T helper cell; Ts, T suppressor cell.

T-lymphocytes and eosinophils had already started to infiltrate the dermis. The mononuclear infiltrate consisted mainly of CD4+ T-lymphocytes and reached its maximum at 24 h. It was mainly present in the dermis and to a lesser extent in the epidermis. These T cells were in an activated state since they expressed activation markers such as class II antigens. In contrast, at 24 h eosinophils had infiltrated in both the dermis and the epidermis. The eosinophils in the dermis stained with the monoclonal antibody (EG2), directed against activated and secreted forms of ECP, indicating activation of those cells. The eosinophils present in the epidermis did not stain positively with this monoclonal antibody, suggesting they were not in an activated state. More careful investigation of the eosinophils present in the epidermis has revealed that these eosinophils regularly contacted IgE-bearing Langerhans cells (Bruijnzeel-Koomen et al., 1988). Electron microscopy studies of this contact did show that secreted eosinophil-derived granules closely contacted IgE-bearing Langerhans cells. Skin biopsies, taken at 72 h, and stained with anti-EPO antibodies, showed a dendritic staining pattern suggestive of EPO-positive Langerhans cells, whereas hardly any intact eosinophils were present in the epidermis at this time point. Altogether, these findings suggest that eosinophils are in an activated state both in the dermis and in the epidermis. Thus, in the dermis these eosinophils are likely to make contact with activated T-lymphocytes, whereas in the epidermis they most likely contact IgE-positive epidermal Langerhans cells.

14.3 Interaction Between T-lymphocytes and Eosinophils from the Circulation of Patients with Allergic Disease

Recent investigations have indicated that certain cytokines can prolong eosinophil survival in vitro (Lopez et al., 1986, 1988; Rothenberg et al., 1988; Owen et al., 1987). The most important cytokines in this respect are IL-3, IL-5 and GM-CSF. These cytokines (but also others) can be synthesized by activated T-lymphocytes, which express interleukin-2 receptors (IL-2R+). Walker et al. (1991) have shown that in patients with allergic disease the degree of IL-2R expression on CD4+ T-lymphocytes closely correlated with the degree of peripheral blood eosinophilia. This correlation did not exist for HLA-DR expression. Since IL-2R expression by T-lymphocytes normally coincides with cytokine production, the cytokine production of these T-lymphocytes was evaluated. It appeared that, in particular, CD4+ T-lymphocytes (IL-2R+) from the blood of allergic individuals, but not from normal individuals, spontaneously secreted IL-3, IL-5 and GM-CSF. Further investigations revealed that even the serum of those patients contained these cytokines. It should be evident that the presence of these cytokines in the circulation may have implications for the kinetics and the functional activity of circulating eosinophils.

In order to be able to understand better the mechanism behind the rather selective infiltration of eosinophils in the dermis after patch testing AD patients with aeroallergens, the influence of the above-mentioned cytokines on the in vitro migration capacity (= chemotaxis) of eosinophils was evaluated.

14.4 Influence of the Cytokines GM-CSF, IL-3 and IL-5 on Eosinophil Chemotaxis

To investigate this, two different Boyden chamber systems were applied (a) a system using two filters with different pore sizes (Bruijnzeel *et al.*, 1990; Warringa *et al.*, 1991) and (b) a system using confluent human umbilical vein endothelial cell (HUVEC) monolayers on a filter (Moser *et al.*, 1989). Using the first system it was investigated whether GM-CSF, IL-3 and IL-5 could modulate chemotactic responses of eosinophils derived from the blood of normal individuals. The chemoattractants used in these studies were platelet-activating factor (PAF), neutrophil-activating factor (NAF-1 or IL-8), leukotriene B4 (LTB4), *N*-formyl-methionyl-leucyl-phenylalanine (FMLP) and the complement fragment C5a. Eosinophils from normal individuals showed a chemotactic response toward PAF, LTB4 and C5a, but not to NAF and FMLP. However, when these eosinophils were pretreated with picomolar concentrations of GM-CSF, IL-3 and IL-5 a significant increase in the response toward PAF and LTB4 occurred, whereas NAF and FMLP became potent chemotaxins. The chemotactic response toward C5a hardly changed. It could also be shown that at nanomolar concentrations GM-CSF, IL-3 and IL-5 acted chemotactically on eosinophils (Yamaguchi *et al.*, 1988; Warringa *et al.*, 1992, manuscript submitted). Eosinophils from the circulation of AD (and allergic asthma) patients showed a significantly enhanced chemotactic response toward PAF, NAF and FMLP compared with eosinophils from normal individuals, whereas the C5a-induced chemotactic response was similar. The observed increase in chemotactic responsiveness of eosinophils from the circulation of AD patients was identical to the one observed in eosinophils from normal individuals pretreated with IL-3, IL-5 or GM-CSF. This observation suggests previous *in vivo* exposure to these cytokines of the eosinophils from the circulation of AD (and allergic asthma) patients (Bruijnzeel *et al.* manuscript submitted; Warringa *et al.*, 1992).

In the Boyden chamber system using confluent HUVEC monolayers eosinophils from AD (and allergic asthma) patients showed a significantly increased capacity to transmigrate across IL-1 or tumour necrosis factor-α (TNF-α) activated HUVEC monolayers compared with eosinophils from normal individuals (Moser *et al.*, 1992). This increased capacity to transmigrate IL-1 or TNF-α activated HUVEC could be induced in eosinophils from normal individuals by pretreatment with IL-3, IL-5 or GM-CSF. This capacity could be inhibited with functional antibodies against CD11a, CD11b and CD18, suggesting a CD11–CD18 mediated mechanism to be involved.

Taken together, these data demonstrate that GM-CSF, IL-3 and IL-5 produced by activated T-lymphocytes, present in the circulation of patients with various allergic diseases, may increase the migration capacity of circulating eosinophils (see Fig. 14.1). Probably these cytokines induce receptor expression changes on the eosinophil, facilitating responsiveness in these migration systems.

14.5 Model for the Interaction Between T-lymphocytes and Eosinophils in Allergic Inflammation

As outlined above our *in vitro* experiments have indicated that in the circulation of individuals suffering from atopic disease T-lymphocytes may be in an activated state and that as a consequence cytokines such as GM-CSF, IL-3 and IL-5 may be released. Circulating eosinophils are exposed to these factors and for example IL-5 may cause them to adhere to endothelium selectively (Walsh *et al.*, 1990). On the other hand, the mentioned cytokines render eosinophils an increased capacity to transmigrate across IL-1 or TNF-α activated HUVEC monolayers, indicating the involvement of adhesion molecules. Once the eosinophils have transmigrated across the endothelial barrier they may respond chemotactically towards factors they are normally not responsive to, e.g. NAF-1 or IL-8, or respond much more strongly than usual, e.g. PAF (Warringa *et al.*, 1991, 1992; Bruijnzeel *et al.*, manuscript submitted). Since cloned allergen-specific T-lymphocytes derived from the skin synthesize IL-3, IL-4, IL-5 and GM-CSF and no IL-2 and γ-interferon (van Reysen *et al.*, 1992), one may expect IL-4 to play a role in the selective tissue mobilization of eosinophils as well. In particular this is so since the expression of VLA-4 (CD49d–CD29) occurs on eosinophils and not on neutrophils (Bochner *et al.*, 1991; Walsh *et al.*, 1991), and IL-4 induces the expression of its counterpart vascular cell adhesion molecule-1 (VCAM-1) on endothelial cells (Elices *et al.*, 1990; Thornhill *et al.*, 1991). IL-4 does not induce the expression of intercellular adhesion molecule-1 (ICAM-1) or endothelial leukocyte adhesion molecule-1 (ELAM-1) on endothelial cells (Thornhill *et al.*, 1990, 1991). Therefore IL-4 and IL-5 may be of particular importance for selective eosinophil mobilization in the patch test reaction model in AD patients and for eosinophil mobilization in allergic inflammation in general.

Taken together, all these findings show that T-cell derived cytokines influence the functional state of the eosinophil. They do not, however, answer the question as to how these cells interact with each other once they have infiltrated into the tissue. Therefore, the answer to this question remains open for speculation.

Recently, we were able to demonstrate that eosinophils which have infiltrated into the tissue do express ICAM-1 and HLA-DR (Hansel *et al.*, 1991). These surface markers may point to different functions of the

eosinophil. Via ICAM-1 it may bind to lymphocytes. Perhaps triggering of
the eosinophil via this receptor leads to the release of ECP. ECP may
inhibit the lymphoproliferative response (Peterson *et al.*, 1986). When this
type of interaction indeed takes place this could indicate that the eosinophil could act as an immunomodulatory cell. On the other hand, eosinophils infiltrated into the tissue may express IgE receptors (Capron *et al.*,
1984) and also HLA-DR (Hansel *et al.*, 1991). This would equip them to
act as antigen presenting cells like the Langerhans cell. By means of these
surface structures the eosinophil could therefore also induce a lymphoproliferative reaction. When both these eosinophil–T-cell interactions are
accompanied by the release of ECP and as a consequence an inhibition of
the lymphoproliferative response then this eosinophil–T-cell interaction
may point to a beneficial role of the eosinophil in the patch test reaction to
aeroallergens in AD patients described here. However, the release of ECP
and other eosinophil-derived factors mentioned may in addition cause
tissue damage. On the other hand, the activated T-lymphocytes present in
the tissue may produce eosinophil stimulating factors in addition to IL-3,
IL-4, IL-5 and GM-CSF, which cause eosinophils to degranulate even
more rapidly and as a consequence to contribute to tissue damage.

References

Bochner, B. S., Luscinskas, F. W., Gimbrone, M. A., Newman, W., Sterbinsky, S.
   A., Derse-Anthony, C. P., Klunk, D. and Schleimer, R. P. (1991). Adhesion of
   human basophils, eosinophils and neutrophils to interleukin-1 activated human
   vascular endothelial cells: contributions of endothelial cell adhesion molecules.
   J. Exp. Med., **173**, 1553–6.
Bousquet, J., Chanez, P., Lacoste, J. Y., Barneon, G., Chavanian, N., Enander,
   I., Venge, P., Ahlstedt, S., Simony-Lafontaine, J., Godard, P. and Michel, F. B.
   (1990). Inflammation in asthma. *N. Engl. J. Med.*, **323**, 1033–40.
Bruijnzeel, P. L. B. (1989). Contribution of eosinophil-derived mediators in
   asthma. *Int. Arch. Allergy Appl. Immunol.*, **90**, 57–63.
Bruijnzeel, P. L. B., Warringa, R. A. J., Kok, P. T. M. and Kreukniet, J. (1990).
   Inhibition of neutrophil and eosinophil induced chemotaxis by nedocromil
   sodium and sodium cromoglycate. *Br. J. Pharmacol.*, **99**, 798–802.
Bruijnzeel, P. L. B., Kuijper, P. H. M., Rihs, S., Besy, S., Warringa, R. A. Y. and
   Koenderman, L. Eosinophil chemotaxis in Atopic Dermatitis I: Increased che-
   motactic responsiveness to FMLP, NAF/IL-8, PAF and PFY. Submitted to *J.
   Invest. Dermatol.*
Bruijnzeel-Koomen, C. A. F. M. (1986). IgE on Langerhans cells: new insights in
   the pathogenesis of atopic dermatitis. *Dermatologica*, **172**, 181–3.
Bruijnzeel-Koomen, C. A. F. M., van Wichen, D. F., Toonstra, J., Berrens, L.
   and Bruijnzeel, P. L. B. (1986). The presence of IgE on epidermal Langerhans
   cells in patients with atopic dermatitis. *Arch. Dermatol. Res.*, **278**, 199–205.
Bruijnzeel-Koomen, C. A. F. M., van Wichen, D. F., Spry, C. J. F., Venge, P. and
   Bruijnzeel, P. L. B. (1988). Active participation of eosinophils in patch test

reactions to inhalant allergens in patients with atopic dermatitis. *Br. J. Dermatol.*, **18**, 229–38.

Bruijnzeel-Koomen, C. A. F. M., Mudde, G. C. and Bruijnzeel, P. L. B. (1990). The pathogenesis of atopic dermatitis. *Allergologie*, **13**, 325–38.

Capron, M., Spiegelberg, H. L., Prin, L., Bennich, H., Butterworth, A. E., Pierce, R. J., Aliouaissi, P. M. and Capron, A. (1984). Role of IgE receptors in effector function of human eosinophils. *J. Immunol.*, **132**, 462–8.

Elices, M. J., Osborn, L., Takada, Y., Crouse, C., Luhowskyj, S., Hemmler, M. E. and Lobb, R. R. (1990). VCAM-1 on activated endothelium interacts with the leucocyte integrin VLA-4 at a site distinct from the VLA-4/fibronectin binding site. *Cell*, **51**, 577–84.

Frew, A. J. and Kay, A. B. (1990). Eosinophils and T-lymphocytes in late-phase allergic reactions. *J. Allergy Clin. Immunol.*, **85**, 533–9.

Gleich, G. J. (1990). The eosinophils and bronchial asthma: current understanding. *J. Allergy Clin. Immunol.*, **85**, 422–36.

Hansel, T. T., Braunstein, J. B., Walker, C., Blaser, K., Bruijnzeel, P. L. B., Virchow, J.-Chr., Jr, and Virchow, C. (1991). Sputum eosinophils from asthmatics express ICAM-1 and HLA-DR. *Clin. Exp. Immunol.*, **86**, 271–7.

Lopez, A. F., Williamson, D. J., Gamble, J. R., Begley, C. G., Harlan, J. M., Klebanoff, S. J., Waltersdorph, A., Wong, G., Clark, S. C. and Vadas, M. A. (1986). Recombinant human granulocyte–macrophage colony-stimulating factor stimulates *in vitro* mature human neutrophil and eosinophil function, surface receptor expression and survival. *J. Clin. Invest.*, **78**, 1220–6.

Lopez, A. F., Sanderson, C. J., Gamble, J. R., Campbell, H. D., Young, I. G. and Vadas, M. A. (1988). Recombinant human interleukin 5 is a selective activator of human eosinophil function. *J. Exp. Med.*, **167**, 219–24.

Moser, R., Schleiffenbaum, B., Groscurth, P. and Fehr, J. (1989). Interleukin 1 and tumor necrosis factor stimulate human vascular endothelial cells to promote transendothelial neutrophil passage. *J. Clin. Invest.*, **83**, 444–55.

Moser, R., Fehr, J., Olgiati, L. and Bruijnzeel, P. L. B. (1992). Blood eosinophils of allergic asthmatic but not normal individuals possess a spontaneous increased capacity to adhere to and to transmigrate across IL-1 activated human umbilical vein endothelial monolayers. *Blood*, (in the press).

Mudde, G. C., van Reysen, F. C., Boland, G. J., de Gast, G. C., Bruijnzeel, P. L. B. and Bruijnzeel-Koomen, C. A. F. M. (1990). Allergen presentation by epidermal Langerhans cells from patients with atopic dermatitis is mediated by IgE. *Immunology*, **69**, 335–41.

Owen, W. F. (1991). Cytokine regulation of eosinophil inflammatory disease. *ACI News*, **3** (3), 85–9.

Owen, W. F., Rothenberg, M. E., Silberstein, D. S., Gasson, J. C., Stevens, R. L. and Austen, K. F. (1987). Regulation of human eosinophil viability, density, and function by granulocyte–macrophage colony-stimulating factor in the presence of 3T3 fibroblasts. *J. Exp. Med.*, **166**, 129–46.

Peterson, C., Skoog, V. and Venge, P. (1986). Human eosinophil cationic proteins (ECP and EPX) and their suppressive effects on lymphocyte proliferation. *Immunobiology*, **171**, 1–13.

Rothenberg, M. E., Owen, W. F., Silberstein, D. S., Woods, J., Soberman, R. J., Austen, K. F. and Stevens, R. L. (1988). Human eosinophils have prolonged survival, enhanced functional properties and become hypodense when exposed to human interleukin 3. *J. Clin. Invest.*, **81**, 1986–92.

Thornhill, M. H., Kuang-Aung, U. and Haskard, D. O. (1990). IL-4 increases human endothelial cell adhesiveness for T cells but not neutrophils. *J. Immunol.*, **145**, 865–72.

Thornhill, M. H., Wellicome, S. M., Mahiouz, D. L., Lanchbrory, J. S., Kyan-Aung, U. and Haskard, D. O. (1991). Tumor necrosis factor combines with IL-4 or IFN-gamma to selectively enhance endothelial cell adhesiveness for T-cells. The contribution of vascular cell adhesion molecule-1-dependent and independent binding mechanisms. *J. Immunol.*, **146**, 592–8.

van Reysen, F. C., Bruijnzeel-Koomen, C. A. F. M., Kalthoff, F. S., Maggi, E., Romaguani, S., Westland, J. K. T., Mudde, G. C. (1992). Skin-derived aeroallergen specific T cell cloner of the Th phenotype in patients with atopic dermatitis. *J. Allergy Clin. Immunol.* (in the press).

Walker, C., Virchow, J.-Chr., Jr, Bruijnzeel, P. L. B. and Blaser, K. (1991). T cell subsets and their soluble products regulate eosinophilia in allergic and non-allergic asthma. *J. Immunol.*, **146**, 1829–36.

Walsh, G. M., Hartnell, A., Wardlaw, A. J., Kurihara, K., Sanderson, C. J. and Kay, A. B. (1990). IL-5 enhances the *in vitro* adhesion of human eosinophils, but not neutrophils in a leucocyte integrin (CD11/18)-dependent manner. *Immunology*, **71**, 258–65.

Walsh, G. M., Mermod, J. J., Hartnell, A., Kay, A. B. and Wardlaw, A. J. (1991). Human eosinophil, but not neutrophil, adherence to IL-1 stimulated human umbilical vascular endothelial cells is $\alpha_4 \beta_1$ (very late antigen-4) dependent. *J. Immunol.*, **146**, 3419–3423.

Warringa, R. A. J., Koenderman, L., Kok, P. T. M., Kreukniet, J. and Bruijnzeel, P. L. B. (1991). Modulation and induction of eosinophil chemotaxis by granulocyte–macrophage colony stimulating factor and interleukin 3. *Blood*, **77**, 2694–700.

Warringa, R. A. J., Mengelers, H. J. J., Kuijper, P. H. M., Raaymakers, J. A. M., Bruijnzeel, P. L. B., Koenderman, L. (1992). *In vivo* priming of platelet-activating factor-induced eosinophil chemotaxis in allergic asthmatic individuals. *Blood*, **79**, 1836–41.

Yamaguchi, Y., Hayashi, Y., Sugama, Y., Miura, Y., Kasahari, T., Kitamura, S., Torisu, M., Mita, S., Tominaga, A., Takatsu, K. and Suda, T. (1988). Highly purified murine interleukin 5 (IL-5) stimulates eosinophil function and prolongs *in vitro* survival. IL-5 as an eosinophil chemotactic factor. *J. Exp. Med.*, **167**, 1737–43.

15

Interleukin-5 and Eosinophilia

C. J. Sanderson

15.1 Introduction

The demonstration that eosinophils could kill antibody-coated schistoso-mula of *Schistosoma mansoni* (Butterworth *et al.*, 1975) opened up a new era in eosinophil biology (Butterworth, 1984). It was followed by work showing that eosinophils were capable of lysing parasitic protozoa (Sanderson *et al.*, 1977), chicken erythrocytes (Sanderson and Thomas, 1978) and tumour cells (Lopez *et al.*, 1981; Lopez and Sanderson, 1982) *in vitro*. In allergy eosinophils have a chequered history. It was first thought that they modified an allergic reaction in a positive way by neutralizing mast cell products (Goetzl *et al.*, 1975). The reverse seems to be closer to the truth, and eosinophils are now recognized to be the primary cause of tissue damage in the chronic manifestations of allergic disease (Gleich and Adolph-son, 1986). Thus eosinophils have become a therapeutic target for a new generation of anti-asthma drugs.

There are three important features of eosinophilia which provide some interesting but poorly understood clues about the mechanism of control of eosinophil production. Firstly, eosinophilia is under the control of T-lymphocytes (T cells). Thus it is the consequence of an immune response (Basten and Beeson, 1970; Sanderson, 1990). Secondly, increases in eosinophil numbers are frequently observed independently of increases in other blood leukocytes (Strath and Sanderson, 1986; Maxwell *et al.*, 1987). This biological specificity implies a mechanism of control which is indepen-dent from the mechanisms controlling the production of the other leuko-cytes. Thirdly, eosinophilia is observed in a restricted number of diseases, which indicates that the immune system is able to distinguish these particular types of antigenic challenge from the majority which do not induce eosinophils.

Eosinophil production can be induced *in vitro* by IL-3, GM-CSF and IL-5, but only the latter is specific for the eosinophil lineage (Campbell *et al.*, 1988; Clutterbuck and Sanderson, 1988). There is increasing evidence that IL-5 is the major, and possibly the only, cytokine involved in the production of specific eosinophilia. Thus IL-5 antagonists are a potential therapeutic approach in those diseases where eosinophils are involved in tissue damage, and IL-5 or IL-5 agonists are a potential therapeutic approach in situations where the cytotoxic activity of eosinophils could be exploited.

15.2 Biochemistry of IL-5

There appears to be only a single copy of the IL-5 gene per haploid genome. The coding sequence of the IL-5 gene forms four exons (Campbell *et al.*, 1987). The exon sequences are highly conserved between mouse and man (Campbell *et al.*, 1988). The introns show areas of sequence similarity although the mouse has a considerable amount of sequence including repeat sequences, which are not present in the human gene. The mouse gene includes a 738 bp segment in the 3' untranslated region which is not present in the human gene. Each of the exons contains the codons for an exact number of amino acids, and in each case begin with GT and end in AG. These features of gene structure are also shared by IL-3, IL-4 and GM-CSF (Sanderson *et al.*, 1988). All four cytokine genes are located in tandem on chromosome 5 in man (Sutherland *et al.*, 1988; van-Leeuwen *et al.*, 1989; Chandrasekharappa *et al.*, 1990) and chromosome 11 in the mouse (Lee *et al.*, 1989). Although there is no overall sequence homology at either the nucleotide or the amino acid level, between any of these four cytokines, the localization and structural similarities suggest a common evolutionary origin (Sanderson *et al.*, 1988). In addition they are all produced by T cells and show an overlap in some of their biological activities, and thus they may be regarded as members of a gene family.

IL-5 was originally identified as a T cell product, and is produced by certain lymphomas and hybrids of T cells and lymphomas. This production by T cells is consistent with the observation that eosinophilia is a T cell dependent phenomenon. In T cells transcription is induced by antigen, mitogens and phorbol esters and occurs for about 24 h, before the gene becomes silent again (Sanderson *et al.*, 1985). The demonstration that IL-5 as well as other cytokine mRNA are produced by mast cell lines opens the possibility that these cells may serve to induce or amplify the development of eosinophilia (Plaut *et al.*, 1989; Burd *et al.*, 1989). Similarly, the observation that human Epstein–Barr virus transformed B cells produce IL-5 raises the possibility that B cells may be an additional source of this cytokine (Paul *et al.*, 1990).

Interleukin-5 (IL-5) is produced by T lymphocytes as a glycoprotein with an M_r of 40 000 to 45 000 (Sanderson *et al.*, 1985) and is unusual among the T cell-produced cytokines in being a disulphide-linked homodimer (Takahashi *et al.*, 1990; McKenzie *et al.*, 1991).

Mature mouse and human IL-5 have 113 and 115 amino acids respectively. Murine IL-5 is truncated by two amino acids at the *N*-terminus. The two proteins have 81 identical amino acids, a further 25 can be considered as conservative changes, leaving seven (and the two *N*-terminal amino acids of the human polypeptide) as non-conservative changes. This high degree of similarity is reflected in the ability of the two proteins to cross-react with cells of other mammals (Sanderson, 1990).

Native IL-5 or recombinant IL-5 expressed in mammalian cells is heterogeneously glycosylated. Mouse IL-5 has three potential sites for *N*-glycosylation, while one of these is missing in human IL-5. The carbohydrate is unnecessary for biological activity *in vitro* (Tominaga *et al.*, 1990).

Investigations using reduced and alkylated IL-5 suggest that dimerization is essential for biological activity (Tsuruoka *et al.*, 1990). To investigate the role of the individual cysteine residues in dimerization and biological activity, site-directed mutagenesis was used to produce molecular analogues of IL-5 in which the cysteine residues, either singly (C44 or C86) or together (C44/86), were mutated to threonine. Mutant proteins were expressed in COS cells and all three mutants were monomeric (McKenzie *et al.*, 1991). If IL-5 exists in a head-to-head dimer then dimerization should occur in at least one of the single mutants. As this did not happen it was possible that the molecule may form in a head-to-tail conformation. This was confirmed when it was found that co-transfection of cells with the two single-mutant constructs produced biologically active IL-5. An analysis by peptide sequencing has also indicated that IL-5 exists as a head-to-tail dimer (Minamitake *et al.*, 1990), as none of the mutants monomers had biological activity. These results give final proof that the monomeric form of IL-5 has no significant biological activity. Furthermore, none of the mutant monomers had any inhibitory activity, suggesting that they did not form high affinity interactions with the receptor.

15.3 Biological Activities of IL-5

In the mouse IL-5 induces the production of eosinophils in liquid bone marrow cultures. This is lineage specific, as only eosinophil numbers are increased in these cultures (Sanderson et al., 1985, 1988; Sanderson, 1990). In contrast, both IL-3 and GM-CSF induce eosinophils as well as other cell types, most notably neutrophils and macrophages in bone marrow cultures (Campbell et al., 1988). The production of eosinophils is considerably higher when the bone marrow is taken from mice infected with M. corti than it is from normal marrows. This suggests that marrow from infected mice contains more eosinophil precursors than marrow from normal mice (Sanderson et al., 1985). However, when tested in a colony assay with semi-solid agar, both normal and parasitized mice have similar, relatively small numbers of eosinophil colonies (Warren and Sanderson, 1985). We have interpreted this as indicating a low sensitivity of the mouse colony assay for eosinophil precursor cells (eosinophil colony forming cells). The technical basis for this is not clear, as similar conditions give rise to large numbers of eosinophil colonies from human bone marrow cells (Lopez et al., 1986; Clutterbuck and Sanderson, 1988; Strath et al., 1990; Clutterbuck and Sanderson, 1990).

Liquid bone marrow cultures produce neutrophils for extended periods of time without exogenous factors (Dexter et al., 1977). It appears that the microenvironment of these cultures maintains the production of neutrophil precursors. In contrast, no eosinophils are seen in the absence of exogenous factors. IL-5 induces a production of eosinophils which reaches a peak at about 3 weeks, and continues until about 6–8 weeks. This transient production of eosinophils suggests that IL-5 is unable to stimulate the production of eosinophil precursors at least in these bone marrow cultures. This has led to the concept of IL-5 as a late acting factor in eosinophil haemopoiesis (Sanderson et al., 1985, 1988; Sanderson, 1990).

To study the production of the eosinophil progenitor we have used human bone marrow cultures. This has the advantage that these cells can be quantified in a colony assay in semi-solid medium. Both IL-3 and GM-CSF stimulated a greater number of eosinophil colonies than IL-5 (Clutterbuck et al., 1989). As all the cells in these colonies were morphologically mature and there was no obvious difference in colony size, this surprising result suggested that either IL-3 or GM-CSF would be capable of inducing eosinophilia without the action of IL-5. In addition it suggested that there must be a large pool of eosinophil precursors that were unresponsive to IL-5. Similar experiments were carried out with human bone marrow in liquid cultures where the total number of eosinophils produced rather than the number of colonies could be assessed. In these experiments there was a marked difference to the results in the colony assay, in that IL-5 induced a larger number of eosinophils than IL-3 or GM-CSF. There are two possible explanations. Firstly, there is the trivial possibility that IL-5 is simply a poor stimulant of eosinophils in semi-solid cultures. Secondly, it is possible that IL-5 was capable of inducing a larger number of eosinophils from a smaller pool of precursors (Clutterbuck et al., 1989).

The ability of eosinophils to perform in functional assays can be increased markedly by incubation with a number of different agents, including IL-5 (Silberstein and David, 1987). The phenomenon of activation is apparently independent of differentiation.

The first observations on selective activation of human eosinophils by IL-5 showed that the ability of purified peripheral blood eosinophils to lyse antibody coated tumour cells was increased when IL-5 was included in the assay medium (Lopez et al., 1986). Similarly, the phagocytic ability of these eosinophils towards serum opsonized yeast particles was increased in the presence of IL-5. There was a 90% increase in surface C3bi complement receptors, as well as an approximately 50% increase in the granulocyte functional antigens GFA-1 and GFA-2. IL-5 also induced a rapid increase in superoxide anion production by eosinophils (Lopez et al., 1988). In addition, IL-5 increases the survival of peripheral blood eosinophils (Begley et al., 1986).

A further interesting observation in this context was the demonstration that IL-5 was a potent inducer of Ig-induced eosinophil degranulation, as measured by the release of eosinophil-derived neurotoxin (EDN). IL-5 increased EDN release by 48% for secretory IgA and 136% for IgG. This enhancing effect appeared by 15 min and reached a maximum by 4 h (Fujisawa et al., 1990). The finding that secretory IgA could induce eosinophil degranulation is particularly important because eosinophils are frequently found at mucosal surfaces where IgA is the most abundant immunoglobulin.

As eosinophils frequently occur as the predominant inflammatory cell in tissues, it would seem likely that a specific mechanism exists to cause them to migrate out of the blood stream. One hypothetical mechanism would allow for the production of an eosinophil-specific chemotactic factor. IL-5 has been reported to have chemotactic activity (Yamaguchi et al., 1988; Wang et al., 1989); however, this appears to be weak compared with platelet activating factor which raises doubts about its biological significance (Kay, 1990). Although there are reports of other candidate chemotactic factors, none has so far been unequivocally characterized.

Alternatively, specific localization may occur as a result of the up-regulation of adhesion molecules, causing eosinophils to pass through the capillary endothelium. The demonstration that IL-5 induced an increase in the integrin molecule CD11b (Lopez et al., 1986), and increased 'polarization' including membrane ruffling and pseudopod formation (Lopez et al., 1988), is consistent with this. More recently it has been shown that IL-5 increases the adhesion of eosinophils to endothelial cells in vitro. The inhibition of this effect with monoclonal antibodies suggested that adhesion was mediated by the leucocyte integrin family of surface markers (CD11/18) (Walsh et al., 1990). Even more compelling evidence for the importance of adhesion molecules in the tissue localization of eosinophils has come from experiments *in vivo*. The administration of monoclonal antibody to ICAM1 (CD54) blocked the localization of eosinophils to the lung when the animals were challenged with inhaled ascaris antigen (Wegner *et al.*, 1990).

15.4 Control of Eosinophilia

As discussed in section 15.3, experiments *in vitro* have suggested that IL-5 is a late acting factor in the eosinophil lineage, and that other cytokines are required to generate eosinophil precursors. However, the fact that eosinophilia can occur in the absence of comparable increases in other leukocytes makes it seem unlikely that other broadly active cytokines such as GM-CSF or IL-3 should have obligatory roles in the development of eosinophilia.

An alternative approach to understanding the role of IL-5 *in vivo* is to alter the expression of IL-5 in transgenic mice. As IL-5 is normally a T cell product and the gene is transcribed for only a relatively short period of time after antigen stimulation, transgenic mice in which IL-5 is constitutively expressed by all T cells have been produced (Dent *et al.*, 1990). These mice have detectable levels of IL-5 in the serum. They show a profound and lifelong eosinophilia, with large numbers of eosinophils in the blood, spleen and bone marrow. This indicates that the expression of IL-5 is sufficient to induce the full pathway of eosinophil differentiation. If other cytokines are required for the development of eosinophilia, then either they must be expressed constitutively, or their expression is secondary to the expression of the IL-5 gene. This clear demonstration that the expression of the IL-5 gene in transgenic animals is sufficient for the production of eosinophilia provides an explanation for the biological specificity of eosinophilia. It therefore seems likely that because eosinophilia can occur without a concomitant neutrophilia or monocytosis then a mechanism must exist by which IL-5 is the dominant haemopoietic cytokine produced by the T cell system in natural eosinophilia.

It is interesting to note that despite the massive, long-lasting eosinophilia the transgenic mice appear normal. This illustrates that the presence of increased numbers of eosinophils is not itself harmful, and that the tissue damage seen in allergic reactions and other diseases must be due to agents which trigger the eosinophils to degranulate.

A further intriguing insight into the control of eosinophilia came from experiments where these transgenic mice were infected with *M. corti* (Strath *et al.*, 1992). The DNA construct used as the transgene contained a large amount of flanking sequence at both ends of the IL-5 coding sequences; thus, in addition to the constitutive production brought about by the CD2 LCR, the transgenes retained the capacity to be induced when the T cells were activated (Dent *et al.*, 1990). As might be expected, infection of the mice with *M. corti* resulted in very large amounts of circulating IL-5. For example, normal mice show an increase from undetectable levels to a peak of about 20 units of IL-5 at 15–18 days after infection (Strath and Sanderson, 1986; Strath *et al.*, 1992). In contrast, transgenic mice, carrying eight copies of the transgene, have a base level of about 30–40 units of IL-5, increasing to about 1000 units at 18 days after infection. Surprisingly, these mice show a decrease in tissue and blood eosinophils, and a decrease in eosinophil precursors in the bone marrow during the period of high IL-5 production. These results raise the possibility that a control mechanism is operating to limit the number of eosinophils produced when large amounts of IL-5 are produced.

The observation that IL-5 in transgenic mice is capable of inducing the full pathway of eosinophil production leaves unresolved why IL-5 appears unable to induce the production of eosinophil progenitors *in vitro*. One possibility is that the action of IL-5 is uniquely dependent on the stromal cells for the production of the progenitor cells. Although there is no direct evidence for this, there are a number of factors which suggest that IL-5 may be at least partially dependent on stromal cells even in the later stages of eosinophil differentiation. For example, in the mouse system few eosino-phil colonies form in semi-solid medium, whereas large numbers of eosinophils are produced in the adherent layer of stromal cells in liquid culture (Warren and Sanderson, 1985; Sanderson *et al.*, 1985; Strath *et al.*, 1990). Secondly, in human liquid bone marrow cultures more eosinophils are produced in round-bottomed vessels than in flat-bottomed vessels, possibly as a result of better cell–cell interactions (Clutterbuck and Sander-son, 1988). Thirdly, although, in contrast to the mouse, human eosinophil colonies are produced in semi-solid cultures, the number is significantly lower in the presence of IL-5 compared with either IL-3 or GM-CSF. However, in liquid cultures the situation is reversed and IL-5 stimulates the production of more eosinophils than either IL-3 or GM-CSF. This is again consistent with a requirement for stromal cells by IL-5.

Another important approach to the understanding of the biological role of IL-5 comes from the administration of neutralizing antibody. Mice infected with *Trichinella spiralis* develop eosinophilia and increased levels of IgE; however, when treated with an anti-IL-5 antibody no eosinophils were observed (Coffman *et al.*, 1989). Indeed, the number of eosinophils was lower than the numbers seen in control animals. These experiments illustrate the unique role of IL-5 in the control of eosinophilia in this parasite infection. They also show that the apparent redundancy seen *in vitro*, where both IL-3 and GM-CSF are also able to induce eosinophil production, does not operate in these infections. Furthermore, IL-5 played no role in the development of IgE antibody (this activity is controlled by

IL-4), or in the development of the granuloma seen surrounding schistosomes in the tissues (Sher *et al.*, 1990).

Although eosinophils may exacerbate allergic diseases they do not appear to be harmful in normal animals. Mice infected with *Mesocestoides corti* show no ill effects throughout the period of massive eosinophilia. Transgenic mice expressing IL-5 have lifelong high level eosinophilia, but show no obvious ill effects and appear to live a normal life. Individuals with eosinophilia owing to infestations of parasitic helminths do not appear to suffer harmful effects from the eosinophils.

15.5 Conclusion

The demonstration of the central role of IL-5 in the control of eosinophilia and the recognition of the eosinophil as capable of causing host tissue damage in allergic diseases opens up the possibility that IL-5 antagonists may provide a new therapeutic approach to these diseases.

References

Basten, A. and Beeson, P. B. (1970). Mechanism of eosinophilia. II. Role of the lymphocyte. *J. Exp. Med.*, **131**, 1288–305.

Begley, C. G., Lopez, A. F., Nicola, N. A., Warren, D. J., Vadas, M. A., Sanderson, C. J. and Metcalf, D. (1986). Purified colony stimulating factors enhance the survival of human neutrophils and eosinophils *in vitro*: a rapid and sensitive microassay for colony stimulating factors. *Blood*, **68**, 162–6.

Burd, P. R., Rogers, H. W., Gordon, J. R., Martin, C. A., Jayaraman, S., Wilson, S. D., Dvorak, A. M., Galli, S. J. and Dorf, M. E. (1989). Interleukin-3-dependent and -independent mast cells stimulated with IgE and antigen express multiple cytokines. *J. Exp. Med.*, **170**, 245–57.

Butterworth, A. E. (1984). Cell-mediated damage to helminths. *Adv. Parasitol.*, **23**, 143–235.

Butterworth, A. E., Sturrock, R. F., Houba, V., Mahmoud, A. A., Sher, A. and Rees, P. H. (1975). Eosinophils as mediators of antibody-dependent damage to schistosomula. *Nature (London)*, **256**, 727–9.

Campbell, H. D., Tucker, W. Q., Hort, Y., Martinson, M. E., Mayo, G., Clutterbuck, E. J., Sanderson, C. J. and Young, I. G. (1987). Molecular cloning, nucleotide sequence, and expression of the gene encoding human eosinophil differentiation factor (interleukin-5). *Proc. Natl. Acad. Sci. USA*, **84**, 6629–33.

Campbell, H. D., Sanderson, C. J., Wang, Y., Hort, Y., Martinson, M. E., Tucker, W. Q., Stellwagen, A., Strath, M. and Young, I. G. (1988). Isolation, structure and expression of cDNA and genomic clones for murine eosinophil differentiation factor. Comparison with other eosinophilopoietic lymphokines and identity with interleukin-5. *Eur. J. Biochem.*, **174**, 345–52.

Chandrasekharappa, S. C., Rebelsky, M. S., Firak, T. A., Le Beau, M. M. and

Westbrook, C. A. (1990). A long-range restriction map of the interleukin-4 and interleukin-5 linkage group on chromosome 5. *Genomics*, **6**, 94–9.

Clutterbuck, E. J. and Sanderson, C. J. (1988). Human eosinophil hematopoiesis studied *in vitro* by means of murine eosinophil differentiation factor (IL-5): production of functionally active eosinophils from normal human bone marrow. *Blood*, **71**, 646–51.

Clutterbuck, E. J. and Sanderson, C. J. (1990). The regulation of human eosinophil precursor production by cytokines: a comparison of rhIL-1, rhIL-3, rhIL-4, rhIL-6 and GM-CSF. *Blood*, **75**, 1774–9.

Clutterbuck, E. J., Hirst, E. M. and Sanderson, C. J. (1989). Human interleukin-5 (IL-5) regulates the production of eosinophils in human bone marrow cultures: comparison and interaction with IL-1, IL-3, IL-6, and GMCSF. *Blood*, **73**, 1504–12.

Coffman, R. L., Seymour, B. W., Hudak, S., Jackson, J. and Rennick, D. (1989). Antibody to interleukin-5 inhibits helminth-induced eosinophilia in mice. *Science*, **245**, 308–10.

Dent, L. A., Strath, M., Mellor, A. L. and Sanderson, C. J. (1990). Eosinophilia in transgenic mice expressing interleukin-5. *J. Exp. Med.*, **172**, 1425–31.

Dexter, T. M., Allen, T. D. and Lajtha, L. G. (1977). Conditions controlling the proliferation of haemopoietic stem cells in culture. *J. Cell. Physiol.*, **91**, 335–44.

Fujisawa, T., Abu-Ghazaleh, R., Kita, H., Sanderson, C. J. and Gleich, G. J. (1990). Regulatory effect of cytokines on eosinophil degranulation. *J. Immunol.*, **144**, 642–6.

Gleich, G. J. and Adolphson, C. R. (1986). The eosinophilc leukocyte: structure and function. *Adv. Immunol.*, **39**, 177–253.

Goetzl, E. J., Wasserman, S. I. and Austen, K. F. (1975). Eosinophil polymorphonuclear function in immediate hypersensitivity. *Arch. Pathol.*, **99**, 1–4.

Kay, A. B. (1990). In Kay, A. B. (ed.), *Eosinophils, Allergy and Asthma*, Blackwell, Oxford, 31–44.

Lee, J. S., Campbell, H. D., Kozak, C. A. and Young, I. G. (1989). The IL-4 and IL-5 genes are closely linked and are part of a cytokine gene cluster on mouse chromosome 11. *Somat. Cell. Mol. Genet.*, **15**, 143–52.

Lopez, A. F. and Sanderson, C. J. (1982). Antibody-dependent, cell mediated cytotoxicity of nucleated mammalian cells by rat eosinophils and neutrophils. *Int. Arch. Allergy Appl. Immunol.*, **67**, 200–5.

Lopez, A. F., Strath, M. and Sanderson, C. J. (1981). IgG and complement receptors on purified mouse eosinophils and neutrophils. *Immunology*, **43**, 779–86.

Lopez, A. F., Begley, C. G., Williamson, D. J., Warren, D. J., Vadas, M. A. and Sanderson, C. J. (1986). Murine eosinophil differentiation factor. An eosinophil-specific colony stimulating factor with activity for human cells. *J. Exp. Med.*, **163**, 1085–99.

Lopez, A. F., Sanderson, C. J., Gamble, J. R., Campbell, H. D., Young, I. G. and Vadas, M. A. (1988). Recombinant human interleukin-5 is a selective activator of human eosinophil function. *J. Exp. Med.*, **167**, 219–24.

Maxwell, C., Hussain, R., Nutman, T. B., Poindexter, R. W., Little, M. D., Schad, G. A. and Ottesen, E. A. (1987). The clinical and immunologic responses of normal human volunteers to low dose hookworm (*Necator americanus*) infection. *Am. J. Trop. Med. Hyg.*, **37**, 126–34.

McKenzie, A. N. J., Ely, B. and Sanderson, C. J. (1991). Mutated interleukin-5 monomers are biologically inactive. *Mol. Immunol.*, **28**, 155–8.

Minamitake, Y., Kodama, S., Katayama, T., Adachi, H., Tanaka, S. and Tsujimoto, M. (1990). Structure of recombinant human interleukin-5 produced by Chinese hamster ovary cells. *J. Biochem. Tokyo*, **107**, 292–7.

Paul, C. C., Keller, J. R., Armpriester, J. M. and Baumann, M. A. (1990). Epstein–Barr virus transformed B lymphocytes produce interleukin-5. *Blood*, **75**, 1400–3.

Plaut, M., Pierce, J. H., Watson, C. J., Hanley-Hyde, J., Nordan, R. P. and Paul, W. E. (1989). Mast cell lines produce lymphokines in response to cross-linkage of Fc epsilon RI or to calcium ionophores. *Nature (London)*, **339**, 64–7.

Sanderson, C. J. (1990). In Dexter, T. M., Garland, J. M. and Testa, N. G. (eds.), *Colony Stimulating Factors: Molecular and Cellular Biology*, Dekker, New York, 231–56.

Sanderson, C. J. and Thomas, J. A. (1978). A comparison between the cytotoxic activity of eosinophils and other cells by ^{51}Cr release and time lapse microcinematography. *Immunology*, **34**, 771–80.

Sanderson, C. J., Lopez, A. F. and Bunn Moreno, M. M. (1977). Eosinophils and not lymphoid K cells kill *Trypanosoma cruzi* epimastigotes. *Nature (London)*, **268**, 340–1.

Sanderson, C. J., Warren, D. J. and Strath, M. (1985). Identification of a lymphokine that stimulates eosinophil differentiation *in vitro*. Its relationship to IL-3, and functional properties of eosinophils produced in cultures. *J. Exp. Med.*, **162**, 60–74.

Sanderson, C. J., Campbell, H. D. and Young, I. G. (1988). Molecular and cellular biology of eosinophil differentiation factor (interleukin-5) and its effects on human and mouse B cells. *Immunol. Rev.*, **102**, 29–50.

Sher, A., Coffman, R. L., Hieny, S., Scott, P. and Cheever, A. W. (1990). Interleukin-5 is required for the blood and tissue eosinophilia but not granuloma formation induced by infection with *Schistosoma mansoni*. *Proc. Natl. Acad. Sci. USA*, **87**, 61–5.

Silberstein, D. S. and David, J. R. (1987). The regulation of human eosinophil function by cytokines. *Immunol. Today*, **8**, 380–5.

Strath, M. and Sanderson, C. J. (1986). Detection of eosinophil differentiation factor and its relationship to eosinophilia in *Mesocestoides corti*-infected mice. *Exp. Hematol.*, **14**, 16–20.

Strath, M., Clutterbuck, E. J. and Sanderson, C. J. (1990). In Pollard, J. W. and Walker, J. M. (eds.), *Methods in Molecular Biology*, Vol. 5, *Animal Cell Culture*, Humana Press, Clifton, NJ, 361–78.

Strath, M., Dent, L. A. and Sanderson, C. J. (1992). Infection of IL-5 transgenic mice with *Mesocestoides corti* induces very high levels of IL-5 but depressed production of eosinophils. *Exp. Hematol.*, **20**, 229–34.

Sutherland, G. R., Baker, E., Callen, D. F., Campbell, H. D., Young, I. G., Sanderson, C. J., Garson, O. M., Lopez, A. F. and Vadas, M. A. (1988). Interleukin-5 is at 5q31 and is deleted in the 5q⁻ syndrome. *Blood*, **71**, 1150–2.

Takahashi, T., Yamaguchi, N., Mita, S., Yamaguchi, Y., Suda, T., Tominaga, A., Kikuchi, Y., Miura, Y. and Takatsu, K. (1990). Structural comparison of murine T-cell (B151K12)-derived T-cell-replacing factor (IL-5) with rIL-5: dimer formation is essential for the expression of biological activity. *Mol. Immunol.*, **27**, 911–20.

Tominaga, A., Takahashi, T., Kikuchi, Y., Mita, S., Noami, S., Harada, N., Yamaguchi, N. and Takatsu, K. (1990). Role of carbohydrate moiety of IL-5: effect of tunicamycin on the glycosyation of IL-5 and the biologic activity of deglycosylated IL-5. *J. Immunol.*, **144**, 1345–52.

Tsuruoka, N., Funakoshi, K., Kodama, S. and Tsujimoto, M. (1990). Interaction of interleukin-5 with its receptors on murine leukaemic BCL1 cells and its implication in biological activity. *Cell. Immunol.*, **125**, 354–62.

van-Leeuwen, B. H., Martinson, M. E., Webb, G. C. and Young, I. G. (1989). Molecular organization of the cytokine gene cluster, involving the human IL-3, IL-4, IL-5, and GM-CSF genes, on human chromosome. *Blood*, **73**, 1142–8.

Walsh, G. M., Hartnell, A., Wardlaw, A. J., Kurihara, K., Sanderson, C. J. and Kay, A. B. (1990). IL-5 enhances the *in vitro* adhesion of human eosinophils, but not neutrophils, in a leucocyte integrin (CD11/18)-dependent manner. *Immunology*, **71**, 258–65.

Wang, J. M., Rambaldi, A., Biondi, A., Chen, Z. G., Sanderson, C. J. and Mantovani, A. (1989). Recombinant human interleukin-5 is a selective eosinophil chemoattractant. *Eur. J. Immunol.*, **19**, 701–5.

Warren, D. J. and Sanderson, C. J. (1985). Production of a T cell hybrid producing a lymphokine stimulating eosinophil differentiation. *Immunology*, **54**, 615–23.

Wegner, C. D., Gundel, R. H., Reilly, P., Haynes, N., Letts, L. G. and Rothlein, R. (1990). Intercellular adhesion molecule-1 (ICAM-1) in the pathogenesis of asthma. *Science*, **247**, 456–9.

Yamaguchi, Y., Suda, T., Suda, J., Eguchi, M., Miura, Y., Harada, N., Tominaga, A. and Takatsu, K. (1988). Purified interleukin-5 supports the terminal differentiation and proliferation of murine eosinophilic precursors. *J. Exp. Med.*, **167**, 43–56.

16

The Interaction of Interleukin-1 With the Actors of Asthma

J.-M. Cavaillon

16.1 Interleukin-1: A Pivot Molecule in Inflammation and Immune Response

In 1979, the term 'interleukin-1' (IL-1) was proposed to denote what appeared to be the same factor for which different names had been given according to various biological activities. At the time, it was clear that the same molecule could act on very different targets such as lymphocytes, fibroblasts, hepatocytes, the central nervous system, chondrocytes, bone marrow cells, endothelial cells, neutrophils, etc. (see Dinarello, 1991, for a review). As early as 1977, biochemical characterization led to the discovery of two molecules with different isoelectric points. Cloning of the genes in 1984–1985 confirmed the existence of two related molecules, called IL-1α and IL-1β, with 26% homology. The genes (six coding exons and one non-coding exon), located on chromosome 2 in humans, code for two precursor forms of 30.5 kDa molecules (pro-IL-1). Only pro-IL-1α is biologically active. Pro-IL-1 is cleaved to mature forms of 17.5 kDa. Contrary to other cytokines, IL-1 lacks a signal peptide and secretion of the molecule would require special mechanisms (Rubartelli *et al.*, 1990). In fact, following a triggering signal large amounts of IL-1 are accumulated within the cells. A membrane form, only constituted by IL-1α, has also been described (Kurt-Jones *et al.*, 1986; Bailly *et al.*, 1990a). Both precursors and mature forms are found in the supernatants of activated cells (Beuscher *et al.*, 1990); IL-1β is the main form released by human monocytes–macrophages. Cleavage of pro-IL-1 requires the actions of proteolytic enzymes either produced by the activated cells or found in the environment of inflammation (Hazuda et al., 1990). Monocytes and macrophages appear to be the main sources of IL-1; however, many other cell types, including endothelial cells, neutrophils, eosinophils, are able to produce IL-1 upon adequate stimulation. Epidermic cells have been described so far as the only cells able spontaneously to produce IL-1 (mainly IL-1α). An 80 kDa IL-1α/β receptor (IL-1 R type I), of which the gene is localized on chromosome 2, has been cloned (Sims et al., 1988). This belongs to the immunoglobulin superfamily and is mainly found on T cells, fibroblasts and smooth muscle cells. A second IL-1 receptor has been characterized (IL-1 R type II) (Chizzonite et al., 1989). It is a 60–65 kDa glycoprotein shorter in its intracellular region than the IL-1 R type I and which shares 28% homology in its extracellular domain with the type I. Interestingly, an IL-1 receptor antagonist (IL-1 Ra) has been recently cloned (Eisenberg et al., 1990). It shares 26% homology with IL-1β and 19% with IL-1α. So far all tested in vitro and in vivo activities of IL-1 can be blocked by this IL-1 Ra, which binds to the IL-1 receptor but does not initiate IL-1 signal transduction (Dripps et al., 1991).

Interleukin-1 is involved in the modulation of the immune response. Produced in the context of antigen presentation, IL-1 increases the antibody response as well as the anti-infectious immunity. In addition, IL-1 has been shown to possess some anti-tumoral activities, to amplify haematopoiesis, to induce the proliferation of certain types of cells (fibroblasts, synovial cells, keratynocytes, . . .) and to act on the central nervous system, inducing fever, slow wave sleep, anorexia and production of adrenocorticotropic hormone (ACTH) and corticotropin-releasing factor (CRF). Finally, IL-1 is one of the mediators involved in inflammation (Cavaillon, 1990). This last activity reflects the great efficacy of IL-1 in inducing the production of lipid mediators and other cytokines such as interleukin-6 and interleukin-8. IL-1 can trigger the production of prostaglandins by many cell types, of platelet-activating factor (PAF) by monocytes and endothelial cells, and of leukotrienes by neutrophils. Thus, IL-1 favours the production of agents which are directly involved in the process of asthma leading to smooth muscle contraction, mucosal oedema, cellular infiltration and mucus secretion (Fig. 16.1). For example, mucus secretion has been demonstrated to occur in mouse intestinal explants in the presence of IL-1 (Han et al., 1987). However, one should note that IL-1 can modify cell function independently of prostanoid synthesis and acts differently as shown by its ability to inhibit contraction of vascular smooth muscle (Beasley et al., 1989). Indeed, IL-1 acts as a pivot molecule within the cytokine network and, as a key regulatory factor in inflammatory processes, plays a role together with numerous other actors in the asthma reaction.

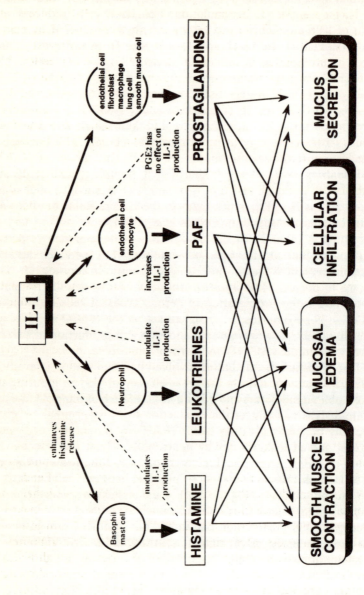

Fig. 16.1 Relationship between IL-1 and the direct mediators of the asthmatic reaction.

16.2 Production of Interleukin-1

Atopy-related Production of IL-1

In *in vitro* studies, endotoxins (lipopolysaccharides, LPS) from Gram-negative bacteria appear to be among the most potent IL-1 inducers, and picograms of LPS are sufficient to induce the synthesis of IL-1 by human monocytes (Cavaillon and Haeffner-Cavaillon, 1990). Thus investigations with other putative inducers should be carefully analysed since low LPS contaminations are very frequent and suffice for the induction of IL-1. Polymyxin B has been widely used to ensure that the observed IL-1 induction was not due to the presence of LPS, although its neutralizing activity depends upon the origin of the LPS (Cavaillon and Haeffner-Cavaillon, 1986). In this context Enk and Mosbech (1988) have established that mite allergen crude extracts could trigger the production of IL-1 by human monocytes. We have also shown that purified allergenic constituents prepared from mite and pollen were able to induce the release of IL-1 (Cavaillon *et al.*, 1984). However, we further observed that LPS contaminations were interfering with the observed phenomenon (unpublished observation) and it was probable that a synergy existed between allergens and endotoxins. Indeed, many signals have been shown to act synergistically with endotoxins, leading to increased IL-1 production. This is for example the case for the anaphylatoxins C3a and C5a (Haeffner-Cavaillon *et al.*, 1987; Cavaillon *et al.*, 1990a), produced following complement activation and well known to induce histamine release. In fact, naturally occurring pneumo-allergens are not 'LPS free', and alveolar macrophages might be exposed to a complex mixture of molecules including LPS. For example, it was reported that the most severe upper airway irritation among poultry farm workers was at sites where levels of dust and endotoxin were high (Thelin *et al.*, 1984). Furthermore, it was suggested that airway hyperreactivity and chronic inflammation observed in cotton workers could be due to the presence of endotoxins in cotton dust (Rylander, 1987). It was also shown that airborne endotoxin in dust may play an important role in the development of symptoms and lung function changes among pig farmers (Heederick *et al.*, 1991). Finally, the role of endotoxin in dust was evaluated in asthma. Michel *et al.* (1989) showed that acute inhalation of lipopolysaccharide induced in asthmatic though not in normal subjects a bronchial obstruction associated with an increase in histamine bronchial responsiveness. Most interestingly, Michel *et al.* (1991) observed among asthmatic patients a significant correlation between high levels of endotoxin in domestic dust and greater bronchodilator and oral corticosteroid intake, greater dyspnea and reduced FEV_1/FVC (forced expired volume/forced vital capacity). Demonstration of *in vivo* production of IL-1 upon allergenic stimulation remains rare. In this context, the work reported by Bochner *et al.* (1990b) is of particular importance. These authors demonstrated that in atopic patients IL-1β could be detected in the fluid of skin chambers after challenge with ragweed, whereas no IL-1β was found in controls. This difference between healthy donors and atopic patients may suggest a role of specific IgE antibodies. Whether monocytes–macrophages can be triggered to produce IL-1 upon activation through their Fc receptors remains an open question. Arend *et al.* (1985) using endotoxin-free immune complexes failed to detect IL-1 activity in the supernatants of human monocytes, whereas Chantry *et al.* (1989) could observe such a production which was not modified upon polymyxin B addition. More recently, Simms *et al.* (1991) have established that FcγR-mediated IL-1 production enhances the phagocytic function of neighbouring neutrophils and monocytes. Triggering of rat macrophages via their Fcε receptor by IgE immune complexes was shown to lead to IL-1 production (Mazingue *et al.*, 1987). A similar observation was reported when monocytes from asthmatic patients were triggered by anti-IgE antibodies (Gosset *et al.*, 1988). Of particular importance was the discovery by Borish *et al.* (1991) that IgE immune complexes can induce the production of IL-1β but not IL-1α by monocytes from asthmatic patients, whereas no activation of monocytes from healthy donors was observed. This phenomenon probably reflects the higher number of Fcε receptor positive (or CD23+) monocytes found in atopic (Melewicz *et al.*, 1981) and asthmatic (Borish *et al.*, 1991) patients.

Human alveolar macrophages differ from blood monocytes in their ability to produce IL-1β upon LPS stimulation (Bernaudin *et al.*, 1988; Wewers and Herzyk, 1989), i.e. IL-1β mRNA production and IL-1β release are lower in LPS-stimulated alveolar macrophages. Gamma interferon can markedly augment this production (Eden and Turino, 1986). Unstimulated alveolar macrophages from healthy donors do not produce IL-1 whereas, as expected, it was found that, during lung infections, IL-1 can be detected in the alveolar lavages or 'spontaneously' produced by alveolar macrophages (Lamontagne *et al.*, 1985; Vacheron *et al.*, 1990). Of particular importance is the work recently published by Pujol *et al.* (1990) who reported that unstimulated alveolar macrophages from patients suffering from allergic or intrinsic asthma were spontaneously releasing IL-1 following a 20 h culture. This observation for alveolar macrophages had not been found by Gosset *et al.* (1988) although these authors reported an elevated spontaneous IL-1 release by monocytes from asthmatic patients. These very crucial observations lead to a new field of investigations. Does this *in vitro* spontaneous production reflect a higher reactivity of the cells to culture conditions? Indeed, it has been shown that adherence itself can trigger IL-1 production (Fuhlbrigge *et al.*, 1987), very probably through the stimulation of adhesion-promoting proteins (Couturier *et al.*, 1990). Alternatively, do freshly isolated cells already contain IL-1? The answers to these questions would definitively establish whether environmental conditions related to the lungs of asthmatic patients can trigger the production of IL-1 by alveolar macrophages or enhance their reactivity. In agreement with the study of Hsieh and Lue (1987) on monocytes, the LPS-induced section of IL-1 by alveolar macrophages was not significantly different between normal and asthmatic patients (Pujol *et al.*, 1990). Upon stimulation by allergen or anti-IgE, Gosset *et al.* (1988) reported that alveolar macrophages from asthmatic patients release an IL-1 inhibitory activity which differs from PGE_2 or serum protease. Last but not least is the recent and fascinating description by Burd *et al.* (1989) of mast cells as IL-1 producer cells in response to IgE and antigen. These authors have shown that, among many other cytokines, mast cell clones and bone marrow derived mast cells which do not express IL-1 mRNA spontaneously are driven to synthesize mRNAs as well as bioactivity for IL-1 upon stimulation by IgE plus antigen. Whether this phenomenon occurs *in vivo* remains to be fully established, but, if it is the case, this might represent an important local source of IL-1 specifically encountered upon allergen activation.

Regulation of IL-1 Production

Histamine, prostaglandins, leukotrienes, and platelet-activating factor (PAF) are among the different mediators responsible for the pathological changes in asthma. Furthermore, cytokines such as IL-3, which primes basophils for histamine release, and IL-4, which favours IgE secretion, might be encountered in the process of asthma. In this section we will analyse whether these agents can modulate the IL-1 production.

As far as histamine is concerned, contradictory results have been reported. Histamine itself was shown by Okamoto *et al.* (1990) and Okamoto and Nakano (1990) to induce the production of IL-1 and to act synergistically with LPS. On the contrary, other authors reported an inhibitory effect on LPS-induced IL-1 production (Manosroi *et al.*, 1987; Dohlsten *et al.*, 1988). One should note that rather non-physiological concentrations were employed in these studies (10^{-5} to 10^{-3} M). Working with purified human monocytes, we have never succeeded in finding any modulatory activity of histamine (10^{-7} to 10^{-5} M) on IL-1 production (unpublished observation). In agreement with our observation, Dinarello and his colleagues (personal communication) have recently observed that histamine had no effect on *in vitro* IL-1 production by purified human monocytes, whereas, when experiments were performed with whole peripheral blood mononuclear cells, histamine reduced the LPS-induced IL-1 production. Interestingly, histamine had suppressive effects on tumour necrosis factor α (TNFα) production whatever the cell population (Vannier *et al.*, 1991). These authors showed that the inhibitory activity was mediated by H_2 receptors.

For a long time the dogma was that prostaglandin E_2 could inhibit the production of IL-1. In fact, artifactual results were behind the interference of prostaglandins in the biological assay for IL-1 (i.e. the so-called thymocyte co-mitogenic assay). Since then, Northern analysis, specific ELISAs or RIAs have been used and it has become clear that, in fact, PGE_2 does not interfere at all with IL-1 production, whereas it suppresses that of TNFα (Scales *et al.*, 1989; Bailly *et al.*, 1990b).

Contradictory results have been published concerning the effect of leukotrienes on IL-1 production. Addition of exogeneous leukotrienes has been shown to augment IL-1 production (Rola-Pleszczynski and Lemavic, 1985; Tatsuno *et al.*, 1990), whereas addition of lipoxygenase inhibitors either did not modify or even enhanced IL-1 synthesis (Parkar *et al.*, 1990; Sirko *et al.*, 1991).

PAF has been unanimously shown by many authors (Pignol *et al.*, 1990; Barthelson *et al.*, 1990; Poubelle *et al.*, 1991) to potentiate, *in vitro*, IL-1 synthesis and to prime cells for a further enhanced IL-1 production. Whether the phenomenon occurs *in vivo* remains to be demonstrated, since PAF which also enhances TNFα production *in vitro* decreases TNFα in the plasma of mice treated with endotoxin (Ferguson-Chanowitz *et al.*, 1990).

Histamine and lipid mediators are not the only factors able to modulate the activation of monocytes–macrophages leading to IL-1 production. Within a rather complex network, other cytokines may enhance or decrease the release of IL-1. This is the case for certain cytokines which can be induced upon T-cell activation by IL-1. For example, together with Weiss *et al.* (1989) we showed that interleukin-4 inhibits the release of IL-1 by LPS-stimulated human monocytes. The inhibitory activity of IL-4 on cytokine production by monocytes–macrophages has also been shown for TNFα and IL-6, and it has been demonstrated that IL-4 suppresses the expression of IL-1 mRNA (Essner *et al.*, 1989; Hart *et al.*, 1989). On the contrary, other cytokines such as γ interferon, granulocyte–macrophage-colony stimulating factor and IL-3 act as 'macrophage activating factors'. We have reported that interleukin-3 enhances the production of IL-1, as well as that of TNF and IL-6, by LPS-stimulated macrophages (Cohen *et al.*, 1991). Frendl *et al.* (1990) showed that IL-3 itself induces IL-1 mRNA in the absence of IL-1 bioactivity expression and heightens IL-1 mRNA and IL-1 bioactivity synergistically with suboptimal doses of LPS.

Altogether these data indicate that IL-1 production depends upon a complex balance between negative and amplificatory signals which might evolve as an asthmatic reaction is occurring.

16.3 Modulation of IgE Synthesis by IL-1

The participation of IL-1 in B-cell activation and IgE production occur at both the B and T cell level. A helper T cell dichotomy (Th1–Th2), as a function of cytokine production, has been described in the mouse model and probably exists in the human system (Mossman and Moore, 1991). Unlike Th1 cells, Th2 cells produce IL-4, IL-5, IL-6, and IL-10 but do not synthesize IL-2, TNFβ and γ interferon (γIFN). Both subpopulations produce IL-3 and GM-CSF granulocyte–macrophage colony stimulating factor). IL-4 is the main cytokine which enables the production of IgE by B-cells (see Ohara, 1989, for a review), whereas γIFN inhibits the IL-4 dependent IgE synthesis (Chrétien *et al.*, 1990). IL-1 favours the proliferation of helper T cells which preferentially secrete IL-4 (Chang *et al.*, 1990), and it was shown that the *in vivo* administration of IL-1 in mice induces the expression of IL-4 mRNA in lymph nodes and the spleen (Killar *et al.*, 1989). Furthermore, IL-1 can potentiate the production of IL-4 by other cell types such as stromal cells (King *et al.*, 1988). The action of IL-1 on Th2 cells reflects that this subpopulation expresses high affinity receptors for IL-1 whereas Th1 cells do not (Lichtman *et al.*, 1988). In addition to its action on T cells, IL-1 can act on B cells as a cell growth and differentiation factor (Pike and Nassal, 1985). Although IL-1 is an important co-factor of B-cell activation it does not seem to interfere with IgE synthesis induced by IL-4 in humans (Maliszewski *et al.*, 1990), although it was shown that IL-1 enhances IgE synthesis by rat lymphocytes (Mazingue *et al.*, 1987). This last observation might reflect the capacity of IL-1 to induce PGE_2 formation and the capacity of these prostaglandins to enhance IL-4 induced IgE synthesis (Roper *et al.*, 1990).

Normal donors and atopic patients have similar lymphocyte proliferative responses to purified allergens (Cavaillon *et al.*, 1988). Interestingly, it has been demonstrated that most allergen-specific T cell clones derived from atopic or asthmatic patients are able to produce IL-4 but not γIFN (Parronchi *et al.*, 1991; Wierenga *et al.*, 1990). The frequency of allergen-specific clones derived from atopic patients and able to secrete IL-4 was higher than among clones derived from a non-atopic donor or among bacteria-specific clones. Similarly, studies by *in situ* hybridization of skin biopsies from allergen-induced late-phase cutaneous reactions revealed that mRNA for IL-4 (as well as for IL-3 and IL-5) was often detectable, whereas no hybridization signals were obtained for γIFN (Kay *et al.*, 1991). However, no differences in IL-4 and γIFN mRNA levels were observed in peripheral blood mononuclear cells of normal donors and allergic donors, following allergen-specific stimulation (Gauchat *et al.*, 1991). Nevertheless, most of the studies support the hypothesis that atopy is associated with preferential activation of cells having a similar cytokine profile to the Th2 subset.

16.4 Activities of IL-1 on Basophils and Mast Cells

Numerous so-called 'histamine-releasing factors' were described before recombinant cytokines became available and were tested for their abilities to induce histamine release. The first studies indicated that IL-1 had the ability to trigger histamine release by basophils and mast cells (Subramanian and Bray, 1987; Haak-Frendscho et al., 1988a; Alam et al., 1989). However, they were often performed in the presence of a rather non-physiological buffer containing D_2O. Using a more accurate medium, we have never succeeded in inducing significant histamine release by human basophils in the presence of recombinant IL-1β (unpublished observation). Similarly, Massey et al. (1989) and Brunner et al. (1991) reported that IL-1 alone failed to induce histamine release whereas it can upregulate the response to IgE-related signals. These results do not exclude the possibility that in vivo IL-1 itself is able to activate basophils or mast cells. Indeed, histological observations of rat skin sections pretreated with IL-1β revealed an increased number of degranulated mast cells (Martin et al., 1988). We have shown that IL-1 can induce the production of IL-3 (Cavaillon et al., 1990b) and many studies have reported that IL-3 can be considered as a histamine-releasing factor (Haak-Frendscho et al., 1988b). IL-3 alone is more active on cells from atopic than from normal donors (MacDonald et al., 1989). Furthermore, IL-3 primes basophils and enhances their histamine release induced by anti-IgE (Hirai et al., 1988; Valent et al., 1989), C5a (Kurimoto et al., 1989) C3a (Bischoff et al., 1990), PAF (Brunner et al., 1991), and IL-8 (Dahinden et al., 1989). In this last context one should remember that IL-1 is a potent inducer of IL-8. Furthermore, IL-1 is also able to induce the production of PAF, a factor which has been shown to lead to histamine release in 60% of the tested donors (Columbo et al., 1990). Altogether these results suggest that IL-1 is able to contribute to the activation of basophils leading to an enhancement of histamine release, although its direct activity is minimal.

16.5 IL-1 and Leukocyte Recruitment

In his elegant review, Schleimer et al. (1991) presented the mechanisms involved in leukocyte recruitment in the lung and overviewed the role of cytokines in the different steps of this phenomenon, i.e. adherence of leukocytes to vascular endothelium, diapedesis, chemotaxis and leukocyte priming. In vivo experiments have demonstrated that IL-1 leads to pulmonary leukostasis (Goldblum et al., 1987; Heidel et al., 1990). The first step of this mechanism is due to an increase of adherence molecules on the surface of endothelial cells upon IL-1 activation. These cell markers include the CD18 complex and particularly the 'leukocyte function-associated antigen-1' (LFA-1) (Pohlman *et al.*, 1986), the 'endothelial leukocyte adhesion molecule-1' (ELAM-1), the 'intercellular adhesion molecule-1' (ICAM-1) (Wellicome *et al.*, 1990; Kyan-Aung *et al.*, 1991) and the 'vascular cell adhesion molecule-1' (VCAM-1) (Carlos *et al.*, 1990). These cell surface antigens are involved not only in neutrophil adherence to endothelium but also in the increased adhesiveness described for B and T lymphocytes (Cavender *et al.*, 1986), monocytes (Carlos *et al.*, 1991) basophils (Bochner *et al.*, 1991), and eosinophils (Kyan-Aung *et al.*, 1991). 'Very late antigen 4' (VLA 4) has been described as a specific ligand for eosinophils involved in their adhesiveness to endothelial cells, though not for neutrophils (Walsh *et al.*, 1991a). Other cytokines such as IL-4 can potentiate the IL-1-induced increased adherence for leukocytes to endothelium (Masinowsky *et al.*, 1990). Furthermore, TNFα, which shares with IL-1 many of its activities, is also able to contribute to an augmentation of adhesion molecules on endothelial cells (Walsh *et al.*, 1991b). IL-3 has also been reported to augment adhesiveness of basophils for endothelium (Bochner *et al.*, 1990a). In addition to IL-1 induced adherence of leukocytes to endothelial cells, IL-1, as well as TNFα, promotes the transendothelial passage of neutrophils (Moser *et al.*, 1989) and increases the vascular endothelial permeability (Royall *et al.*, 1989). Furthermore, IL-1 and TNFα are potent inducers of MCP-1, a chemoattractant factor for monocytes and basophils, and IL-8, which is a well-known chemotactic factor for neutrophils and basophils (see Oppenheim *et al.*, 1991, for a review). IL-8 is also a potent activator of neutrophil functions including enhancement of respiratory burst, induction of LTB_4, release of elastase and lactoferrin. IL-8 is a member of the so-called 'small cytokine super-family' which includes many similar cytokines. One of them might be the neutrophil chemotactic factor described by Corrigan *et al.* (1991) as being different from IL-8 and spontaneously synthesized by peripheral blood mononuclear cells from patients with acute asthma.

16.6 Conclusion

We have summarized in Fig. 16.2 some of the activities of IL-1 which are relevant to the allergic and/or asthmatic reaction. We have reviewed above that IL-1 can be produced in the context of an allergic response. Endocrine activities of IL-1 can be observed on many different target organs and paracrine activities within its local site of production can modulate the functions of surrounding cells. In addition to its ability to induce the synthesis of lipid mediators by many cell types (see Fig. 16.1), IL-1 can directly trigger endothelial cells, neutrophils, eosinophils, basophils, and

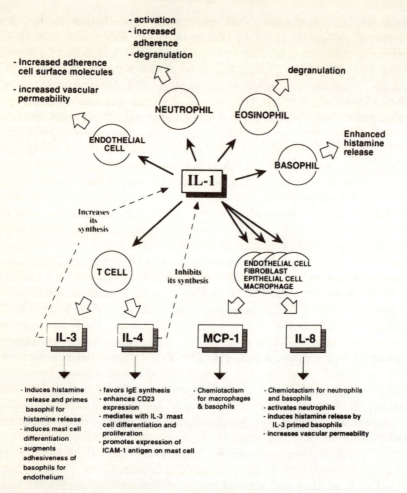

Fig. 16.2 Summary of the activities of IL-1 which are relevant to the allergic and/or asthmatic reaction.

thus, favours an inflammatory response. Furthermore, IL-1, as an initiator of the cytokine cascade, induces the production of IL-3, IL-4, MCP-1, IL-8 (etc.) which might be involved in an amplificatory loop favouring the asthma reaction. The purpose of this review was not to describe IL-1 as a main agent of asthma but rather to illustrate how a cytokine which is involved in both immune and inflammatory responses may contribute to a pathological reaction.

References

Alam, R., Welter, J. B., Forsythe, P. A., Lett-Brown, M. A. and Grant, J. A. (1989). Comparative effect of recombinant IL-1, -2, -3, -4, and -6, IFN-γ granulocyte–macrophage-colony-stimulating factor, tumor necrosis factor-α, and histamine-releasing factors on the secretion of histamine from basophils. *J. Immunol.*, **142**, 3431–5.

Arend, W. P., Joslin, F. G. and Massoni, R. J. (1985). Effects of immune complexes on production by human monocytes of interleukin-1 or an interleukin-1 inhibitor. *J. Immunol.*, **134**, 3868–75.

Bailly, S., Ferrua, B., Fay, M. and Gougerot-Pocidalo, M. A. (1990a). Paraformaldehyde fixation of LPS stimulated human monocytes: technical parameters permitting the study of membrane IL-1 activity. *Eur. Cytokine Network*, **1**, 47–51.

Bailly, S., Ferrua, B., Fay, M. and Gougerot-Pocidalo, M. A. (1990b). Differential regulation of IL-6, IL-1α, IL-1β and TNFα production in LPS-stimulated human monocytes: role of cyclic AMP. *Cytokine*, **2**, 205–10.

Barthelson, R. A., Potter, T. and Valone, F. H. (1990). Synergistic increases in IL-1 synthesis by the human monocytic cell line THP-1 treated with PAF and endotoxin. *Cell. Immunol.*, **125**, 142–50.

Beasley, D., Cohen, R. A. and Levinsky, N. G. (1989). Interleukin-1 inhibits contraction of vascular smooth muscle. *J. Clin. Invest.*, **83**, 331–5.

Bernaudin, J.-F., Yamauchi, K., Wewers, M. D., Tocci, M. J., Ferrans, V. J. and Crystal, R. G. (1988). Demonstration by *in situ* hybridization of dissimilar IL-1β gene expression in human alveolar macrophages and blood monocytes in response to lipopolysaccharide. *J. Immunol.*, **140**, 3822–9.

Beuscher, H. U., Günther, C. and Röllinghoff, M. (1990). IL-1β is secreted by activated murine macrophages as biologically inactive precursor. *J. Immunol.*, **144**, 2179–83.

Bischoff, S. C., De Weck, A. L. and Dahinden, C. A. (1990). Interleukin-3 and granulocyte/macrophage-colony-stimulating factor render human basophils responsive to low concentrations of complement component C3a. *Proc. Natl. Acad. Sci. USA*, **87**, 6813–17.

Bochner, B. S., McKelvey, A. A., Sterbinsky, S. A., Hildreth, J. E. K., Derse, C. P., Klunk, D. A., Lichtenstein, L. M. and Schleimer, R. P. (1990a). IL-3 augments adhesiveness for endothelium and CD11b expression in human basophils but not neutrophils. *J. Immunol.*, **145**, 1832–7.

Bochner, B. S., Charlesworth, E. N., Lichtenstein, L. M. and Derse, C. P. (1990b). Interleukin-1 is released at sites of human cutaneous allergic reactions. *J. Allergy Clin. Immunol.*, **86**, 830–9.

Bochner, B. S., Luscinskas, F. W., Gimbrone, M. A., Jr, Newman, W., Sterbinsky, S. A., Derse-Anthony, C. P., Klunk, D. and Schleimer, R. P. (1991). Adhesion of human basophils, eosinophils, and neutrophils to interleukin 1-activated human vascular endothelial cells: contributions of endothelial cell adhesion molecules. *J. Exp. Med.*, **173**, 1553–6.

Borish, L., Mascali, J. J. and Rosenwasser, L. J. (1991). IgE-dependent cytokine production by human peripheral blood mononuclear phagocytes. *J. Immunol.*, **146**, 63–7.

Brunner, T., De Weck, A. L. and Dahinden, C. A. (1991). Platelet-activating factor induces mediator release by human basophils primed with IL-3, granulocyte macrophage colony stimulating factor, or IL-5. *J. Immunol.*, **147**, 237–42.

Burd, P. R., Rogers, H. W., Gordon, J. R., Martin, C. A., Jayaraman, S., Wilson, S. D., Dvorak, A. M., Galli, S. J. and Dorf, M. E. (1989). Interleukin-3 dependent and -independent mast cells stimulated with IgE and antigen express multiple cytokines. *J. Exp. Med.*, **170**, 245–57.

Carlos, T. M., Schwartz, B. R., Kovach, N. L., Yee, E., Rosso, M., Osborn, L., Chi-Rosso, G., Newman, B., Lobb, R. and Harlan, J. M. (1990). Vascular cell adhesion molecule-1 mediates lymphocyte adherence to cytokine-activated cultured human endothelial cells. *Blood*, **76**, 965–70.

Carlos, T., Kovach, N., Schwartz, B., Rosa, M., Newman, B., Wayner, E.,

Benjamin, C., Osborn, L., Lobb, R. and Harlan, J. (1991). Human monocytes bind to two cytokine-induced adhesive ligands on cultured human endothelial cells: endothelial-leukocyte adhesion molecule-1 and vascular cell adhesion molecule-1. *Blood*, **77**, 2266–71.

Cavaillon, J. M. (1990). Interleukines et inflammation. *Path. Biol.*, **38**, 36–42.

Cavaillon, J. M. and Haeffner-Cavaillon, N. (1986). Polymyxin-B inhibition of LPS-induced interleukin-1 secretion by human monocytes is dependent upon the LPS origin. *Mol. Immunol.*, **23**, 965–9.

Cavaillon, J. M. and Haeffner-Cavaillon, N. (1990). Signals involved in interleukin-1 synthesis and release by lipopolysaccharide-stimulated monocytes/macrophages. *Cytokine*, **2**, 313–29.

Cavaillon, J. M., Dandeu, J. P., Mécheri, S. and David, B. (1984). Presence of IL-1 activity in the supernatant of human monocytes challenged with purified allergenic constituents. *Int. Arch. Allergy Appl. Immunol.*, **75**, 113–19.

Cavaillon, J. M., Fitting, C., Guinnepain, M. T., Rassemont, R. and David, B. (1988). Lymphocyte proliferative responses to the purified *Dermatophagoïdes farinae* major allergen in untreated and hyposensitized atopic patients. *Allergy*, **43**, 146–51.

Cavaillon, J. M., Fitting, C. and Haeffner-Cavaillon, N. (1990a). Recombinant C5a enhances interleukin-1 and tumor necrosis factor release by lipopolysaccharide-stimulated monocytes and macrophages. *Eur. J. Immunol.*, **20**, 253–7.

Cavaillon, J. M., Vidard, L., Boudaly, S., Fitting, C., Cohen, L., Seman, M. and David, B. (1990b). Induction of interleukin-3 by interleukin-1 in the absence of other exogenous stimuli. *Cell. Immunol.*, **129**, 176–88.

Cavender, D. E., Haskard, D. O., Joseph, B. and Ziff, M. (1986). Interleukin-1 increases the binding of human B and T lymphocytes to endothelial cell monolayers. *J. Immunol.*, **136**, 903–7.

Chang, T. L., Shea, C. M., Urioste, S., Thompson, R. C., Boom, W. H. and Abbas, A. K. (1990). Heterogeneity of helper/inducer T lymphocytes. III. Responses of IL-2 and IL-4-producing (Th1 and Th2) clones to antigens presented by different accessory cells. *J. Immunol.*, **145**, 2803–8.

Chantry, D., Winearls, C. G., Maini, R. N. and Feldmann, M. (1989). Mechanism of immune complex-mediated damage: induction of interleukin-1 by immune complexes and synergy with interferon-γ and tumor necrosis factor-α. *Eur. J. Immunol.*, **19**, 189–92.

Chizzonite, R., Truitt, T., Kilian, P. L., Stern, A. S., Nunes, P., Parker, K. P., Kaffka, K. L., Chua, A. O., Lugg, D. K. and Gubler, U. (1989). Two high-affinity interleukin-1 receptors represent separate gene products. *Immunology*, **86**, 8029–33.

Chrétien, I., Pène, J., Brière, F., De Waal Malefijt, R., Rousset, F. and De Vries, J. E. (1990). Regulation of human IgE synthesis. I. Human IgE synthesis *in vitro* is determined by the reciprocal antagonistic effects of interleukin-4 and interferon-γ. *Eur. J. Immunol.*, **20**, 243–51.

Cohen, L., David, B. and Cavaillon, J. M. (1991). Interleukin-3 enhances cytokine production by LPS-stimulated macrophages. *Immunol. Lett.*, **28**, 121–6.

Columbo, M., Casolaro, V., Warner, J. A., MacGlashan, D. W., Jr, Sobotka-Kagey, A. and Lichtenstein, L. M. (1990). The mechanism of mediator release from human basophils induced by platelet-activating factor. *J. Immunol.*, **145**, 3855–61.

Corrigan, C. J., Collard, P., Nagy, L. and Kay, A. B. (1991). Cultured peripheral blood mononuclear cells derived from patients with acute severe asthma ('status asthmaticus') spontaneously elaborate a neutrophil chemotactic activity distinct from interleukin-8. *Am. Rev. Respir. Dis.*, **143**, 538–44.

Couturier, C., Haeffner-Cavaillon, N., Weiss, L., Fischer, E. and Kazatchkine, M. D. (1990). Induction of cell-associated interleukin-1 through stimulation of the adhesion-promoting proteins LFA-1 (CD11a/CD18) and CR3 (CD11b/CD18) of human monocytes. *Eur. J. Immunol.*, **20**, 999–1005.

Dahinden, C. A., Kurimoto, Y., De Weck, A. L., Lindley, I., Dewald, B. and Baggiolini, M. (1989). The neutrophil-activating peptide NAF/NAP-1 induces histamine and leukotriene release by interleukin-3-primed basophils. *J. Exp. Med.*, **170**, 1787–92.

Dinarello, C. A. (1991). Interleukin-1 and interleukin-1 antagonism. *Blood*, **77**, 1627–52.

Dohlsten, M., Kalland, T., Sjögren, H.-O. and Carlsson, R. (1988). Histamine inhibits interleukin-1 production by lipopolysaccharide-stimulated human peripheral blood monocytes. *Scand. J. Immunol.*, **27**, 527–32.

Dripps, D. J., Brandhuber, B. J., Thompson, R. C. and Eisenberg, S. P. (1991). Interleukin-1 (IL-1) receptor antagonist binds to the 80-kDa IL-1 receptor but does not initiate IL-1 signal transduction. *J. Biol. Chem.*, **266**, 10331–6.

Eden, E. and Turino, G. M. (1986). Interleukin-1 secretion by human alveolar macrophages stimulated with endotoxin is augmented by recombinant immune (gamma) interferon. *Am. Rev. Respir. Dis.*, **133**, 455–60.

Eisenberg, S. P., Evans, R. J., Arend, W. P., Verderber, E., Brewer, M. T., Hannum, C. H. and Thompson, R. C. (1990). Primary structure and functional expression from complementary DNA of a human interleukin-1 receptor antagonist. *Nature (London)*, **343**, 341–6.

Enk, C. and Mosbech, H. (1988). Interleukin-1 production by monocytes from patients with allergic asthma after stimulation *in vitro* with lipopolysaccharide and *Dermatophagoïdes pteronyssinus* mite allergen. *Int. Arch. Allergy Appl. Immunol.*, **85**, 308–11.

Essner, R., Rhoades, K., McBride, W. H., Morton, D. L. and Economou, J. S. (1989). IL-4 down-regulates IL-1 and TNF gene expression in human monocytes. *J. Immunol.*, **142**, 3857–61.

Ferguson-Chanowitz, K. M., Katocs, A. S., Jr, Pickett, W. C., Kaplan, J. B., Sass, P. M., Oronsky, A. L. and Kerwar, S. S. (1990). Platelet-activating factor or a platelet-activating factor antagonist decreases tumor necrosis factor in the plasma of mice treated with endotoxin. *J. Infect. Dis.*, **162**, 1081–6.

Frendl, G., Fenton, M. J. and Beller, D. I. (1990). Regulation of macrophage activation by IL-3. II. IL-3 and lipopolysaccharide act synergistically in the regulation of IL-1 expression. *J. Immunol.*, **144**, 3400–10.

Fuhlbrigge, R. C., Chaplin, D. D., Kiely, J. M. and Unanue, E. R. (1987). Regulation of interleukin-1 gene expression by adherence and lipopolysaccharide. *J. Immunol.*, **138**, 3799–802.

Gauchat, J. F., Gauchat, D., Qiu, G., Mandallaz, M. and Stadler, B. M. (1991). Detection of cytokine mRNA in polyclonally-, antigen- or allergen-stimulated mononuclear cells. *Immunol. Rev.*, **119**, 147–61.

Goldblum, S. E., Cohen, D. A., Gillespie, M. N. and McClain, C. J. (1987). Interleukin-1-induced granulocytopenia and pulmonary leukostasis in rabbits. *J. Appl. Physiol.*, **62**, 122–8.

Gosset, Ph., Lassalle, P., Tonnel, A. B., Dessaint, J. P., Wallaert, B., Prin, L., Pestel, J. and Capron, A. (1988). Production of an interleukin-1 inhibitory factor by human alveolar macrophages from normals and allergic asthmatic patients. *Am. Rev. Respir. Dis.*, **138**, 40–6.

Haak-Frendscho, M., Dinarello, C. and Kaplan, A. P. (1988a). Recombinant human interleukin-1 beta causes histamine release from human basophils. *J. Allergy Clin. Immunol.*, **82**, 218–23.

Haak-Frendscho, M., Arai, N., Arai, K.-i, Baeza, M. L., Finn, A. and Kaplan, A. P. (1988b). Human recombinant granulocyte–macrophage colony-stimulating factor and interleukin-3 cause basophil histamine release. *J. Clin. Invest.*, **82**, 17–20.

Haeffner-Cavaillon, N., Cavaillon, J. M., Laude, M. and Kazatchkine, M. D. (1987). C3a (C3adesArg) induces production and release of interleukin-1 by cultured human monocytes. *J. Immunol.*, **139**, 794–9.

Han, V., Resau, J., Prendergast, R., Scott, A. and Levy, D. A. (1987). Interleukin-1 induces mucus secretion from mouse intestinal explants. *Int. Arch. Allergy Appl. Immunol.*, **82**, 364–5.

Hart, P. H., Vitti, G. F., Burgess, D. R., Whitty, G. A., Piccoli, D. S. and Hamilton, J. A. (1989). Potential antiinflammatory effects of interleukin-4: suppression of human monocyte tumor necrosis factor α, interleukin-1, and prostaglandin-E_2. *Proc. Natl. Acad. Sci. USA*, **86**, 3803–7.

Hazuda, D. J., Strickler, J., Kueppers, F., Simon, P. L. and Young, P. R. (1990). Processing of precursor interleukin-1β and inflammatory disease. *J. Biol. Chem.*, **265**, 6318–22.

Heederik, D., Brouwer, R., Biersteker, K. and Boleij, J. S. M. (1991). Relationship of airborne endotoxin and bacteria levels in pig farms with the lung function and respiratory symptoms of farmers. *Int. Arch. Occup. Environ. Health*, **62**, 595–601.

Heidel, J. R., Sassenfeld, H. M., Maliszewdki, C. R., Silflow, R. M., Baker, P. E., Taylor, S. M. and Wes Leid, R. (1990). Functional studies of bovine alveolar neutrophils elicited with recombinant bovine IL-1β. *J. Immunol.*, **144**, 1037–41.

Hirai, K., Morita, Y., Misaki, Y., Ohta, K., Takaishi, T., Suzuki, S., Motoyoshi, K. and Miyamoto, T. (1988). Modulation of human basophil histamine release by hemopoietic growth factors. *J. Immunol.*, **141**, 3958–64.

Hsieh, K.-H. and Lue, K.-H. (1987). Defective monokine production and decreased responsiveness of polymorphonuclear leukocytes to recombinant interleukin-1 in asthmatic patients. *J. Clin. Immunol.*, **7**, 203–9.

Kay, A. B., Ying, S., Varney, V., Gaga, M., Durham, S. R., Moqbel, R., Wardlaw, A. J. and Hamid, Q. (1991). Messenger RNA expression of the cytokine gene cluster, interleukin 3 (IL-3), IL-4, IL-5, and granulocyte/ macrophage colony-stimulating factor, in allergen-induced late-phase cutaneous reactions in atopic subjects. *J. Exp. Med.*, **173**, 775–8.

Killar, L. M., Hatfield, C. A., Carding, S. R., Pan, M., Winterrowd, G. E. and Bottomly, K. (1989). *In vivo* administration of interleukin-1 elicits increased Ia antigen expression on B cells through the induction of interleukin-4. *Eur. J. Immunol.*, **19**, 2205–10.

King, A. G., Wierda, D. and Landreth, K. S. (1988). Bone marrow stromal cell regulation of B-lymphopoiesis. I. The role of macrophages, IL-1, and IL-4 in pre-B cell maturation. *J. Immunol.*, **141**, 2016–26.

Kurimoto, Y., De Weck, A. L. and Dahinden, C. A. (1989). Interleukin-3-dependent mediator release in basophils triggered by C5a. *J. Exp. Med.*, **170**, 467–79.

Kurt-Jones, E. A., Virgin, I. V. H. W. and Unanue, E. R. (1986). *In vivo* and *in vitro* expression of macrophage membrane interleukin-1 in response to soluble and particulate stimuli. *J. Immunol.*, **137**, 10–14.

Kyan-Aung, U., Haskard, D. O., Poston, R. N., Thornhill, M. H. and Lee, T. H. (1991). Endothelial leukocyte adhesion molecule-1 and intercellular adhesion molecule-1 mediate the adhesion of eosinophils to endothelial cells *in vitro* and are expressed by endothelium in allergic cutaneous inflammation *in vivo*. *J. Immunol.*, **146**, 521–8.

Lamontagne, L., Gauldie, J., Stadnyk, A., Richards, C. and Jenkins, E. (1985). *In vivo* initiation of unstimulated *in vitro* interleukin-1 release by alveolar macrophages. *Am. Rev. Resp. Dis.*, **131**, 326–30.

Lichtman, A. H., Chin, J., Schmidt, J. A. and Abbas, A. K. (1988). Role of interleukin-1 in the activation of T lymphocytes. *Proc. Natl. Acad. Sci. USA*, **85**, 9699–703.

MacDonald, S. M., Schleimer, R. P., Kagey-Sobotka, A., Gillis, S. and Lichtenstein, L. M. (1989). Recombinant IL-3 induces histamine release from human basophils. *J. Immunol.*, **142**, 3527–32.

Maliszewski, C. R., Sato, T. A., Vanden Bos, T., Waugh, S., Dower, S. K., Slack, J., Beckmann, M. P. and Grabstein, K. H. (1990). Cytokine receptors and B cell functions. I. Recombinant soluble receptors specifically inhibit IL-1- and IL-4-induced B cell activities *in vitro*. *J. Immunol.*, **144**, 3028–33.

Manosroi, J., Manosroi, A. and Vithayasai, V. (1987). Effect of histamine and antihistamines on interleukin-1 production by human monocytes. *Microbiol. Immunol.*, **31**, 1217–30.

Martin, S., Maruta, K., Burkart, V., Gillis, S. and Kolb, H. (1988). IL-1 and IFN-γ increase vascular permeability. *Immunology*, **64**, 301–5.

Masinovsky, B., Urdal, D. and Gallatin, W. N. (1990). IL-4 acts synergistically with IL-1β to promote lymphocyte adhesion to microvascular endothelium by induction of vascular cell adhesion molecule-1. *J. Immunol.*, **145**, 2886–95.

Massey, W. A., Randall, T. C., Kagey-Sobotka, A., Warner, J. A., MacDonald, S. M., Gillis, S., Allison, A. C. and Lichtenstein, L. M. (1989). Recombinant human IL-1α and -1β potentiate IgE-mediated histamine release from human basophils. *J. Immunol.*, **143**, 1875–80.

Mazingue, C., Carrière, V., Dessaint, J. P., Detoeuf, F., Turz, T., Auriault, C. and Capron, A. (1987). Regulation of IgE synthesis by macrophages expressing Fc-receptors: role of interleukin-1. *Clin. Exp. Immunol.*, **67**, 587–93.

Melewicz, F. M., Zeiger, R. S., Mellon, M. H., O'Connor, R. D. and Spiegelberg, H. L. (1981). Increased peripheral blood monocytes with Fc receptors for IgE in patients with severe allergic disorders. *J. Immunol.*, **126**, 1592–5.

Michel, O., Duchateau, J. and Sergysels, R. (1989). Effect of inhaled endotoxin on bronchial reactivity in asthmatic and normal subjects. *J. Appl. Physiol.*, **66**, 1059–64.

Michel, O., Ginanni, R., Duchateau, J., Vertongen, F., Le Bon, B. and Sergysels, R. (1991). Domestic endotoxin exposure and clinical severity of asthma. *Clin. Exp. Allergy*, **21**, 441–8.

Moser, R., Schleiffenbaum, B., Groscurth, P. and Fehr, J. (1989). Interleukin-1 and tumor necrosis factor stimulate human vascular endothelial cells to promote transendothelial neutrophil passage. *J. Clin. Invest.*, **83**, 444–55.

Mosmann, T. R. and Moore, K. W. (1991). The role of IL-10 in crossregulation of T_H1 and T_H2 responses. *Immunol. Today*, **12**, A49–A53.

Ohara, J.-i. (1989). Interleukin-4: molecular structure and biochemical characteristics, biological function, and receptor expression. *Year Immunol.*, **5**, 126–59.

Okamoto, H. and Nakano, K. (1990). Regulation of interleukin-1 synthesis by histamine produced by mouse peritoneal macrophages *per se*. *Immunology*, **69**, 162–5.

Okamoto, H., Oh, C. and Nakano, K. (1990) Possible involvement of adenosine 3':5'-cyclic monophosphate and extracellular calcium ions in histamine stimulation of interleukin-1 release from macrophage-like P388D1 cells. *Immunology*, **70**, 186–90.

Oppenheim, J. J., Zachariae, C. O. C., Mukaida, N. and Matsushima, K. (1991). Properties of the novel proinflammatory supergene "intercrine" cytokine family. *Annu. Rev. Immunol.*, **9**, 617–48.

Parkar, B. A., McCormick, M. E. and Foster, S. J. (1990). Leukotrienes do not regulate interleukin-1 production by activated macrophages. *Biochem. Biophys. Res. Commun.*, **169**, 422–9.

Parronchi, P., Macchia, D., Piccinni, M. P., Biswas, P., Simonelli, C., Maggi, E., Ricci, M., Ansari, A. A. and Romagnani, S. (1991). Allergen- and bacterial antigen-specific T-cell clones established from atopic donors show a different profile of cytokine production. *Proc. Natl. Acad. Sci.*, *USA*, **88**, 4538–42.

Pignol, B., Henane, S., Sorlin, B., Rola-Pleszczynski, M., Mencia-Huerta, J. M. and Braquet, P. (1990). Effect of long-term treatment with platelet-activating factor on IL-1 and IL-2 production by rat spleen cells. *J. Immunol.*, **145**, 980–4.

Pike, B. L. and Nossal, G. J. V. (1985). Interleukin-1 can act as a B-cell growth and differentiation factor. *Proc. Natl. Acad. Sci. USA*, **82**, 8153–7.

Pohlman, T. H., Stanness, K. A., Beatty, P. G., Ochs, H. D. and Harlan, J. M. (1986). An endothelial cell surface factor(s) induced *in vitro* by lipopolysaccharide, interleukin-1, and tumor necrosis factor-α increases neutrophil adherence by a CDw18 dependent mechanism. *J. Immunol.*, **136**, 4548–53.

Poubelle, P. E., Gingras, D., Demers, C., Dubois, C., Harbour, D., Grassi, J. and Rola-Pleszczynski, M. (1991). Platelet-activating factor (PAF-acether) enhances the concomitant production of tumour necrosis factor-alpha and interleukin-1 by subsets of human monocytes. *Immunology*, **72**, 181–7.

Pujol, J. L., Cosso, B., Daurès, J. P., Clot, J., Michel, F. B. and Godard, P. (1990). Interleukin-1 release by alveolar macrophages in asthmatic patients and healthy subjects. *Int. Arch. Allergy Appl. Immunol.*, **91**, 207–10.

Rola-Pleszczynski, M. and Lemaire, I. (1985). Leukotrienes augment interleukin-1 production by human monocytes. *J. Immunol.*, **135**, 3958–61.

Roper, R. L., Conrad, D. H., Brown, D. M., Warner, G. L. and Phipps, R. P. (1990). Prostaglandin-E promotes IL-4-induced IgE and IgG1 synthesis. *J. Immunol.*, **145**, 2644–51.

Royall, J. A., Berkow, R. L., Beckman, J. S., Cunningham, M. K., Matalon, S. and Freeman, B. A. (1989). Tumor necrosis factor and interleukin-1α increase vascular endothelial permeability. *Am. J. Physiol.*, **257**, L399–L410.

Rubartelli, A., Cozzolino, F., Talio, M. and Sitia, R. (1990). A novel secretory pathway for interleukin-1β, a protein lacking a signal sequence. *EMBO J.*, **9**, 1503–10.

Rylander, R. (1987). The role of endotoxin for reactions after exposure to cotton dust. *Am. J. Ind. Med.*, **12**, 687–97.

Scales, W. E., Chensue, S. W., Otterness, I. and Kunkel, S. L. (1989). Regulation of monokine gene expression: prostaglandin-E_2 suppresses tumor necrosis factor but not interleukin-1α or β-mRNA and cell-associated bioactivity. *J. Leuk. Biol.*, **45**, 416–21.

Schleimer, R. P., Benenati, S. V., Friedman, B. and Bochner, B. S. (1991). Do cytokines play a role in leukocyte recruitment and activation in the lungs? *Am. Rev. Respir. Dis.*, **143**, 1169–74.

Simms, H. H., Gaither, T. A., Fries, L. F. and Frank, M. M. (1991). Monokines released during short-term Fcγ receptor phagocytosis up-regulate polymorphonuclear leukocytes and monocyte-phagocytic function. *J. Immunol.*, **147**, 265–72.

Sims, J. E., March, C. J., Cosman, D., Widmer, M. B., MacDonald, H. R., McMahan, C. J., Grubin, C. E., Wignall, J. M., Jackson, J. L., Call, S. M., Friend, D., Alpert, A. R., Gillis, S., Urdal, D. L. and Dower, S. K. (1988). cDNA expression cloning of the IL-1 receptor, a member of the immunoglobulin superfamily. *Science*, **241**, 585–8.

Sirko, S. P., Schindler, R., Doyle, M. J., Weisman, S. M. and Dinarello, C. A. (1991). Transcription, translation and secretion of interleukin-1 and tumor necrosis factor: effects of tebufelone, a dual cyclooxygenase/5-lipoxygenase inhibitor. *Eur. J. Immunol.*, **21**, 243–50.

Subramanian, N. and Bray, M. A. (1987). Interleukin-1 releases histamine from human basophils and mast cells *in vitro*. *J. Immunol.*, **138**, 271–5.

Tatsuno, I., Saito, H., Chang, K.-J., Tamura, Y. and Yoshida, S. (1990). Comparison of the effect between leukotriene-B_4 and leukotriene-B_5 on the induction of interleukin-1-like activity and calcium mobilizing activity in human blood monocytes. *Agents Actions*, **29**, 3–4.

Thelin, A., Tegler, O. and Rylander, R. (1984). Lung reactions during poultry handling related to dust and bacterial endotoxin levels. *Eur. J. Respir. Dis.*, **65**, 266–71.

Vacheron, F., Rudent, A., Perin, S., Labarre, C., Quero, A. M. and Guenounou, M. (1990). Production of interleukin-1 and tumour necrosis factor activities in bronchoalveolar washings following infection of mice by influenza virus. *J. Gen. Virol.*, **71**, 477–9.

Valent, P., Besemer, J., Nuhm, M., Majdic, O., Lechner, K. and Bettelheim, P. (1989). Interleukin-3 activates human blood basophils via high-affinity binding sites. *Proc. Natl. Acad. Sci.*, *USA*, **86**, 5542–6.

Vannier, E., Miller, L. C. and Dinarello, C. A. (1991). Histamine suppresses gene expression and synthesis of tumor necrosis factor α via histamine H_2 receptors, *J. Exp. Med.*, **174**, 281–4.

Walsh, G. M., Mermod, J. J., Hartnell, A., Kay, A. B. and Wardlaw, A. J. (1991a). Human eosinophil, but not neutrophil, adherence to IL-1-stimulated human umbilical vascular endothelial cells is $\alpha_4\beta_1$ (very late antigen-4) dependent. *J. Immunol.*, **146**, 3419–23.

Walsh, L. J., Trinchieri, G., Waldorf, H. A., Whitaker, D. and Murphy, G. F. (1991b). Human dermal mast cells contain and release tumor necrosis factor which induces endothelial leukocyte adhesion molecule-1. *Proc. Natl. Acad. Sci. USA*, **88**, 4220–4.

Weiss, L., Haeffner-Cavaillon, N., Laude, M., Cavaillon, J. M. and Kazatchkine, M. D. (1989). Human T cells and interleukin-4 inhibit the release of interleukin-1 induced by lipopolysaccharide in serumfree cultures of autologous monocytes. *Eur. J. Immunol.*, **19**, 1347–50.

Wellicome, S. M., Thornhill, M. H., Pitzalis, C., Thomas, D. S., Lanchbury, J. S. S., Panayi, G. S. and Haskard, D. O. (1990). A monoclonal antibody that detects a novel antigen on endothelial cells that is induced by tumor necrosis factor, IL-1, or lipopolysaccharide. *J. Immunol.*, **144**, 2558–65.

Wewers, M. D. and Herzyk, D. J. (1989). Alveolar macrophages differ from blood monocytes in human IL-1 β release. Quantitation by enzyme-linked immunoassay. *J. Immunol.*, **143**, 1635–41.

Wierenga, E. A., Snoek, M., de Groot, C., Chretien, I., Bos, J. D., Jansen, H. M. and Kapsenberg, M. L. (1990). Evidence for compartmentalization of functional subsets of CD4$^+$ T lymphocytes in atopic patients. *J. Immunol.*, **144**, 4651–6.

17

Endothelial Cells and Asthma

P. Lassalle, Y. Delneste, P. Gosset and
A.-B. Tonnel

Summary

In bronchial asthma, interest has been mainly focused on inflammatory
cells such as eosinophils, mononuclear phagocytes but also activated T
lymphocytes. However, other cells such as vascular endothelial cells
(VECs) belonging to the bronchial tissue structure itself are also susceptible to participation in the inflammatory processes of asthma.

As it is impossible to access the bronchial endothelium directly, two
different ways of investigation have been explored.

(a) Circulating antibodies to VEC components can be detected. By West-
    ern blotting, the presence of antibodies against a 55 kD protein was
    demonstrated in patients suffering from severe chronic asthma. Inci-
    dence of anti 55 kD antibodies was clearly enhanced in corticosteroid-
    dependent asthmatics and in patients with aspirin intolerance.
(b) Adhesion molecules (ICAM-1 and ELAM-1) present at the surface of
    human VEC can be modulated by cytokines. Among cytokines,
    tumour necrosis factor α (TNFα) is known to be able to up-regulate
    adhesion molecule expression on endothelial cells (ECs). When added
    on EC cultures, alveolar macrophage supernatants obtained from
    patients exhibiting a late asthmatic reaction (LAR) induced a highly
    significant increase of ICAM-1 and ELAM-1 expression, specifically
    inhibited in the presence of anti-TNF antibodies but not with anti-IL-6
    or anti-IFNγ immune sera.

Therefore these results suggest that VECs may perhaps represent a target for specific autoantibodies in some cases of chronic severe asthma but also are susceptible to participation, namely during the LAR to adhesion and subsequently of cell infiltration processes.

17.1 Introduction

Current concepts on the pathogenesis of asthma emphasize the role of inflammatory cells such as mast cells, eosinophils, mononuclear phagocytes but also T lymphocytes, recruited on the site of the allergen conflict and responsible for cell and tissue alterations occurring in the bronchial tree (Beasley *et al.*, 1989; Azzawi *et al.*, 1990; Djukanovic *et al.*, 1990; Kay *et al.*, 1991). However, other cells belonging to the tissue structure itself seem to have been relatively neglected in the general scheme of the asthmatic reaction. Among these structural components, the vascular endothelial cells (VECs) are directly involved in the local cellular migration. They act as a barrier that selectively regulates the transfer of cells and fluids between circulating blood and surrounding tissue structures.

In addition, pathological studies proved that the airway vasculature, in human bronchi, is particularly developed with a very dense network of microvessels present in the submucosa (Persson, 1991). More recently, ultrastructural studies pointed to the fact that, in the bronchial mucosa of asthmatics, eosinophils, monocytes and platelet plugs were found in close contact with the vascular endothelium, by contrast to the data observed in control subjects where only some intravascular neutrophils could be seen (Beasley *et al.*, 1989). Another study also indicated a participation of bronchial microvessels through the finding of an enhanced detection of immunoreactive endothelin both in the small vessels and in the bronchial epithelium (Springall *et al.*, 1991). All these findings suggest that VECs might actively participate in the development of the inflammatory reaction in asthma.

17.2 Vascular Endothelial Cell Activation in Asthma

Functions of endothelial cells have been recently re-evaluated. Beside their basic role of blood-tissue barrier, the VECs tend to regulate actively various biological processes. VECs release vasoactive mediators such as endothelium-derived relaxing factor (Furchgott and Zawadzki, 1980) and endothelin (Yanagisawa *et al.*, 1988) that act on smooth muscle cells not only from the vessels (endothelial derived releasing factor (EDRF) and endothelin) but also from the bronchial tree (Nomura *et al.*, 1989a, b). They also release several other mediators such as interleukin 1 (IL-1) IL-6, IL-8, and PAF that act on various inflammatory and immune processes (Miossec and Ziff, 1986; Jirik *et al.*, 1989; Streiter *et al.*, 1989; Zimmerman *et al.*, 1990). Indeed, there is increasing evidence that interactions between vascular endothelium and cytokines are of major importance in the development of the inflammatory response (Mantovani and Dejana, 1989). For example, cytokines such as IL-1, tumour necrosis factor α (TNFα) and interferen Nγ (IFNγ) have been found to enhance the production and the release of several VEC-derived cytokines such as IL-1, IL-6, IL-8, and growth factors such as platelet derived growth factor (PDGF) and granulocyte–macrophage colony stimulating factor (GM-CSF). Cytokines also increase cell surface expression on VECs of molecules involved in cell–cell adherence such as CD54 (ICAM-1), ELAM-1, and VCAM-1 (Dustin *et al.*, 1986; Bevilacqua *et al.*, 1989; Osborn *et al.*, 1989). Lastly, VECs that produce factors modify eosinophil survival and maturation (Rothenberg *et al.*, 1987). These factors have been related to GM-CSF (Lamas *et al.*, 1989).

Bearing in mind the concept that asthma is mainly an inflammatory disease, it is possible to consider the involvement of endothelial cells in the bronchial response to allergens, namely through the complex network of cytokines released *in situ*. One of the putative cell sources of cytokines is represented by mononuclear phagocytes. There is now evidence *in vitro* that these cells can release TNFα and IL-6 upon immunoglobulin E (IgE) dependent stimulation (Gosset *et al.*, 1989). This release was amplified in case of costimulation with IFNγ. In asthmatics, alveolar macrophages (AMs), recovered by bronchoalveolar lavage 18 h following bronchial challenge with the relevant allergen, demonstrated a high production level of TNFα and IL-6. This production was exclusively observed with AMs from patients who have experienced a dual reaction (Gosset *et al.*, 1991). TNFα production was lacking in the case of a single early reaction or in asthmatics who did not shown any significant bronchial response to allergen challenge.

In order to investigate intercellular communication signals between VECs and alveolar macrophages, AM supernatants were studied in the presence of VECs: AM supernatants were incubated with VEC cultures and the expression of adhesion molecules such as CD54 and ELAM-1 was analysed (Lassalle, 1992). These cell surface adhesion molecules were highly expressed with AM supernatants provided from patients exhibiting a late or dual reaction. Neutralization assays with anti-sera against TNFα, IL-6 and IFNγ have been performed demonstrating that TNFα represents the major AM-derived cytokine involved in the expression of endothelial cell adhesion molecules (Fig. 17.1). So, these results indicate that in asthmatics who experienced a dual reaction (i.e. immediate and late reac-

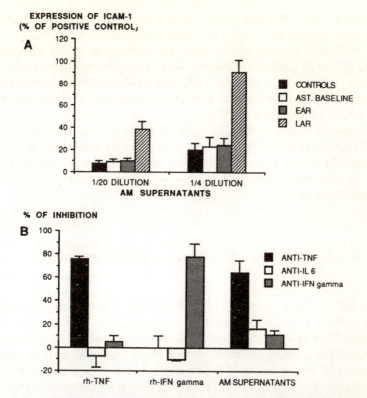

Fig. 17.1 (A) Modulation of ICAM-1 expression on endothelial cells by alveolar macrophage (AM) supernatants from controls and from asthmatic patients at baseline or after bronchial challenge: patients exhibiting a single early asthmatic reaction (EAR) or an EAR followed by a late asthmatic reaction (LAR). Results were expressed as percentage of optical density (OD) = [(OD AM supernatant − OD medium) / (OD rhTNF − OD medium)] × 100. The means of OD obtained with medium alone and after addition of rh-TNF or rh-IFNγ were respectively 0.361 ± 0.105, 0.955 ± 0.240 and 1.061 ± 0.257 ($n = 5$). (B) Effect of different neutralizing antibodies on ICAM-1 expression induced by rh-TNF, rh-IFNγ and by the 5 AM supernatants from patients developing a LAR. These experiments were repeated three times. Results are expressed as the percentage of inhibition obtained in the presence of the different antibodies compared with the inducer alone.

tion), AMs were activated to release TNFα and IL-6, and consecutively to activate VECs through the expression of adhesion molecules involved in the recruitment of inflammatory cells.

These *ex vivo* studies have to be put in parallel with data obtained both in experimental models and in allergic patients. The role of VEC adhesion molecules has been clearly identified by Wegner. In monkeys exposed to repeated allergen inhalations, the treatment by monoclonal anti-CD54 decreased both eosinophil infiltration and airway responsiveness (Wegner *et al.*, 1990). In man, ELAM-1 expression in skin biopsies occurred concurrently with the development of the late phase cutaneous reaction, with a maximal intensity between 3 and 6 h (Leung *et al.*, 1991). The increased expression of VEC adhesion molecules was clearly related to the production of TNFα. First, the treatment by neutralizing antibodies to TNFα of cutaneous tissue section challenged with anti-IgE inhibited ELAM-1 expression (Klein *et al.*, 1989). Second, mast cells from the cutaneous tissue represent, the major cell source of TNFα, able to induce ELAM-1 expression on VECs (Walsh *et al.*, 1991).

All these data indicate that, after IgE-dependent triggering, mast cells as well as mononuclear phagocytes are able via TNFα production to cause endothelial cell activation. One of the consequences of this pathway is the control of the recruitment of inflammatory cells, especially those observed in allergic diseases.

17.3 Endothelial Cells as a Source of Autoantigens in Asthma

There are a number of items of evidence that the pathogenesis of non-atopic asthma is, in part, linked to T-cells and T-cell mediators (Corrigan and Kay, 1990; Walker *et al.*, 1991; Lassalle *et al.*, 1992b). Bearing in mind the particular clinical features of non-atopic asthma, asthma may be hypothesized as the result of T-cell hyperreactivity against an unknown antigen present in bronchial mucosa. Because endothelial cells represent the first resident cell type in the bronchial tissues, we have searched for an endothelial cell-derived component, which might act as a target antigen for T and B cells in asthmatics. Antibodies directed against VEC components with a molecular weight of 120 kD and 55 kD were detected in subsets of patients with asthma.

In the group of patients with anti 120 kD antibodies, the isotype was defined as IgG. Indirect immunofluorescence on VECs using a fluorescent cell sorter demonstrated a high IgG binding activity in sera containing the anti 120 kD antibodies (Lassalle *et al.*, 1989).

In the group of patients with anti 55 kD antibodies, the isotype was defined as IgE in two cases, and as IgG isotype in the 24 others. No IgM or IgA isotypes were detected. Indirect immunofluorescence of endothelial cells did not allow us to distinguish a significant binding whatever the strongest reactive sera used. The preclearing of the positive sera on endothelial cells or platelets did not remove the anti 55 kD antibodies, suggesting thus that this antigen was not expressed on the cell surface (Lassalle, 1992c).

Among the patients with other autoantibody-associated diseases, five have shown specific binding to the 55 kD antibodies (three patients with systemic lupus erythematosus (SLE), and two patients with rheumatoid arthritis(RA)). 15 have shown specific binding to 120 kD antibodies (seven patients with SLE, and eight patients with RA). All other patients were negative (patients with chronic bronchitis, and healthy subjects).

Among all cell types tested for the presence of an immunoreactive antigen of 55 kD, only platelets and cultured SV40-transfected endothelial cells shared a 55 kD antigen similar to the VEC-derived antigen (Lassalle *et al.*, 1992a). By contrast, no such antigen could be detected on fibroblasts, neutrophils, mononuclear phagocytes, red blood cells, and K562 cell line.

The detection of these anti-VEC antibodies was evaluated according to the clinical, biological and therapeutic characteristics of the asthmatic population (Table 17.1): distribution of the positive skin prick-tests and total IgE levels were found similar in both groups of asthmatics, indicating that atopy alone was not associated with the presence of such antibodies.

Table 17.1   Clinical, biological, and therapeutic characteristics of the asthmatic population

	Presence of anti 120 kD antibody	Presence of anti 55 kD antibody	Absence of antibodies	Significance
Number of patients	13	26	51	
Age				
Mean ± s.d.	37 ± 21	41.2 ± 13	42.2 ± 14	
Range	18–71	17–59	18–62	
Sex ratio (female/male)	5/8	14/12	27/24	
Cutaneous prick-tests				
Positive	2	13	29	
Negative	11	13	22	
IgE levels (iu/ml)				
Mean ± s.e.m.	714 ± 281	388 ± 91	478 ± 67	
Range	217–1621	8–1055	32–1620	
Allergic granulomatosis and angiitis	7	0	4	$p < 0.001$
History of aspirin-induced asthma	3	14	6	$p < 0.001$
Corticodependent asthma	10 (77%)	18 (79%)	19 (37%)	$p < 0.01$

Characteristics of the asthmatic population classified upon the detection of anti-endothelial cell antibodies. The presence of these antibodies has been determined by Western blot. All patients were subjected to skin prick-tests under standard method at the Department of Pneumology (Hopital Calmette, Lille). Total IgE levels were determined by PRIST (Professor J. P. Dessaint, Department of Immunology, Lille). Corticodependence was assumed when control of asthma required daily oral steroids for at least one year despite usual anti-asthma therapy and daily inhaled 2000 μg beclomethasone. Aspirin sensitivity was defined on either typical clinical history or a bronchospastic adverse reaction after oral provocation. Statistical analysis was performed with the χ^2 test and the Wilcoxon rank sum test for unpaired data as described in material and methods.

In contrast, anti 55 kD antibodies were present, mainly in corticodependent asthma ($p<0.01$), and in aspirin-induced asthma ($p<0.001$). Anti 120 kD antibodies were mainly present in patients with allergic granulomatosis and angiitis, also called Churg–Strauss syndrome ($p<0.01$).

In order to search for reactive T-lymphocytes, we used a [³H]thymidine incorporation assay with peripheral blood mononuclear cells (PBMCs) from patients in the presence or in the absence of 55 kD antigen, resuspended from nitrocellulose sheets. A specific [³H]thymidine incorporation was observed in four out of seven patients with circulating anti 55 kD antibodies, with index values ranging from 12 to 3.8. In one case, this test was performed during an acute severe asthma attack, before any treatment, showing index values of 4.9 with a fall of index values to 2.3 during a remission period, 3 weeks later, indicating that the proliferative index to the 55 kD antibody might perhaps be related to the subsequent evolution of the disease.

This point is of interest and is worth being connected to other studies demonstrating that T-cell activation is more marked in non-atopic asthma than in atopics. First, the number of blood T-cell activation phenotypes such as CD25 was increased in acute severe asthma and the highest numbers were provided from non-atopic asthmatics (Corrigan and Kay, 1990). Second, a significant number of T-cells expressing HLA DR was found only in non-atopic asthmatics (Walker *et al.*, 1991). Third, the level of soluble IL-2 receptor was found to be increased in non-atopic asthmatics despite the use of long-term corticosteroid therapy (Lassalle *et al.*, 1992b). These observations suggest a possible link between the severity of asthma and an enhanced T cell activation. At present no direct proof exists for the involvement of endothelial components; however, there is some evidence that such a mechanism needs to be more completely investigated (Lassalle *et al.*, 1990). Using an SV40-transfected human endothelial cell line, the molecular cloning of these molecules should provide powerful tools to explore this hypothetical mechanism in asthma.

References

Azzawi, M., Bradley, B., Jeffrey, P. K., Frew, A. J., Wardlaw, A. J., Knowles, G., Assoufi, B., Collins, J. V., Durham, S. and Kay, A. B. (1990). Identification of activated T-lymphocytes and eosinophils in bronchial biopsies in stable atopic asthma. *Am. Rev. Respir. Dis.*, **142**, 1407–13.

Beasley, R., Roche, W. R., Roberts, J. A. and Holgate, S. T. (1989). Cellular events in the bronchi in mild asthma and after bronchial provocation. *Am. Rev. Respir. Dis.*, **139**, 806–17.

Bevilacqua, M. P., Stengelin, S., Gimbrone, M. A. Jr., and Seed, B. (1989). Endothelial leukocyte adhesion molecule 1: an inducible receptor for neutrophils related to complement regulatory proteins and lectins. *Science*, **243**, 1160–5.

Corrigan, C. J. and Kay, A. B. (1990). CD4 T-lymphocyte activation in acute severe asthma. Relationship to disease severity and atopic status. *Am. Rev. Respir. Dis.*, **141**, 970–7.

Djukanovic, R., Wilson, J. W., Britten, K. M., Wilson, S. J., Walls, A. F., Roche, W. R., Howarth, P. H. and Holgate, S. T. (1990). Quantitation of mast cells and eosinophils in the bronchial mucosa of symptomatic atopic asthmatics and healthy control subjects in immunohistochemistry. *Am. Rev. Respir. Dis.*, **142**, 863–71.

Dustin, M. L., Rothlein, R., Bhan, A. K., Dinarello, C. A. and Springer, T. A. (1986). Induction by IL-1 and interferon gamma: tissue distribution, biochemistry, and function of a natural adherence molecule (ICAM-1). *J. Immunol.*, **137**, 245–54.

Furchgott, R. F. and Zawadzki, J. V. (1980). The obligatory role of endothelial cells in the relaxation of arterial smooth muscle by acetylcholine. *Nature (London)*, **288**, 373–6.

Gosset, P., Lassalle, P., Pestel, J., Tonnel, A. B. and Capron, A. (1989). Production of TNFα by alveolar macrophages and blood monocytes from allergic asthmatics. *J. Allergy Clin. Immunol.*, **83**, 222A.

Gosset, P., Tsicopoulos, A., Wallaert, B., Joseph M., Tonnel, A. B. and Capron, A. (1991). Increased secretion of tumor necrosis factor alpha and interleukin-6 by alveolar macrophages consecutive to the development of the late asthmatic reaction. *J. Allergy Clin. Immunol.* (in press).

Jirik, F. R., Podor, T. J., Hirano, T., Kishimoto, T., Loskutoff, D. J., Carson, D. A. and Lotz, M. (1989). Bacterial lipopolysaccharide and inflammatory mediators augment IL-6 secretion by human endothelial cells. *J. Immunol.*, **142**, 144–7.

Kay, A. B., Ying, S., Varney, V., Gaga, M., Durham, S. R., Moqbel, R., Wardlaw, A. J. and Hamid, Q. (1991). Messenger RNA expression of the cytokine gene cluster, interleukin 3 (IL-3), IL-4, IL-5, and granulocyte–macrophage colony-stimulating factor, in allergen-induced late phase cutaneous reactions in atopic subjects. *J. Exp. Med.*, **173**, 775–8.

Klein, L. M., Lavker, R. M., Matis, W. L. and Murphy, G. F. (1989). Degranulation of human mast cells induces an endothelial antigen central to leukocyte adhesion. *Proc. Natl. Acad. Sci. USA*, **86**, 8972–6.

Lamas, A. M., Marcotte, G. V. and Schleimer, R. P. (1989). Human endothelial cells prolong eosinophil survival. Regulation by cytokines and glucocorticoides. *J. Immunol.*, **142**, 3978–84.

Lassalle, P., Gosset, P., Tonnel, A. B., Dessaint, J. P. and Capron, A. (1989). Serum antibodies to endothelial cells in allergic granulomatosis and angiitis (AGA). *J. Allergy Clin. Immunol.*, **83**, 227A.

Lassalle, P., Joseph, M., Ramon, P., Dracon, P., Tonnel, A. B. and Capron, A. (1990). Plasmapheresis in a patient with severe asthma associated with autoantibodies to platelets. *Clin. Exp. Allergy*, **20**, 707–12.

Lassalle, P., Lagrou C., Delneste, Y., Sanceau, Y., Coll, J., Wietzerbin, J., Stehelin, D., Tonnel, A. B. and Capron, A. (1992a). Human endothelial cells transfected by SV40: characterization and potent use as a source of normal endothelial factors. *Eur. J. Immunol.*, **22**, 425–31.

Lassalle, P., Sergant, M., Delneste, Y., Wallaert, B., Zandecki, M., Capron, A., Joseph, M., and Tonnel, A. B. (1992b). High levels of soluble IL-2 receptor in plasma from asthmatics. Correlations with blood eosinophilia, lung function, and corticosteroid therapy. *Clin. Exp. Immunol.*, **87**, 266–71.

Lassalle, P., Delneste, Y., Wallaert, B., Capron, A. and Tonnel, A. B. (1992c). Cross-reactive anti-platelet and anti-endothelial cell antibodies in bronchial asthma: a plea for an autoimmune process in the pathogenesis of asthma. Submitted for publication.

Leung, D. Y. M., Pober, J. S. and Cotran, R. S. (1991). Expression of endothelial-leukocyte adhesion molecule-1 in elicited late phase allergic reactions. *J. Clin. Invest.*, **87**, 1805–9.

Mantovani, A. and Dejana, E. (1989). Cytokines as communication signals between leukocytes and endothelial cells. *Immunol. Today*, **10**, 370–5.

Miossec, P. and Ziff, M. (1986). Immune interferon enhances the production of interleukin-1 by human endothelial cells stimulated with lipopolysaccharide. *J. Immunol.*, **137**, 2848–52.

Nomura, A., Uchida, Y., Kameyama, M., Saotome, M., Oki, K. and Hasegawa, S. (1989a). Endothelin and bronchial asthma. *Lancet*, **2**, 747–8.

Nomura, A., Uchida, Y., Ohtsuka, M., Hamada, M., Ishii, Y., Ninomiya, H., Saotome, M. and Hasegawa, S. (1989b). Endothelium-derived polypeptide potently constricts human bronchi. *Am. Rev. Respir. Dis.*, **139**, A468.

Osborn, L., Hession, C., Tisard, R., Vassallo, C., Luhowskyj, S., Chi-Rosso, G. and Lobb, R. (1989). Direct expression cloning of vascular cell adhesion molecule 1, a cytokine-induced endothelial protein that bind to lymphocytes. *Cell*, **59**, 1203–11.

Persson, C. G. A. (1991). Tracheobronchial microcirculation in asthma. In Kalirer, M. A., Barnes, P. J. and Persson, C. G. A. (eds.), *Asthma: its Pathology and Treatment*, Dekker, New York, 209–29.

Rothenberg, M. E., Owen, W. F. Jr., Silberstein, D. S., Soberman, R. J., Austen, K. F. and Stevens, R. L. (1987). Eosinophils cocultured with endothelial cells have increased survival and functional properties. *Science*, **237**, 645–7.

Springall, D. R., Howarth, P. H., Counihan, H., Djukanovic, R., Holgate, S. T. and Polak, J. M. (1991). Endothelin immunoreactivity of airway epithelium in asthmatic patients. *Lancet*, **337**, 697–701.

Strieter, R. M., Kunkel, S. L., Showell, H. J., Remick, D. G., Phan, S. H., Ward, P. A. and Marks, R. M. (1989). Endothelial cell gene expression of a neutrophil chemotactic factor by TNF-α, LPS, and IL-1β. *Science*, **243**, 1467–9.

Walker, C. Virchow, J. C., Bruijnzeel, P. L. B. and Blaser, K. (1991). T cell subsets and their soluble products regulate eosinophilia in allergic and non allergic asthma. *J. Immunol.*, **146**, 1829–35.

Walsh, L. J., Trinchieri, G., Waldorf, H. A., Whitaker, D. and Murphy, G. F. (1991). Human dermal mast cells contain and release tumor necrosis factor alpha, which induces endothelial leukocyte adhesion molecule 1. *Proc. Natl. Acad. Sci. USA*, **88**, 4220–4.

Wegner, C. G., Gundel, R. H., Reilly, P., Haynes, N., Letts, L. G. and Rothlein, R. (1990). Intercellular adhesion molecule-1 (ICAM-1) in the pathogenesis of asthma. *Science*, **247**, 456–8.

Yanagisawa, M., Kurihara, H., Kimura, S., Tomobe, Y., Kobayashi, M., Mitsui, Y., Yazaki, Y., Goto, K. and Masaki, T. (1988). A novel potent vasoconstrictor peptide produced by vascular endothelial cells. *Nature (London)*, **332**, 411–15.

Zimmerman, G. A., McIntyre, T. M., Mehra, M. and Prescott, S. M. (1990). Endothelial cell-associated platelet-activating factor: a novel mechanism for signaling intercellular adhesion. *J. Cell. Biol.*, **110**, 529–40.

18

Intercellular Adhesion Molecules in the Pathogenesis of Airway Hyperresponsiveness

C. D. Wegner, R. H. Gundel and L. G. Letts

18.1 Introduction

The importance of airway hyperresponsiveness in asthma is underscored by reports correlating its severity with the intensity of symptoms (Boulet *et al.*, 1983; Chan-Yeung *et al.*, 1982; Hargreave *et al.*, 1981), diurnal variations in airway caliber (Ryan *et al.*, 1982) and therapy required (Juniper *et al.*, 1981). Once established, airway hyperresponsiveness can remain stable for years (Juniper *et al.*, 1982; Townley *et al.*, 1975), persist apparently in the absence of allergen inhalation (Becker, *et al.*, 1989; Chan-Yeung *et al.*, 1982), airway inflammation and epithelial desquamation (Lundgren *et al.*, 1988; Jeffery *et al.*, 1989), and, thus, possibly become permanent as a result of irreversible alterations in airway ultrastructure (Bellofiore *et al.*, 1989; Etienne *et al.*, 1989; Macklem, 1989; Brewster *et al.*, 1990). However, results from several studies indicate that the onset or development of airway hyperresponsiveness is induced by repeated allergen inhalation (Boulet *et al.*, 1983; Wegner *et al.*, 1991b; Sotomayor *et al.*, 1984; Chan-Yeung *et al.*, 1982; Cockcroft *et al.*, 1989) and linked to the activation of lymphocytes (Azzawi *et al.*, 1990), the infiltration of eosinophils (Wardlaw *et al.*, 1988; Frigas and Gleich, 1986; Gundel *et al.*, 1989; Beasley *et al.*, 1989), and their damage and/or desquamation of airway epithelium (Gleich *et al.*, 1988; Laitinen *et al.*, 1985; Lam *et al.*, 1987). Consequently, understanding of the molecule basis for the development of airway hyperresponsiveness is critical to the clinical management of asthma early in its history (i.e. before airway hyperresponsiveness becomes persistent).

Intimate cell–cell contact or 'adhesion' is crucial to many aspects of an immune or inflammatory response including antigen presentation and antibody production, leukocyte margination and migration, leukocyte activation and degranulation, and cell-mediated cytotoxicity (Springer, 1990; Leff et al., 1991; Albelda, 1991). The cell surface glycoproteins that specifically mediate adhesion control both the strength of the intercellular contact as well as transducing signals that control intracellular activation, degranulation and probably motility. Thus, these molecules are principal regulators of inflammatory reactions.

Using monoclonal antibodies (MAbs) to individual adhesion glycoproteins, we have begun to investigate the expression and possible roles of specific cell adhesion molecules in a primate model of antigen-induced airway hyperresponsiveness. The results not only confirm the importance of cell adhesion in the pathogenesis of lung disease–dysfunction but also indicate that the contribution of each specific adhesion molecule is determined by the conditions and components of the inflammatory reaction. We begin with an introduction to some of the endothelial, epithelial and granulocyte adhesion molecules as well as concepts on how they might regulate inflammatory reactions.

18.2 Adhesion: Molecules and Concepts

Adhesion of leukocytes to the microvascular endothelium is primary to their infiltration into tissue (Colditz, 1985; Anderson et al., 1985). This adhesion is also essential to leukocyte (e.g. neutrophil) retention within the pulmonary circulation (margination) and mediation of endothelial damage that characterize many acute lung injuries (Harlan, 1985; Crapo et al., 1983). Likewise, adhesion of leukocytes to lung tissue components, including airway and alveolar epithelium, is integral to both their retention within and their destruction of lung tissue. The initiation of these adhesions is apparently through the upregulated expression of adhesion molecules on the endothelium or epithelium, and/or the activating of adhesion molecules on leukocytes (see below and Rampart and Williams, 1988).

Endothelial–Epithelial Adhesion Molecule Expression

Activation of endothelial cells with inflammatory mediators upregulates or induces the expression of several adhesion 'ligands' including granulocyte membrane protein with an M_r of 140 kD (GMP-140), endothelial-

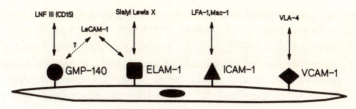

Inflamed Endothelial Cell

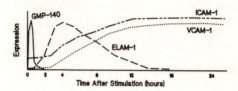

Fig. 18.1 Endothelial adhesion molecules, as well as their receptors and time course of expression, that direct the margination, and then diapedesis, of granulocytes to blood vessels at sites of inflammation (Bevilacqua *et al.*, 1987; Pober *et al.*, 1986; Smith *et al.*, 1989; Osborn *et al.*, 1989; Johnston *et al.*, 1989; Kishimoto *et al.*, 1991; Elices *et al.*, 1990; Lowe *et al.*, 1990; Larsen *et al.*, 1990).

leukocyte adhesion molecule-1 (ELAM-1), intercellular adhesion molecule-1 (ICAM-1), and vascular cell adhesion molecule-1 (VCAM-1) (Fig. 18.1). The inducible expression of these molecules seems to be important for directing the focal adhesion of leukocytes to blood vessels at sites of inflammation (Rampart and Williams, 1988; Argenbright and Barton, 1992).

ICAM-1 (CD54) and VCAM-1 are members of the immunoglobulin supergene family (Staunton *et al.*, 1988; Osborn *et al.*, 1989). Their induction requires *de novo* protein synthesis, is slow in onset but prolonged in term (onset 2 to 4 h with a peak of 8 to 24 h post-stimulation), and consequently thought to mediate chronic inflammation–infiltrations. The leukocyte 'receptors' for these two ligands are members of the integrin supergene family: LFA-lα (CD11a/CD18) and Mac-1 (CD11b/CD18) for ICAM-1 (Smith *et al.*, 1989; Springer, 1990), and VLA-4 (CD49d/CD29) for VCAM-1 (Elices *et al.*, 1990).

GMP-140 (CD62) and ELAM-1 are members of the selectin family indicative of their amino-terminal carbohydrate-binding (lectin) domain (Bevilacqua *et al.*, 1989; Johnston *et al.*, 1989). Their induction is more rapid and transient and consequently thought to mediate more acute infiltrations. The storage of GMP-140 in Weibel–Palade bodies of endothelial cells allows for its mobilization to the surface in less than five minutes of endothelial activation. The leukocyte receptors for GMP-140 and ELAM-1 are not yet well defined but are apparently also selectins, for example LeCAM-1 (Kishimoto *et al.*, 1991). ELAM-1 binds specifically to the carbohydrate group sialyl Lewis X, a terminal structure found on cell surface glycoproteins and glycolipids of neutrophils, monocytes and some tumour cells (Lowe *et al.*, 1990), while GMP-140 binds to the CD15 antigen, lacto-*N*-fucopentaose III (LNF III), on neutrophils and monocytes (Larsen *et al.*, 1990).

In addition to endothelium, ICAM-1 is inducible on airway and alveolar epithelial cells by inflammatory stimuli–mediators including cytokines, eosinophil major basic protein, and hyperoxia (Wegner *et al.*, 1990, 1992b). In contrast, GMP-140, ELAM-1 and VCAM-1 are not expressed or inducible on lung epithelial cells.

Granulocyte Adhesion Molecules

The major adhesion 'receptors' on granulocytes seem to be members of one of two supergene families: (1) the selectins, represented by lectin cell adhesion molecule-1 (LeCAM-1), the human homolog of the mouse MEL-14 antigen, and other yet undefined sialyl Lewis X and LNF III (CD15) containing glycoproteins (Lasky, 1991), and (2) the integrins, represented by the lymphocyte function-associated antigen-1 (LFA-1) family (β_2, CD18) (Kishimoto *et al.*, 1989a) and the very late antigen (VLA) family (β_1, CD29) (Hemler, 1990). Besides adhesion, these receptors possess additional properties that aid in their regulation, fine tuning, of immune–inflammatory responses. As the result of neutrophil stimulation with a chemoattractant (Kishimoto *et al.*, 1989b), or possibly ELAM-1 mediated adhesion (Lo *et al.*, 1991), LeCAM-1 is rapidly proteolytically shed from the cell membrane presumably to cause a de-adhesion necessary for migration and diapedesis, or de-margination. Integrin receptors are transmembrane glycoprotein heterodimers (α and β chains) whose interaction with an intact cytoskeleton is required for adhesion. Their interaction with the cytoskeleton, possibly via talin, is believed to regulate both avidity for ligand binding and signalling (priming or activation) of the leukocyte on ligand binding (Springer, 1990; Dustin and Springer, 1989; Regnier-Vigouroux *et al.*, 1986; Shappell *et al.*, 1990).

Granulocyte Infiltration, Activation and Mediated Tissue Injury

Several lines of evidence suggest that the initial adhesion (rolling or margination) of granulocytes to endothelium is mediated by selectins (Lawrence and Springer, 1991; Ley *et al.*, 1991) (Fig. 18.2). The marginated neutrophil is then activated, via this adhesion (Lo *et al.*, 1991) or chemoat-

a. Rolling/Margination

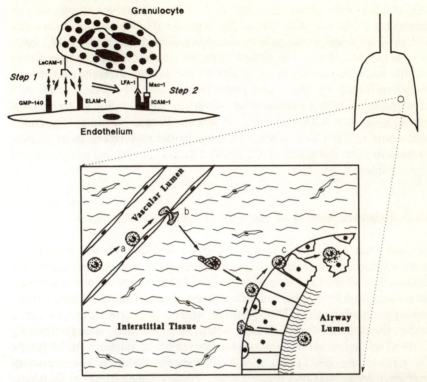

b. Transendothelial Migration   c. Epithelial Desquamation

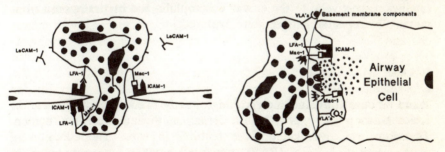

Fig. 18.2 Adhesion molecules believed to regulate granulocyte extravasation, activation and mediated tissue injury.

tractants (Kishimoto *et al.*, 1989b), causing the shedding of LeCAM-1 and activation (increased avidity) of Mac-1 (CD11b/CD18). LFA-1α to ICAM-1 and Mac-1 to ICAM-1 interactions then mediate neutrophil diapedesis (Smith *et al.*, 1989). Although less frequently studied, the presence of these same molecules and processes on eosinophils suggests that eosinophil infiltration is similarly regulated (Kyan-Aung et al., 1991; Wegner et al., 1989). However, unlike neutrophils, eosinophils also express notable amounts of VLA-4 (CD49d/CD29) that via its binding to endothelial VCAM-1 may also participate in eosinophil diapedesis (Walsh et al., 1991; Bochner et al., 1991). The adhesion of the activated granulocytes (neutrophils and presumably eosinophils) to the airway–alveolar epithelium, mediated largely by Mac-1 and partially by epithelial ICAM-1, then governs epithelial killing (Simon et al., 1986) or the retention of the primed granulocytes just adjacent to the air spaces (Wegner et al., 1990). Adhesion via Mac-1 has been shown to enhance the respiratory burst of neutrophils in vitro (Shappell et al., 1990).

18.3 Primate Model of Airway Hyperresponsiveness

In adult, male cynomolgus monkeys with a naturally occurring hypersensitivity of Ascaris suum extract, we have reported that Ascaris inhalation induces a prolonged airway eosinophilia and that chronic airway eosinophilia is associated with a marked airway hyperresponsiveness (Wegner et al., 1991a; Gundel et al., 1990). Multiple (three alternate day), but not a single, inhalations of antigen were found to produce an increase (usually more than eightfold) in airway responsiveness to inhaled methacholine (Wegner et al., 1991b) whose severity was correlated to the degree of epithelial desquamation (Wegner et al., 1991a). Using MAbs to ICAM-1, ELAM-1 and Mac-1 (CD11b/CD18), the contributions of these cell adhesion molecules, of the immunoglobulin, selectin and integrin supergene families respectively, to the airway eosinophilia and hyperresponsiveness induced by repeated antigen were explored.

ICAM-1

When we began our studies on ICAM-1, its role in eosinophil adherence to endothelium or its expression on airway epithelium were not known. Therefore, we investigated these features in vitro. The adhesion of platelet-activating factor (PAF) stimulated monkey lung eosinophils to human umbilical vein endothelial cells previously stimulated with lipopolysaccharide (LPS; for 4 h) was found to be partially (~50%) inhibited by a MAb to ICAM-1 (Wegner et al., 1989, 1990). Using an enzyme-linked immunosorbent assay (ELISA), ICAM-1 was found to be constitutively expressed and impressively upregulated by 16 h of stimulation with inflammatory cytokines on confluent monlayers of cultured monkey bronchus epithelial cells (Wegner et al., 1990). Immunohistochemical staining for ICAM-1 confirmed its expression and upregulation on antigen-inflamed airways *in vivo*. A marked increase in ICAM-1 staining was found on both the vascular endothelium and airway epithelium (basilateral portion only) of a tracheal section taken 20 min after the third of three alternate day *Ascaris* inhalations compared with a similar section obtained after a single inhalation (Wegner *et al.*, 1990).

With these results as background, the role of ICAM-1 on the airway eosinophilia and hyperresponsiveness induced by multiple antigen inhalations was determined using two mouse anti-human MAbs: one R6.5 that inhibits function and another CL203 that binds to a separate epitope (domain) on ICAM-1 not involved in leukocyte adhesion (Wegner *et al.*, 1990, 1991a). Airway cell composition (assayed by BAL) and responsiveness (inhaled methacholine PC_{100}) were determined three days prior to (day 0) and three days after (day 10) three alternate day (day 3, 5, 7) inhalations of *Ascaris* extract. R6.5 and CL203 were administered intravenously at 1.76 mg/kg daily (days 2–9) and compared with bracketing control studies in each animal. The monkeys were rested five or more weeks between each study to allow the induced airway inflammation and hyperresponsiveness to resolve. R6.5, but not CL203, attenuated the eosinophil infiltration (60 ± 8% and −3 ± 38%, respectively). More importantly, the increase in airway responsiveness was markedly inhibited by R6.5 (Fig. 18.3), but not CL203 (92 ± 34% and −15 ± 39%, respectively).

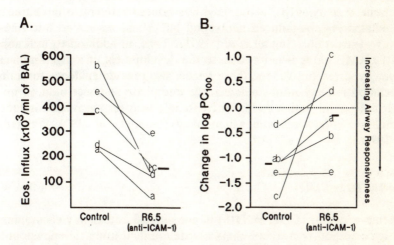

Fig. 18.3 Effects of the mouse anti-human ICAM-1 MAb R6.5 (1.76 mg/kg, i.v., daily) on (A) the airway eosinophil infiltration and (B) the hyperresponsiveness induced by three alternate day antigen inhalations in cynomolgus monkeys. Values are treatment compared with the mean of bracketing control studies for each animal. Bars are means of all animals (see Wegner *et al.*, 1990).

ELAM-1

Like ICAM-1, ELAM-1 expression is enhanced on inflamed endothelium and contributes to both neutrophil and eosinophil adhesion to endothelium *in vitro* (Luscinskas *et al.*, 1989; Pober *et al.*, 1986; Kyan-Aung *et al.*, 1991; Bochner *et al.*, 1991). However, ELAM-1 upregulation occurs more rapidly (peak at 4 h) and is more transient (gone by 16 h) (Wegner *et al.*, 1991a; Kishimoto *et al.*, 1991). In addition, while immunohistochemical staining for ICAM-1 is enhanced on airway and alveolar epithelium and vascular endothelium, ELAM-1 staining was only evident on airway vascular endothelium in sections obtained from monkey lungs 4 h after the third of three alternate day *Ascaris* inhalations (Wegner *et al.*, 1992a). The lack of ELAM-1 induction on airway epithelium was confirmed *in vitro* using the above-mentioned ELISA on cytokine (including IL-1β) stimulated confluent monolayers of cultured monkey bronchus epithelial cells (Wegner *et al.*, 1991a).

Using the mouse anti-human ELAM-1 MAb CL2 as well as the same protocol and dosing regimen as for the anti-ICAM-1 MAbs, the role of ELAM-1 in antigen-induced airway inflammation and hyperresponsiveness was evaluated. CL2 treatment did not significantly inhibit the eosinophil infiltration ($\times 10^3$/ml BAL: 507 ± 118 in control vs 430 ± 114 in CL2 treated) or the increase in airway responsiveness (change in log(PC_{100}): −1.16 ± 0.27 in controls vs − 1.24 ± 0.29 in CL2 treated). In contrast, functional activity of CL2 in monkeys was demonstrated by its inhibition of the inhaled *Ascaris*-induced neutrophil influx and associated late phase airway obstruction (Gundel *et al.*, 1991). Thus, in addition to indicating that ELAM-1 alone is not critical to the development of antigen-induced airway hyperresponsiveness, these results also provide evidence for a disassociation in mechanisms between the late phase response induced by a single antigen inhalation and the increase in airway responsiveness induced by multiple antigen inhalations in monkeys (Gundel *et al.*, 1991; Wegner *et al.*, 1992a).

Mac-1 (CD11b/CD18)

The role of Mac-1 (CD11b/CD18) in antigen-induced airway eosinophilia and hyperresponsiveness was similarly determined using the mouse anti-human Mac-1 MAb LM2. We have previously reported that LM2 impressively inhibits the adhesion of PAF stimulated monkey lung eosinophils to (i) protein-coated plastic (90–100%), and (ii) LPS stimulated monolayers of human umbilical vein endothelial cells (~75%) (Wegner *et al.*, 1989). LM2 treatment did not reduce the eosinophil infiltration but significantly inhibited their activation within the airways (BAL eosinophil peroxidase (EPO) activity) as well as the increase in airway responsiveness (Fig. 18.4).

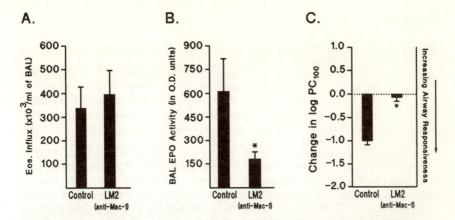

Fig. 18.4   Effects of the mouse anti-human Mac-1 (CD11b/CD18) MAb LM2 (2 mg/kg, i.v., daily) on (A) the airway eosinophil infiltration, (B) the eosinophil activation/degranulation, and (C) the hyperresponsiveness induced by three alternate day antigen inhalations in cynomolgus monkeys. Values are mean ± SEM of six animals, with treatment compared with the mean of the bracketing control studies for these animals.

18.4 Summary

We have found that both ICAM-1 and Mac-1, but not ELAM-1, contribute to the airway hyperresponsiveness induced by repeated allergen inhalations in primates. Our results are consistent with (i) endothelial ICAM-1 binding to eosinophil LFA-1α (CD11a/CD18) to partially mediate eosinophil diapedesis, and (ii) eosinophil Mac-1 binding its ligand(s) within the airways (including epithelial ICAM-1) to mediate eosinophil activation and probably epithelial desquamation (refer to Fig. 18.2). These postulates are supported by our recent results demonstrating that targeting epithelial ICAM-1 via the daily (day 2–9) inhalation of R6.5 (anti-ICAM-1) reduced the antigen-induced increases in eosinophil activation (BAL EPO activity), epithelial desquamation (histopathologic scoring of epithelial shedding) and airway hyperresponsiveness (Wegner *et al.*, 1991c).

Acknowledgements

The experimental and intellectual inputs provided by C. Clarke, N. Haynes, A. LaPlante, P. Reilly, R. Rothlein, and C. Torcellini are greatly appreciated. Special thanks are also extended to R. Rothlein for supplying the mouse anti-human ICAM-1 MAb R6.5, S. Ferrone for the mouse anti-human ICAM-1 MAb CL203, C. W. Smith for the mouse anti-human ELAM-1 MAb CL2, and T. A. Springer for the mouse anti-human Mac-1 MAb LM2.

References

Albelda, S. M. (1991). Endothelial and epithelial cell adhesion molecules. *Am. J. Respir. Cell Mol. Biol.*, **4**, 195–203.

Anderson, D. C., Schmalstieg, F. C., Finegold, M. J., Hughes, B. J., Rothlein, R., Miller, L. J., Kohl, S., Tosi, M. F., Jacobs, R. L., Waldrop, T. C., Goldman, A. S., Shearer, W. T. and Springer, T. A. (1985). The severe and moderate phenotypes of heritable Mac-1, LFA-1 deficiency: their quantitative definition and relation to leukocyte dysfunction and clinical features. *J. Infect. Dis.*, **152**, 668–89.

Argenbright, L. W. and Barton, R. W. (1992). Interactions of leukocyte integrins with intercellular adhesion molecule-1 in the production of inflammatory vascular injury *in vivo*: the Shwartzman reaction revisited. *J. Clin. Invest.*, **89**, 259–72.

Azzawi, M., Bradley, B., Jeffery, P. K., Frew, A. J., Wardlaw, A. J., Knowles, G., Assoufi, B., Collins, J. V., Durham, S. and Kay, A. B. (1990). Identification of activated T lymphocytes and eosinophils in bronchial biopsies in stable atopic asthma. *Am. Rev. Respir. Dis.*, **142**, 1407–13.

Beasley, R., Roche, W. R., Roberts, J. A. and Holgate, S. T. (1989). Cellular events in the bronchi in mild asthma and after bronchial provocation. *Am. Rev. Respir. Dis.*, **139**, 806–17.

Becker, A. B., Hershkovich, J. Simons, F. E. R., Simons, K. J., Lilley, M. K. and Kepron, M. W. (1989). Development of chronic airway hyperresponsiveness in ragweed-sensitized dogs. *J. Appl. Physiol.*, **66**, 2691–7.

Bellofiore, S., Eidelman, D. H., Macklem, P. T. and Martin, J. G. (1989). Effects of elastase-induced emphysema on airway responsiveness to methacholine in rats. *J. Appl. Physiol.*, **66**, 606–12.

Bevilacqua, M. P., Pober, J. S., Mendrick, D. L., Cotran, R. S. and Gimbrone, M. A. (1987). Identification of an inducible endothelial-leukocyte adhesion molecule. *Proc. Natl. Acad. Sci. USA*, **84**, 9238–42.

Bevilacqua, M. P., Stengelin, S., Gimbrone, M. A., Jr, and Seed, B. (1989). Endothelial leukocyte adhesion molecule-1: an inducible receptor for neutrophils related to complement regulatory proteins and lectins. *Science*, **243**, 1160–5.

Bochner, B. S., Luscinskas, F. W., Gimbrone, M. A., Newman, W., Sterbinsky, S. A., Derse-Anthony, C. P., Klunk, D. and Schleimer, R. P. (1991). Adhesion of human basophils, eosinophils, and neutrophils to interleukin-1-activated human vascular endothelial cells: contribution of endothelial cell adhesion molecules. *J. Exp. Med.*, **173**, 1553–6.

Boulet, L.-P., Cartier, A., Thomson, N. C., Roberts, R. S., Dolovich, J. and Hargreave, F. E. (1983). Asthma and increases in nonallergic bronchial responsiveness from seasonal pollen exposure. *J. Allergy Clin. Immunol.*, **71**, 399–406.

Brewster, C. E., Howarth, P. H., Djukanovic, R., Wilson, J., Holgate, S. T. and Roche, W. R. (1990). Myofibroblasts and subepithelial fibrosis in bronchial asthma. *Am. J. Respir. Cell Mol. Biol.*, **3**, 507–11.

Chan-Yeung, M., Lam, S. and Koener, S. (1982). Clinical features and natural history of occupational asthma due to western red cedar (*Thuja plicata*). *Am. J. Med.*, **72**, 411–15.

Cockcroft, D. W., Ruffin, R. E. and Hargreave, F. E. (1989). Appearance of allergen-induced increases in airway responsiveness only after repeated allergen inhalations in two subjects. *Clin. Exp. Allergy*, **19**, 225–7.

Colditz, I. G. (1985). Margination and emigration of leukocytes. *Surv. Synth. Pathol. Res.*, **4**, 44–68.

Crapo, J. D., Freeman, B. A., Barry, B. E., Turrens, J. F. and Young, S. L. (1983). Mechanisms of hyperoxic injury to the pulmonary microcirculation. *Physiologist*, **26**, 170–6.

Dustin, M. L. and Springer, T. A. (1989). T-cell receptor cross-linking transiently stimulates adhesiveness through LFA-1. *Nature (London)*, **341**, 619–24.

Elices, M. J., Osborn, L., Takada, Y., Crouse, C., Luhowskyj, S., Hemler, M. E. and Lobb, R. R. (1990). VCAM-1 on activated endothelium interacts with the leukocyte integrin VLA-4 at a site distinct from the VLA-4/fibronectin binding site. *Cell*, **60**, 577–84.

Etienne, A., Soulard, C., Thonier, F. and Braquet, P. (1989). Modulation of eosinophil recruitment in the rat by the platelet-activating factor (PAF) antagonist, BN 52021, the somatostatin analog, BIM 23014, and by cyclosporin A. *Prostaglandins*, **37**, 345–57.

Frigas, E. and Gleich, G. J. (1986). The eosinophil and the pathophysiology of asthma. *J. Allergy Clin. Immunol.*, **77**, 527–37.

Gleich, G. J., Flavanhan, N. A., Fujisawa, T. and VanHoutte, P. M. (1988). The eosinophil as a mediator of damage to respiratory epithelium: a model for bronchial hyperreactivity. *J. Allergy Clin. Immunol.*, **81**, 776–81.

Gundel, R. H., Gerritsen, M. E. and Wegner, C. D. (1989). Antigen-coated sepharose beads induce airway eosinophilia and airway responsiveness in cynomolgus monkeys. *Am. Rev. Respir. Dis.*, **140**, 629–33.

Gundel, R. H., Gerritsen, M. E., Gleich, G. J. and Wegner, C. D. (1990). Repeated antigen inhalation results in a prolonged airway eosinophilia and airway hyperresponsiveness in primates. *J. Appl. Physiol.*, **68**, 779–86.

Gundel, R. H., Wegner, C. D., Torcellini, C. A., Clarke, C. C., Haynes, N., Rothlein, R., Smith, C. W. and Letts, L. G. (1991). Endothelial-leukocyte adhesion molecule-1 mediates antigen-induced acute airway inflammation and late-phase bronchoconstriction in monkeys. *J. Clin. Invest.*, **88**, 1407–11.

Hargreave, F. E., Ryan, G., Thomson, N. C., O'Byrne, P. M., Latimer, K., Juniper, E. F. and Dolovich, J. (1981). Bronchial responsiveness to histamine or methacholine in asthma: measurement and clinical significance. *J. Allergy Clin. Immunol.*, **68**, 347–55.

Harlan, J. M. (1985). Leukocyte-endothelial cell interactions. *Blood*, **65**, 513–25.

Hemler, M. E. (1990). VLA proteins in the integrin family: structures, functions, and their role on leukocytes. *Annu. Rev. Immunol.*, **8**, 365–400.

Jeffery, P. K., Wardlaw, A.J., Nelson, F.C., Collins, J.V. and Kay, A.B. (1989). Bronchial biopsies in asthma. An ultrastructural, quantitative study and correlation with hyperreactivity. *Am. Rev. Respir. Dis.*, **140**, 1745–53.

Johnston, G. I., Cook, R. G. and McEver, R. P. (1989). Cloning of GMP-140, a granule membrane protein of platelets and endothelium: sequence similarity to proteins involved in cell adhesion and inflammation. *Cell*, **56**, 1033–44.

Juniper, E. F., Frith, P. A. and Hargreave, F. E. (1981). Airway responsiveness to histamine and methacholine: relationship to minimum treatment to control symptoms of asthma. *Thorax*, **36**, 575–9.

Juniper, E. F., Frith, P. A. and Hargreave, F. E. (1982). Long-term stability of bronchial responsiveness to histamine. *Thorax*, **37**, 288–91.

Kishimoto, T. K., Larson, R. S., Corbi, A. L., Dustin, M. L., Staunton, D. E. and Springer, T. A. (1989a). The leukocyte integrins. *Adv. Immunol.*, **46**, 149–82.

Kishimoto, T. K., Jutila, M. A., Berg, E. L. and Butcher, E. C. (1989b). Neutrophil Mac-1 and MEL-14a adhesion proteins inversely regulated by chemotactic factors. *Science*, **245**, 1238–41.

Kishimoto, T. K., Warnock, R. A., Jutila, M. A., Butcher, E. C., Lane, C.,

Anderson, D. C. and Smith, C. W. (1991). Antibodies against human neutrophil LeCAM-1 (LAM-1/Leu-8/DREG-56 antigen) and endothelial cell ELAM-1 inhibit a common CD18-independent adhesion pathway *in vitro*. *Blood*, **78**, 805–11.

Kyan-Aung, U., Haskard, D. O., Poston, R. N., Thornhill, M. H. and Lee, T. H. (1991). Endothelial leukocyte adhesion molecule-1 and intercellular adhesion molecule-1 mediate the adhesion of eosinophils to endothelial cells *in vitro* and are expressed by endothelium in allergic cutaneous inflammation *in vivo*. *J. Immunol.*, **146**, 521–8.

Laitinen, L. A., Heino, M., Laitinen, A., Kava, T. and Haahtela, T. (1985). Damage of the airway epithelium and bronchial reactivity in patients with asthma. *Am. Rev. Respir. Dis.*, **131**, 599–606.

Lam, S., LeRiche, J., Phillips, D. and Chan-Yeung, M. (1987). Cellular and protein changes in bronchial lavage fluid after late asthmatic reaction in patients with red cedar asthma. *J. Allergy Clin. Immunol.*, **80**, 44–50.

Larsen, E., Palabrica, T., Sajer, S., Gilbert, G. E., Wagner, D. D., Furie, B. C. and Furie, B. (1990). PADGEM-dependent adhesion of platelets to monocytes and neutrophils is mediated by a lineage-specific carbohydrate, LNF III (CD15). *Cell*, **63**, 467–74.

Lasky, L. A. (1991). Lectin cell adhesion molecules (LEC-CAMs): a new family of cell adhesion proteins involved with inflammation. *J. Cell Biochem.*, **45**, 139–46.

Lawrence, M. B. and Springer, T. A. (1991). Leukocytes roll on a selectin at physiologic flow rates: distinction from and prerequisite for adhesion through integrins. *Cell*, **65**, 859–73.

Leff, A. R., Hamann, K. and Wegner, C. D. (1991). Inflammation and cell–cell interactions in airway hyperresponsiveness. *Am. J. Physiol. (Lung Cell. Mol. Physiol.)*, **260**, L189–L206.

Ley, K., Gaehtgens, P., Fennie, C., Singer, M. S., Lasky, L. A. and Rosen, S. D. (1991). Lectin-like cell adhesion molecule-1 mediates leukocyte rolling in mesenteric venules *in vivo*. *Blood*, **77**, 2553–5.

Lo, S. K., Lee, S., Ramos, R. A., Lobb, R., Rosa, M., Chi-Rosso, G. and Wright, S. D. (1991). Endothelial-leukocyte adhesion molecule 1 stimulates the adhesive activity of leukocyte integrin CR3 (CD111b/CD18, Mac-1, alpha-m, beta-2) on human neutrophils. *J. Exp. Med.*, **173**, 1493–500.

Lowe, J. B., Stoolman, L. M., Nair, R. P., Larsen, R. D., Berhend, T. L. and Marks, R. M. (1990). ELAM-1-dependent cell adhesion to vascular endothelium determined by a transfected human fucosyltransferase cDNA. *Cell*, **63**, 475–84.

Lundgren, R., Soderberg, M., Horstedt, P. and Stenling, R. (1988). Morphological studies of bronchial mucosal biopsies from asthmatics before and after ten years of treatment with inhaled steroids. *Eur. Respir. J.*, **1**, 883–9.

Luscinskas, F. W., Brock, A. F., Arnaout, M. A. and Gimbrone, M. A., Jr (1989). Endothelial-leukocyte adhesion molecule-1-dependent and leukocyte (CD11/CD18)-dependent mechanisms contribute to polymorphonuclear leukocyte adhesion to cytokine-activated human vascular endothelium. *J. Immunol.*, **142**, 2257–63.

Macklem, P. T. (1989). Mechanical factors determining maximum bronchoconstriction. *Eur. Respir. J.*, **2**, 516s–519s.

Osborn, L., Hession, C., Tizard, R., Vassallo, C., Luhowskyj, S., Chi-Rosso, G. and Lobb, R. (1989). Direct expression cloning of vascular cell adhesion molecule-1, a cytokine-induced endothelial protein that binds to lymphocytes. *Cell*, **59**, 1203–11.

Pober, J. S., Gimbrone, M. A., Jr, LaPierre, L. A., Mendrick, D. L., Fiers, W., Rothlein, R. and Springer, T. A. (1986). Overlapping patterns of activation of human endothelial cells by interleukin-1, tumor, necrosis factor, and immune interferon. *J. Immunol.*, **137**, 1893–6.

Rampart, M. and Williams, T. J. (1988). Evidence that neutrophil accumulation induced by interleukin-1 requires both local protein biosynthesis and neutrophil CD18 antigen expression *in vivo. Br. J. Pharmacol.*, **94**, 1143–8.

Regnier-Vigouroux, A., Blanc, D., Pont, S., Marchetto, S. and Pierres, M. (1986). Accessory molecules and T cell activation I. Antigen receptor avidity differentially influences T cell sensitivity to inhibition by monoclonal antibodies to LFA-1 and L3T4. *Eur. J. Immunol.*, **16**, 1385–90.

Ryan, G., Latimer, K., Dolovich, J. and Hargreave, F. E. (1982). Bronchial responsiveness to histamine: relationship to diurnal variation of flow rates and improvement after bronchodilation. *Thorax*, **37**, 423–8.

Shappell, S. B., Toman, C., Anderson, D. C., Taylor, A. A., Entman, M. L. and Smith, C. W. (1990). Mac-1 (CD11b/CD18) mediates adherence-dependent hydrogen peroxide production by human and canine neutrophils. *J. Immunol.*, **144**, 2702–11.

Simon, R. H., DeHart, P. D. and Todd III, R. F. (1986). Neutrophil-induced injury of rat pulmonary alveolar epithelial cells. *J. Clin. Invest.*, **78**, 1375–86.

Smith, C. W., Marlin, S. D., Rothlein, R., Toman, C. and Anderson D. C. (1989). Cooperative interactions of LFA-1 and Mac-1 with intercellular adhesion molecule-1 in facilitating adherence and transendothelial migration of human neutrophils *in vitro. J. Clin. Invest.*, **83**, 2008–17.

Sotomayor, H., Badier, M., Vervloet, D. and Orehek, J. (1984). Seasonal increase of carbachol airway responsiveness in patients allergic to grass pollen. *Am. Rev. Respir. Dis.*, **130**, 56–8.

Springer, T. A. (1990). Adhesion receptors of the immune system. *Nature (London)*, **346**, 425–34.

Staunton, D. E., Marlin, S. D., Stratowa, C., Dustin, M. L. and Springer, T. A. (1988). Primary structure of ICAM-1 demonstrates interaction between members of the immunoglobulin and integrin supergene families. *Cell*, **52**, 925–33.

Townley, R. G., Ryo, U. Y., Kolotkin, B. M. and Kang, B. (1975). Bronchial sensitivity to methacholine in current and former asthmatics and allergic rhinitis patients and control subjects. *J. Allergy Clin. Immunol.*, **56**, 429–42.

Walsh, G. M., Mermod, J.-J., Hartnell, A., Kay, A. B. and Wardlaw, A. J. (1991). Human eosinophil, but not neutrophil, adherence to IL-1-stimulated human umbilical vascular endothelial cells is alpha-4–beta-1 (very late antigen-4) dependent. *J. Immunol.*, **146**, 3419–23.

Wardlaw, A. J., Dunnette, S., Gleich, G. J., Collins, J. V. and Kay, A. B. (1988). Eosinophils and mast cells in bronchoalveolar lavage in subjects with mild asthma: relationship to bronchial hyperreactivity. *Am. Rev. Respir. Dis.*, **137**, 62–9.

Wegner, C. D., Smith, C. W. and Rothlein, R. (1989). CD18 dependence of primate eosinophil adherence *in vitro*. In Springer, T. A., Anderson, D. C., Rosenthal, A. S. and Rothlein, R. (eds.), *Leukocyte adhesion molecules: Structure, Function, and Regulation*, Springer, New York, 208–14.

Wegner, C. D., Gundel, R. H., Reilly, P., Haynes, N., Letts, L. G. and Rothlein, R. (1990). Intercellular adhesion molecule-1 (ICAM-1) in the pathogenesis of asthma. *Science*, **247**, 456–9.

Wegner, C. D., Rothlein, R. and Gundel, R. H. (1991a). Adhesion molecules in the pathogenesis of asthma. *Agents Actions*, **34**, *Suppl.*, 529–44.

Wegner, C. D., Torcellini, C. A., Clarke, C. C., Letts, L. G. and Gundel, R. H. (1991b). Effects of single and multiple inhalations of antigen on airway responsiveness in monkeys. *J. Allergy Clin. Immunol.*, **87**, 835–41.

Wegner, C. D., Rothlein, R., Clarke, C. C., Haynes, N., Torcellini, C. A., LaPlante, A. M., Averill, D. R., Letts, L. G. and Gundel, R. H. (1991c). Inhaled anti-intercellular adhesion molecule-1 (ICAM-1) reduces antigen-induced airway hyperresponsiveness in monkeys. *Am. Rev. Respir. Dis.*, **143**, A418 (Abstract).

Wegner, C. D., Gundel, R. H., Rothlein, R. and Letts, L. G. (1992a). Expression and probable roles of cell adhesion molecules in lung inflammation. *Chest*, **101**, 34S–39S.

Wegner, C. D., Wolyniec, W. W. LaPlante, A. M., Marschman, K., Lubbe, K., Haynes, N., Rothlein, R. and Letts, L. G. (1992b). Intercellular adhesion molecule-1 (ICAM-1) contributes to pulmonary oxygen toxicity in mice: role of leukocytes revised. *Lung*, **170** (in the press).

19

Cells and Mediators Involved in Airway Hyperresponsiveness

G. Folkerts and F. P. Nijkamp

19.1 Introduction

Inflammation of the airways has long been recognized as a prominent feature of fatal asthma attacks, and recently, similar changes have been found in bronchial biopsies of even mild asthmatics. There is now abundant experimental evidence that inflammation of the airways may lead to bronchial hyperresponsiveness, which is a characteristic feature of asthma (Barnes *et al.*, 1988b; Djukanovic *et al.*, 1990; Postma *et al.*, 1989). These changes are likely to be induced by the release of various mediators, and the aim of this chapter is to discuss some of the cells and mediators that have been implicated.

19.2 Monocytes and Macrophages

The macrophage is part of a family of mononuclear cells found in virtually all organs. Traditionally, the classification of lung macrophages divides them into two categories based on their anatomic distribution: alveolar or interstitial.

Alveolar macrophages reside predominantly in the alveoli on the top of epithelial cells. Because of this strategic location, and because of their pronounced phagocytic capabilities, alveolar macrophages are an important component of the first line of defence of the body and the first phagocytic cells to encounter inhaled particles (Herscowitz, 1985; Sibille and Reynolds, 1990). Interstitial macrophages reside in the interstitium of the lung and may have either similar or different characteristics from alveolar macrophage counterparts. Studies are limited, but the available data support the notion that these cells have characteristics of both their precursors, peripheral blood monocytes, and their descendant alveolar macrophages.

Monocytes and macrophages release a vast array of molecules in response to various stimuli. Many of the molecules produced and released by mononuclear phagocytes have no known role in asthma syndromes at this time (Fels and Cohn, 1986; Herscowitz, 1985). Evidence supporting a putative role for some of these products, however, does exist (Rankin, 1989). For instance, six chemotaxins are identified: leukotriene (LT) B_4 (Fels et al., 1982; MacDermot et al., 1984), platelet activating factor (PAF) (Arnoux et al., 1980), tumour necrosis factor (TNF) (Beutler and Cerami, 1987), complement factor C_{5a} (Nathan, 1987), and platelet derived growth factor (Martinet et al., 1987). Interestingly, prostaglandin (PG) D_2, a putative macrophage product, potentiates LTB_4-induced chemotaxis (Soter et al., 1983). Further, products can be formed that will stimulate mucus secretion such as $PGF_{2\alpha}$, LTB_4, and 5-hydroxyeicosatetraenoic acid (HETE) (Raphael and Metcalfe, 1986). In addition, mediators are formed such as LTC_4/D_4, PAF, histamine releasing factors (HRF), enzymes, prostaglandin $F_{2\alpha}$, and thromboxanes (Tx), which can modulate airway contraction or can induce bronchial hyperresponsiveness (Barnes et al., 1988b; Djukanovic et al., 1990; Postma et al., 1989; Raphael and Metcalfe, 1986; Sibille and Reynolds, 1990).

Moreover, macrophages (and other inflammatory cells) can release reactive oxygen species (Fels and Cohn, 1986; Herscowitz, 1985; Nijkamp and Henricks, 1988). These products increase basal pulmonary resistance and the increase in pulmonary resistance induced by acetylcholine in vivo (Katsumata et al., 1990). They can contract guinea pig tracheas in vitro (Rhoden and Barnes, 1989), deteriorate tracheal β-adrenoceptor function (Engels et al., 1987), and are involved in the LTD_4-induced tracheal hyperresponsiveness (Weiss and Bellino, 1986). Further, oxygen species can release histamine from mast cells (Mannaioni and Masini, 1988).

A number of mediators mentioned above have been proved to be formed during phagocytosis of particles by alveolar macrophages. Alveolar macrophages can also be activated through the interaction of immunglobulin E (IgE) immune complexes with an IgE Fc receptor on the macrophage surface (Fels and Cohn, 1986; Herscowitz, 1985). It is now known that the IgE Fc receptor expressed on the surface of macrophages is similar, if not identical, to that on T and B lymphocytes, platelets and eosinophils. This receptor is referred to as IgE $Fc_\varepsilon RII$ receptor and differs both structurally and functionally from the IgE Fc receptor on mast cells and basophils, which is referred to as IgE $Fc_{\varepsilon}RI$ receptor. The most important functional difference is that the IgE $Fc_{\varepsilon}RII$ on macrophages is a low-affinity receptor (Rankin, 1989).

Finally, one of the main functions of mononuclear phagocytes is the initiation of immune responses. Macrophages accomplish this complex task by presenting antigen to lymphocytes, and by elaborating monokines, such as interleukin-1, that in turn stimulate lymphocytes for diverse effector functions.

19.3 Lymphocytes

Lymphocytes can roughly be divided into T-cells and B-cells. T-cells are produced in the thymus; hence the name T cells. In birds, B-cells differentiate in the bursa of Fabricius; hence the name B cells. Mammals have no bursa: instead, islands of haemopoietic cells in the foetal liver and in the foetal and adult bone marrow give rise directly to B lymphocytes. As well as being a site of B-cell generation, the adult bone marrow contains many mature T-cells and plasma cells. In man bone marrow is also an important secondary lymphoid organ like the spleen and lymph nodes.

B lymphocytes represent about 5–10% of the circulating lymphoid pool and are classically defined by the presence of endogenously produced immunoglobulins (antibodies). These molecules are inserted into the surface membrane where they act as specific antigen receptors. T-cells can be subdivided into $T_{helper/inducer}$-cells ($T_{h/i}$, $CD4^+$), which recognize antigens in association with major histocompatibility complex (MHC) class II molecules, and $T_{cytotoxic/suppressor}$ cells ($T_{c/s}$, $CD8^+$) which recognize antigens in association with MHC class I molecules. The subscripts are indicative of the functions of the T-cells in the immune system.

Lymphocytes are mononuclear cells with a diameter of 6–8 μm and can be found throughout airway tissue. Particularly prominent in bronchioles are discrete aggregates of lymphatic tissue subjacent to morphologically specialized lympho-epithelium. Intra-epithelial lymphocytes are mainly T-cells (Fournier et al., 1989). Among these T-cells the suppressor–cytotoxic subtypes usually predominate in humans. Several studies have demonstrated a disturbance of cell-mediated immunity in asthma. A relative deficiency in the number of T-suppressor cells has been observed in both allergic and non-allergic asthma. It has been shown recently that T-helper lymphocytes are activated, as measured by membrane activation markers, in acute asthma (Corrigan et al., 1988). Lymphocytes from patients with allergic asthma produce more IL-2 than do those from healthy persons after allergen stimulation in vitro (Hseih, 1985). Moreover, viral respiratory tract infections in asthmatic patients can additionally enhance IL-2 production after allergen stimulation (Lin *et al.*, 1988). Interestingly, IL-2, the principal lymphokine responsible for lymphocyte proliferation, induces airway hyperresponsiveness to methacholine in rats *in vivo* when administered intraperitoneally twice a day during 4.5 days (Renzi, 1991). Further, lymphocytes from patients with allergic and non-allergic asthma spontaneously produce histamine releasing factor (HRF) *in vitro* (Alam *et al.*, 1987). Interestingly, the magnitude of the spontaneous HRF release correlated with the state of bronchial hyperresponsiveness in asthmatic patients. This lymphokine induces the release of histamine and LTC_4 from basophils and mast cells *in vitro* and induces bronchoconstriction and skin, weal and flare reactions *in vivo*. Besides HRF, lymphocytes from asthmatic patients spontaneously produce a factor with chemokinetic, chemotactic and complement receptor-inducing activities on eosinophils (Parish and Luckhurst, 1982). The effect of this factor is specific for eosinophils as neutrophils do not respond to it. This factor might be IL-5, as this lymphokine is a selective stimulator of eosinophil but not neutrophil function in humans (Lopez *et al.*, 1988). IL-5 stimulates eosinophil phagocytosis, cytotoxicity and superoxide production. It also stimulates the growth and differentiation of eosinophils and enhances IgE antibody production by B-lymphocytes (Miyajima *et al.*, 1988).

Upon stimulation of lymphocytes, interferon-(INF) γ is released, which is the key lymphokine in the activation of monocytes and macrophages. INF-γ enhances the phagocytic and microbicidal activity as well as the production of superoxide and hydrogen peroxide by macrophages (Black *et al.*, 1987). In addition, INF-γ releases PAF from human monocytes (Valone and Epstein, 1988). Alveolar macrophages activated by INF-γ release more LTB_4, TxB_2, and $PGF_{2\alpha}$ after stimulation by zymosan than do non-activated alveolar macrophages (O'Sullivan *et al.*, 1988). So, a number of lymphokines could contribute to the induction of airway hyperresponsiveness.

19.4 Eosinophils

Eosinophils constitute 1–4% of the leukocytes in normal blood and have a diameter of about 9 μm. The nucleus is usually bilobate and the main identifying characteristic of eosinophils is the presence of ovoid granulations (0.5–1.5 μm) (along the main axis) that can be stained with eosin (acidophilic granules).

In allergic and non-allergic asthma the number of eosinophils is increased (eosinophilia) in the peripheral blood and in sputum (Franklin, 1974; Horn *et al.*, 1975; Lowell, 1967). Investigations of the putative role of eosinophils in asthma have mostly been restricted to blood and BAL studies in asthmatic subjects. With allergen challenge, a transient decrease in the number of eosinophils (eosinopenia) occurs at 6 h post-challenge (Durham *et al.*, 1989) followed by a progressive eosinophilia continuing up to 24 h post-challenge (Durham and Kay, 1985). In animal studies, the selective trapping of these cells by the bronchial vascular endothelium suggests an important role for adherence in cell recruitment (Dunn *et al.*, 1988) and provides a mechanism for transient eosinopenia. The eosinophilia can be explained by release of eosinophils from the reticuloendothelial system in response to cytokines released into the circulation from the airways.

Several factors are capable of stimulating eosinophil growth, including those released by epithelial (Ohnishi *et al.*, 1989) and mast cells, granulocyte–macrophage colony-stimulating factor (GM-CSF) (Metcalf *et al.*, 1986), IL-3 (Yang *et al.*, 1986) and IL-5 (Campbell *et al.*, 1987). In addition to supporting colony growth and maturation of eosinophils, these factors also liberate cells from the bone marrow and preactivate (prime) them (Lopez *et al.*, 1986). Eosinophils have to be primed before they release their preformed and newly generated mediators maximally. Besides the cytokines mentioned above, LTB_4, and PAF are also capable of priming eosinophils (Lopez *et al.*, 1986).

Circulating eosinophils display a range of densities upon separation by discontinuous density contrifugation, with predominance of hypodense cells. In asthmatic patients, the hypodense eosinophils are in an activated state, as shown by their increase in oxygen consumption, phagocytosis and cytotoxic capacity, and their spontaneous release of their granule contents (Wardlaw *et al.*, 1988b). The capacity of activated eosinophils to generate LTC_4 surpasses that of many other cells considered to be involved in the inflammatory process in asthma (Shaw *et al.*, 1985). Further, eosinophils can generate reactive oxygen radicals (Agosti *et al.*, 1987), PAF (Lee *et al.*, 1984), LTB_4 and 5- and 15-HETE (Shaw *et al.*, 1985; Wardlaw *et al.*, 1988b). Besides these products, four highly charged arginine-rich proteins have been located in the granules of human eosinophils; major basic protein (MBP), eosinophilic cationic protein (ECP), eosinophil peroxidase (EPO), and eosinophil-derived neurotoxin (EDN).

MBP is cytotoxic for guinea pig tracheal epithelial cells at concentrations as low as 9×10^{-7} M which is well below the 1×10^{-5} M found in asthmatic sputum (Gleigh *et al.*, 1979). High concentrations of MBP lead to extensive damage of guinea pig tracheal epithelial cells and at lower concentrations (10 µg/ml) ciliostasis is found (Frigas *et al.*, 1980). MBP is also cytotoxic in human bronchial tissue explants (Frigas *et al.*, 1981) and decreases ciliary function, possibly by inhibiting axonomal activity (Hastie *et al.*, 1987). The concentration of MBP has been shown to correlate with indices of airway responsiveness and the number of ciliated epithelial cells recovered by broncho-alveolar lavage (BAL). The concentration of MBP in BAL of symptomatic asthmatics has been documented in relation to disease exacerbations, with a decrease after appropriate treatment (Frigas *et al.*, 1981). Finally, MBP deposition in bronchial wall and mucus has been demonstrated by immunofluorescent techniques (Filley *et al.*, 1982). Other eosinophil proteins, active radicals of oxygen, and neutral proteases may damage the epithelium as well. The combination of epithelial damage and the release of mediators that will stimulate mucus secretion and broncho-constriction may contribute to airway hyperresponsiveness.

However, a protective role of the eosinophil cannot be excluded since the cell is able to degrade histamine, to inactivate leukotrienes and PAF, and to suppress histamine release (Bass, 1979; Goetzl *et al.*, 1975; Hubscher, 1975; Wasserman *et al.*, 1975; Zeiger and Colten, 1977). A defect in this balance could be the central point in asthma.

19.5 Neutrophils

Neutrophils, which constitute 60–70% of circulating leukocytes, develop in the bone marrow and are released into the circulation. They are about 12 μm in diameter, with a nucleus consisting of 2–5 sausage-shaped lobes linked to each other by threads of chromatin. Neutrophils are part of the primary defence of the body against infections and contain two types of granules: the primary azurophilic granules which contain acid hydrolase (e.g. acid phosphatase, β-glucuronidase), neutral proteases (elastase) and myeolperoxydase; the specific granules which contain lysozyme, lactoferrin, cathepsin G and collagenase and a protease that generates reactive oxygen metabolites and the phospholipid mediators LTB_4, TxA_2, 5-HETE and PAF (Djukanovic *et al.*, 1990; Herscowitz, 1985).

There is no convincing evidence to suggest a role for neutrophils in asthma.

BAL performed 4 h post-allergen challenge has shown an increase in both neutrophil and eosinophil number, with neutrophils subsiding and the eosinophil counts remaining elevated 24 h post-challenge (Joseph *et al.*, 1986). In another study the number of neutrophils in BAL in asthmatics and non-asthmatics demonstrated widely different values (Collins *et al.*, 1986). In one report there was an increase in neutrophils in asthma; in another report their numbers were similar in asthmatics and non-asthmatics. Also the reports about the role of the neutrophils in non-allergic airway hyperresponsiveness are contradictory.

In humans (Seltzer *et al.*, 1986) and dogs (Holtzman *et al.*, 1983b) exposed to ozone, an increase in airway hyperresponsiveness is observed in association with an increase of neutrophils in BAL. Dogs that were made neutropenic did not show an increased airway response after ozone treatment (O'Byrne *et al.*, 1984).

In contrast, hyperresponsiveness induced by ozone in rats (Evans *et al.*, 1988a) and guinea pigs (Murlas and Roum, 1985a, b) was neutrophil independent. In addition, increased airway response induced by cigarette smoke (Hulbert *et al.*, 1985) and toluene diisocyanate (Thompson *et al.*, 1986) in guinea pigs was not associated with an influx of neutrophils into the lung. Moreover, a marked increase of neutrophils in the airways, induced by sulphur dioxide in dogs (Shore *et al.*, 1987) and by endotoxin nebulization in guinea pigs (Folkerts *et al.*, 1988), caused a hyporesponsiveness of the respiratory tract, rather than a hyperresponsiveness.

These results taken together make it seem unlikely that neutrophils play a crucial role in asthma.

19.6 Basophils and Mast Cells

Ehrlich identified mast cells in human connective tissue on the basis of the metachromatic staining properties of their prominent cytoplasmic granules (Ehrlich, 1878). Ehrlich also described the basophil, a circulating leukocyte containing cytoplasmic granules similar in staining properties to those of mast cells (Ehrlich, 1879). Both cell types express plasma membrane receptors ($Fc_\varepsilon RI$) that specifically bind, with high affinity, the Fc portion of IgE antibody (Blank *et al.*, 1989; Michell *et al.*, 1983; Miller *et al.*, 1989). Basophils and mast cells can be actively or passively sensitized with IgE (Galli, 1990). After exposure to the specific antigen both cell types release preformed mediators stored in the cytoplasmic granules (such as histamine, heparin, or other sulphated proteoglycans, and certain proteases) and the *de novo* synthesis and release of mediators such as prostaglandins and leukotrienes (Galli, 1990). Interestingly, degranulation of metachromatic cells is not only induced by stimulation of Fc receptors but can be induced by a number of non-specific agents such as hypoxia, cytokines, C_{3a}, C_{4a}, C_{5a}, heat–cold–trauma, osmotic changes, substance P, neuropeptides Y and K, somatostatin, adenosine triphosphate, PAF, oxygen intermediates, and arachidonic acid metabolism (Djukanovic *et al.*, 1990; Galli, 1990).

Despite the many remarkable similarities, mammalian mast cells and basophils are clearly not identical.

Basophils constitute only 0–1% of blood leukocytes. They measure 5–7 μm in diameter and have a large nucleus with an irregular twisted shape, generally in the form of an S. Basophils are not primarily found in connective tissue but they mainly circulate in blood. They mature in bone marrow and share a common precursor with other granulocytes and monocytes. Basophils may share more similarities with eosinophils than with neutrophils (Denburg *et al.*, 1986; Slifman *et al.*, 1988). The recruitment of basophils into the tissues can be established during IgE-dependent reactions and by a variety of inflammatory, immunologic and pathologic responses (Galli and Askenase, 1986; Galli *et al.*, 1984). Basophils are exquisitely sensitive to anti-IgE. Maximal release of basophil mediators can be achieved by 0.05 to 0.1 µg/ml of anti-IgE, and that is about 1% as much as is required to activate mast cells maximally (Ehrlich, 1879). Further, basophils are sensitive to cytokines, especially to HRF which can be formed by many cells (macrophages, mononuclear cells, platelets and endothelial cells) (Lett-Brown *et al.*, 1989). Basophils can also be activated by a variety of secretagogues such as F-met-leu-phe, C5a, and phorbol esters (TPA), and various polyamines (e.g. polyarginine and polylysine, but not compound 48/80) that fail to activate mast cells (Cohan *et al.*, 1989; Galli, 1990). Upon stimulation basophils release primarily histamine and LTC_4, but probably not metabolites of the cyclooxygenase pathway (Cohan *et al.*, 1989; Galli, 1990).

In addition, a number of autacoids can modulate mediator release negatively by stimulating adenylyl cyclase, for instance by histamine, prostanoids and beta-adrenergic agonist (Cohen *et al.*, 1989; Galli, 1990).

Mast cells are large (6–12 µm) and have an ovoid structure. Their cytoplasm is filled with smaller and more granules than occur in basophils. The nucleus of the mast cell is spherical, non-segmented and centrally situated. In contrast to basophils, mast cells are ordinarily distributed throughout normal connective tissue where they are often situated adjacent to blood and lymphatic vessels, near to or within nerves, and beneath epithelial surfaces, such as those of the respiratory and gastrointestinal system and skin, areas that are exposed to environmental stimuli. Mammalian mast cells are probably derived from precursors that originate in the bone marrow. In contrast to basophils, there are no mature mast cells in the circulation. The life span of mast cells is weeks to months and that of basophils days like other granulocytes.

Mast cells can be divided into subtypes. In 1895 Hardy and Wesbrook published evidence for morphological differences among mast cells, observed in different anatomical locations in the rat. On the basis of detailed conditions of fixation and histochemical staining, mast cells were discriminated into 'atypical' or 'mucosal' mast cells (MMCs) observed in the intestinal lamina propria and the 'connective tissue type' mast cell (CTMC) of the skin, peritoneal cavity and other sites in the rat (Enerback, 1981, 1986). Later MMCs and CTMCs were found to differ in many other aspects of biochemistry, function and role in inflammation and immunity (Aldenborg and Enerback, 1985; Bienenstock *et al.*, 1986; Jarrett, 1984). It is not possible to define completely human mast cell subpopulations that are analogous in all respects to MMCs and CTMCs of different animal species. The most attractive available potential 'marker' to differentiate human mast cell subpopulations is now the cytoplasmic granule protease content (Galli, 1990). Like rats and mice, humans have mast cells that differ in neutral protease content. Some human mast cells contain measurable levels of both tryptase and chymase (MC^{tc}) (Craig et al., 1986; Irani et al., 1986; Schwatz, 1989) whereas other human mast cells contain tryptase but no detectable chymase (MC^{t}) (Irani et al., 1986; Schwatz, 1989). MC^{t}s predominate in lung and small intestinal mucosa and MC^{tc} predominate in skin and small intestinal submucosa, however, all of these sites contain representatives of both mast cells subtypes (Schwatz, 1989).

MC^{t}s seem similar to rat and mouse MMCs, and MC^{tc}s resemble murine CTMCs. However, we must be cautious in predicting properties of MC^{t}s and MC^{tc}s on the bases of the properties of MMCs and CTMCs respectively (Galli, 1990).

In general some remarks can be made about MC^{t}–MMCs and MC^{tc}–CTMCs.

When stimulated, MC^{t}–MMCs release histamine and products of both pathways of arachidonic acid metabolism, LTC_4 and PGD_2. Contradictory results have been obtained about the release of PAF in vitro after stimulation of human MC^{t}–MMCs (Schleimer et al., 1986). It is clear, however, that PAF and its lyso derivative have been characterized after challenge by antigen of the human airways in vivo (Peters et al., 1986). F-met-leu-phe, C_{5a} and TPA are not as active in these MC^{t}–MMCs as in basophils, and human MC^{t}–MMCs fail to respond to substance P or other neuropeptides studied. Further, human lung and gut mast cells do not respond to compound 48/80, which is a favoured secretagogue used for murine mast cells (Cohan et al, 1989). MC^{t}–MMCs are exquisitely sensitive to changes in osmolarity (Eggleston et al., 1987), a stimulus that is believed to be responsible for the contraction of the airways during inhalation of cold and dry air in vivo (Togias et al., 1988b). In contrast to the basophil, this type of MC^{t}–MMC is unresponsive to corticosteroids, but has beta-adrenergic and prostanoid receptors linked to adenylyl cyclase (Peters et al., 1982). There are no functional histamine H_2-receptors.

MC^{tc}–CTMCs are as sensitive to anti IgE as are MC^{t}–MMCs and in contrast to MC^{t}–MMCs they are not sensitive to the inhibitory effect of cromolyn sodium. MC^{tc}–CTMCs do not respond to C_{5a} or F-met-leu-phe but can be activated by compound 48/80, tachykinins, basic polyamines and opiates (Cohan et al., 1989). Further, it is the only cell containing histamine that responds to bradykinin. The major inflammatory mediators released by this cell type are histamine and PGD_2.

Recently, a third mast cell type has been characterized, namely the mast cell in broncho-alveolar lavage fluid (MC^{bal}) (Pearce et al., 1987). In healthy human lung washings 0.04–0.6% of the total population of nucleated cells comprises mast cells (Flint et al., 1985a, b; Pearce et al., 1987; Tomioka et al., 1984; Wilson et al., 1986) whereas, in ashmatics, the numbers can be increased three- to five-fold (Pearce et al., 1987; Wilson *et al.*, 1986). The MC^{bal}s from both healthy persons, and allergic or asthmatic patients are about 10–30-fold more sensitive than are human basophils and almost a thousand times more reactive to anti-IgE than are human lung mast cells (Bleecker *et al.*, 1988). In addition, MC^{bal}s respond to HRF, which is present in bronchial secretions *in vivo*. It is suggested that the presence of HRF, the responsiveness to HRF of MC^{bal}s and the extreme sensitivity of these cells to anti IgE may be interrelated (Gittlen *et al.*, 1988). MC^{bal}s produce histamine and PGD_2; the release of LTC_4 is not clear. They do not react to the protein kinase inhibitor staurosporine, but are very sensitive to inhibition by isoproterenol and theophylline (Cohan *et al.*, 1989).

Besides the type, the stimulation, and mediator release of the mast cell, the proliferation can be of importance in disease. In the murine system two distinct T-cell factors, IL-3 and IL-4, are known to stimulate proliferation of cultured mast cells (Hmamguchi *et al.*, 1986). IL-3 induces development of MMCs while IL-4 stimulates clonal growth of CTMCs in the presence of IL-3. In a recent study the effects of IL-3 and IL-4 were investigated on cultured human mast cells obtained by broncho-alveolar lavages (Tanno *et al.*, 1990). The results suggested that T-cell factors, including IL-3 and IL-4, and fibroblasts influence the phenotype and the survival of these mast cells in BAL, whereas there was no evidence for the presence of mast cell precursors in BAL fluid.

Interestingly, some mast cells may be able to release factors with both positive and negative effects on their own proliferation. For instance, the mast cell can be stimulated by and can produce IL-3 (Bressler *et al.*, 1989). Upon appropriate stimulation, mast cells can produce GM-CSF (Bressler *et al.*, 1989) and GM-CSF can subsequently suppress the growth of mast cells *in vitro* (Gordon *et al.*, 1990). The mast cell contains messenger RNA for a number of other cytokines, and the formation of TNFα and IL-6 is evident (Gordon *et al.*, 1990).

Increases in the number of mast cells in the airways and/or changes in mediator release can contribute to airway hyperresponsiveness. The causal relationship between mediators and their biological effect in the respiratory tract has therefore been studied extensively. When compared with the BAL mast cells of healthy control subjects, those from atopic asthmatics contain and release more histamine, both spontaneously and when stimulated with anti-IgE or allergen (Tomioka *et al.*, 1984; Wilson *et al.*, 1986). An inverse correlation between both the percentage of mast cells in the recovered BAL fluid and their histamine content and baseline spirometry suggests that histamine and other mediators derived from mast cells contribute to airflow obstruction (Wilson *et al.*, 1986). Histamine causes contraction of bronchial smooth muscle through stimulation of H_1-receptors. Other actions that may be relevant to bronchoconstriction of this mediator are its capacity to dilate and increase the permeability of the bronchial vascular bed (Evans *et al.*, 1988b; Persson, 1987; White *et al.*, 1987). Through stimulation of histamine H_2-receptors, mucus is secreted (White *et al.*, 1987) and, by activation of H_1-receptors, mucus viscosity can be modulated (Marin *et al.*, 1977), contributing further to airway obstruction. A positive correlation is found between airway responsiveness and the relative numbers of mast cells recovered by BAL (Flint *et al.*, 1985a; Kirby *et al.*, 1987). Further, an increased spontaneous histamine release by BAL mast cells is seen only in those subjects with enhanced bronchial responsiveness (Wardlaw *et al.*, 1988a). Moreover, the concentration of histamine in the cell-free supernatant of BAL is related to the level of methacholine responsiveness (Casale *et al.*, 1987). Recently, we demonstrated (Folkerts, 1991) that the virus-induced airway hyperresponsiveness in guinea pigs can be inhibited by pretreatment of the animals with H_1-receptor antagonists or mast cell stabilizers. In addition, mast cell morphology and number were changed and the histamine content was increased in BAL of guinea pigs infected with parainfluenza 3 virus. The mechanism by which histamine modulates airway smooth muscle responsiveness is probably a general phenomenon since it has been shown that coronary arteries from hearts of cardiac patients contain significantly higher concentrations of histamine than do those from non-cardiac patients, and the coronary artery vessels of cardiac patients are also hyperresponsive to histamine and serotonin (Kalsner and Richards, 1984).

Other mast cell mediators that are likely to play important roles as effectors of bronchoconstriction and inflammation are PGD_2, tryptase, and the sulphidopeptide leukotrienes. In addition to being a direct spasmogen, approximately 30 times more potent than histamine, PGD_2 is a potent vasodilator and increases vascular permeability (Beasley *et al.*, 1988). Tryptase has recently been shown to augment airway smooth muscle response in dogs (Proud *et al.*, 1988), being able to degrade bronchodilator neuropeptides such as VIP and to cleave complement components to form anaphylatoxins and kininogen to yield bradykinin and lysylbradykinin (Caughey *et al.*, 1988; Sekizawa *et al.*, 1989). In addition to increasing vascular leakage, the suphidopeptide leukotrienes are reported to be 100 to 1000 times more potent than histamine or methacholine as contractile agonists (Adelroth *et al.*, 1986; Schwartz *et al.*, 1983).

The mast cell may be the key cell, in concert with other inflammatory cells, in the induction of airway hyperresponsiveness.

19.7 Epithelial Cells

The respiratory airways, like the skin and gut, are covered by an epithelial layer. All epithelial cells adhere with their basal surface to the basement membrane. The lining of the trachea and bronchi down to the region of the bronchioles is composed of pseudostratified columnar ciliated epithelium, which contains numerous goblet cells. At least thirteen cell types (eleven epithelial and two mesenchymal) can be recognized in the tracheo-bronchial epithelium. The six most important will be discussed in short.

The ciliated cells are columnar and have a broad luminal surface covered by numerous cilia and microvilli (250–300/cell). They are present until the level of the respiratory bronchioles. Their main function is to transport the tracheo-bronchial secretions towards the pharynx. The goblet cells are interspersed among the ciliated cells and are present until the level of the terminal bronchioles. They secrete mucus, which is a heterogeneous substance, consisting mainly of water (95%), salts (1%), glycoproteins (1–3%), and small amounts of protein. The function of mucus is to clear the airways of particles and to humidify the incoming air. Clara cells (non-ciliated bronchiolar secretory cells) are most abundant in the bronchioles and secrete a material which is not mucoid, but possibly a lipoprotein, which may serve as a kind of surfactant. Brush cells are covered by numerous microvilli. They can be divided into two types. The first type has the characteristics of an immature cell and presumably is a replacement of ciliated or goblet cells that have died. The second type possesses synapses at the basal surface. Because of this morphologic feature, which is a characteristic of neural cells, it is regarded as a sensory receptor cell. K cells or small granulated cells contain 'neurosecretory' granules. These granules contain small amounts of serotonin and catecholamines. They are part of the so-called APUD (amine precursor uptake and degradation) system and are involved in mucous and serous secretory processes. Basal cells are rounded or triangular cells, in close contact with the basement membrane. They are thought to be the regenerative cells of the epithelium, from which all other types of cells differentiate.

In patients with asthma, epithelial desquamation and sloughing are characteristic findings in bronchial tissue obtained at autopsy (Dunnill, 1960) and biopsy (Salvato, 1968). Laitinen and coworkers (Laitinen et al., 1985) have found extensive damage of the epithelium and areas in which only basal cells were present in biopsies of airways of asthmatics. In addition it has been demonstrated that the intercellular spaces are widened and that the size and number of epithelial goblet cells are increased. In two studies, a positive relation was found between the epithelial cell number in broncho-alveolar lavage (BAL) and airway hyperresponsiveness (Beasley et al., 1989; Wardlaw et al., 1988a). Further, in the study of Laitinen et al. (1985) it was shown that, in asthmatic patients, the degree of airway hyperresponsiveness was associated with the degree of epithelial damage.

This could be due to a number of factors (Hogg and Eggleston, 1984). First, damage of the epithelial layer may result in mediator release (Nadel, 1988). Epithelial cells are able to produce leukotriene B_4 (Holtzman et al.,

1983a) which predominantly attracts neutrophils. However, leukotriene B_4 also contracts airway smooth muscle in some species (Lawson et al., 1986) and causes airway hyperresponsiveness in dogs after aerosol inhalation, which is associated with an increase in the tromboxane B_2 concentration in broncho-alveolar lavage fluid (O'Byrne et al., 1985). Epithelial cells also release prostaglandin $F_{2\alpha}$ which contracts smooth muscle and enhances mucus secretion and airway reactivity (Barnes et al., 1988). The chemotactic agent 5-hydroxyeicosatraenoic acid (HETE) is synthesized by epithelial cells and 15-HETE and 8,15-di-HETE which are likely to be important to airway homeostasis (Hunter et al., 1985). In addition it was recently found that guinea pig tracheal epithelial cells could produce 9- and 13-hydroxyoctadecadienoic acid (HODE) after incubation with [^{14}C]linoleic acid (Oosthuizen et al., 1990). Interestingly, 13-HODE can induce bronchial hyperresponsiveness in the guinea pig in vitro and in vivo (Henricks et al., 1991).

Secondly, the epithelial layer could be just a diffusion barrier. It has been shown in animal studies that drugs when applied to the serosal side of the airways were 35–115-fold more active than applied to the luminal side of the airways (Mitchell et al., 1989; Munakata et al., 1989). This difference disappeared after epithelial denudation. Further, it was demonstrated that epithelium-derived factors that could inhibit airway contractions were not involved (Sparrow and Mitchell, 1991). So, they argued that the epithelium was a diffusion barrier. In contrast, a number of authors provided evidence that the epithelial layer can release factors that suppress airway contractions (Aizawa et al., 1988; Barnett et al., 1988; Goldie et al., 1990; Vanhoutte, 1989). We demonstrated (Nijkamp and Folkerts, 1986) in an in vitro study that KCl precontracted tracheas relaxed after arachidonic acid stimulation. This relaxation was associated with an increase in the prostaglandin E_2 concentration in the organ bath. Tracheas denuded of epithelium, in contrast, responded with a contraction that was mediated by leukotrienes and was associated with a diminished production of prostaglandin E_2. Further, it was shown (Folkerts et al., 1989) that the increased airway contraction to histamine after removal of epithelium was accompanied by a decreased prostaglandin E_2 concentration. Therefore, a decreased production of relaxing factors derived from the epithelium may also contribute to airway hyperresponsiveness.

Thirdly, the epithelium contains neutral metallo-endopeptidase (Jacques et al., 1989), which rapidly degrades (neuro)-peptides. A number of peptides (endothelin, neurokinins A and B, substance P) have potent contractile effects on airway smooth muscle (Black et al., 1988; Naline et al., 1989). The diminished breakdown of these peptides could enhance airway contractility.

Fourthly, unmyelinated afferent nerve endings (located between the epithelial cells) exposed by epithelial damage can be more easily stimulated by inflammatory mediators or inhaled air and particles. This leads to an axon reflex and liberation of neuro-peptides that in turn can contract airway smooth muscle and can stimulate mast cells (Barnes, 1987; McDonald, 1987).

Finally, a dysfunction of the cilia and/or goblet cells may not only lead to airway obstruction (Cutz *et al.*, 1978) but also influence the osmolarity, humidity and temperature of the lining fluid covering the airways which in turn can result in mast cell activation (Finnerty and Holgate, 1990; Togias *et al.*, 1988a). It has been shown that the inhalation of dry air resulted in a bronchoconstriction that was induced by mediators from mast cells. In addition, a dysfunction of the ciliated cells can lead to infections of the deeper airways, since the mucus blanket with the inhaled particles will not be transported to the pharynx but will sink into the peripheral airways (Macklam *et al.*, 1970; Wanner, 1977).

In conclusion, by a number of ways inflammatory – and epithelial – cells can be involved in the induction of airway hyperresponsiveness.

References

Adelroth, E., Morris, M. M., Hargreave, F. E. and O'Byrne, P. M. (1986). Airway responsiveness to leukotrienes C4 and D4 and to methacholine in patients with asthma and normal controls. *N. Eng. J. Med.*, **315**, 480–4.

Agosti, J. M., Altman, L. C., Ayars, G. M., Loegering, D. A., Gleich, G. H. and Klebanoff, S. J. (1987). The injurious effect of eosiniphil, peroxidase, hydrogen peroxide and halides on pneumocytes *in vitro*. *J. Allergy Clin. Immunol.*, **79**, 496–504.

Aizawa, H., Miyazaki, N., Shigematsu, N. and Tomooka, M. (1988). A possible role of airway epithelium in modulating hyperresponsiveness. *Br. J. Pharmacol.*, **93**, 139–45.

Alam, R., Kuna, P., Rozniecki, J. and Kuzminska, B. (1987). The magnitude of the spontaneous production of histamine-releasing factor (HRF) by lymphocytes *in vitro* correlates with the state of bronchial hyperreactivity in patients with asthma. *J. Allergy Clin. Immunol.*, **79**, 103–8.

Aldenborg, F. and Enerback, L. (1985). Thymus dependence of connective tissue mast cells: a quantitative cytofluorometric study of the growth of peritoneal mast cells in normal and athymic rats. *Int. Allergy Appl. Immunol.*, **78**, 277–80.

Arnoux, B., Duval, D. and Benveniste, J. (1980). Release of platelet activating factor (PAF-acether) from alveolar macrophages *in vitro*. *J. Clin. Invest.*, **10**, 437–41.

Barnes, P. J. (1987). Airway neuropeptides and asthma. *Trends Pharmacol. Sci.*, **8**, 24–7.

Barnes, P. J., Chung, K. F. and Page, C. P. (1988). Inflammatory mediators and asthma, *Pharmacol. Rev.*, **40**, 49–84.

Barnett, K., Jacoby, D. B., Nadel, J. A. and Lazarus, S. C. (1988). The effects of epithelial cell supernatants on contractions of isolated canine tracheal smooth muscle. *Am. Rev. Respir. Dis.*, **138**, 780–3.

Bass, D. A. (1979). The functions of eosinophils. *Ann. Intern. Med.*, **91**, 120–1.

Beasley, R., Hovel, C., Mani, R., Robinson, C., Varley, J. and Holgate, S. T. (1988). Comparative effects of histamine, prostaglandin (PG)D2, and its metabolite 9alpha, 11beta-PGF2 in human skin. *Clin. Allergy*, **18**, 619–27.

Beasley, R., Roche, W. R., Roberts, J. A. and Holgate, S. T. (1989). Cellular events in the bronchi in mild asthma and after bronchial provocation. *Am. Rev. Respir. Dis.*, **139**, 806–17.

Corrigan, C. J., Hartnell, A. and Kay, A. B. (1988). T-lymphocyte activation in acute severe asthma. *Lancet*, **i**, 1129–32.

Craig, S. S., DeBlois, G. and Schwartz, L. B. (1986). Mast cells in human keloid, small intestine, and lung by an immunoperoxidase technique using a murine monoclonal antibody. *Am. J. Pathol.*, **124**, 427–34.

Cutz, E., Levison, H. and Cooper, D. M. (1978). Ultrastructure of airways in children with asthma. *Histopathology*, **2**, 407–21.

Denburg, J. A., Tanno Y. and Bienenstock, J. (1986). Growth and differentiation of human basophils, eosinophils, and mast cells. In Befus, A. D., Bienenstock, J. and Denburg, J. A. (eds.), *Mast Cell Differentiation and Heterogeneity*, Raven Press, New York, 71–103.

Djukanovic, R., Roche, W. R., Wilson, J. W., Beasley, C. R. W., Twentyman, O. P., Howarth, P. H. and Holgate, S. T. (1990). Mucosal inflammation in asthma. *Am. Rev. Respir. Dis.*, **142**, 434–57.

Dunn, C. J., Elliot, G. A., Oostven, J. A. and Richards, I. M. (1988). Development of a prolonged eosinophil-rich inflammatory leukocyte infiltration in the guinea pig asthmatic response to ovalbumin inhalation. *Am. Rev. Respir. Dis.*, **137**, 541–7.

Dunnill, M. S. (1960). The pathology of asthma with special reference to changes in the bronchial mucosa. *J. Clin. Pathol.*, **13**, 27–33.

Durham, S. R. and Kay, A. B. (1985). Eosinophils, bronchial hyperreactivity and late-phase asthmatic reactions. *Clin. Allergy*, **15**, 411–18.

Durham, S. R., Cookson, W. O., Faux, J., Craddock, C. F. and Benson, M. K. (1989). Basic mechanisms in allergen-induced late asthmatic responses. *Clin. Exp. Allergy*, **19**, 117A.

Eggleston, P. A., Kagey-Sobotka, A. and Lichtenstein, L. M. (1987). A comparison of the osmotic activation of basophils and human lung mast cells. *Am. Rev. Respir. Dis.*, **135**, 1043–8.

Ehrlich, P. (1878). *Beiträge zur Theorie and Praxis der histologischen Färbung.* Dissertation.

Ehrlich, P. (1879). Uber die spezifischen Granulationen des Blutes. *Arch. Anat. Physiol. Abt.*, 571–7.

Enerback, L. (1981). The gut mucosal mast cell. *Monogr. Allergy*, **17**, 222–6.

Enerback, L. (1986). Mast cell heterogeneity: the evolution of the concept of a specific mucosal mast cell. In Befus, A. D., Bienenstock, J. and Denburg, J. A. (eds.), *Mast Cell Differentiation and Heterogeneity*, Raven Press, New York, 1–32.

Engels, F., Oosting, R. and Nijkamp, F. P. (1987). Dual effects of *Haemophilus influenzae* on guinea pig tracheal beta-adrenergic receptor function: involvement of oxygen-centered radicals from pulmonary macrophages. *J. Pharmacol. Exp. Ther.*, **241**, 994–9.

Evans, T. W., Brokaw, J. J., Chung, K. F., Nadel, J. A. and McDonald, D. M. (1988a). Ozone-induced bronchial hyperresponsiveness in the rat is not accompanied by neutrophil influx or increased vascular permeability in the trachea. *Am. Rev. Respir. Dis.*, **138**, 140–4.

Evans, T., Rogers, D. F., Aursudkij, B., Chung, K. F. and Barnes, P. J. (1988b). Differential effect of inflammatory mediators on microvascular permeability in different parts of the guinea pig airways. *Clin. Sci.*, **74**, 46P.

Fels, A. and Cohn, Z. A. (1986). The alveolar macrophage, *J. Appl. Physiol.*, **60**, 353–69.

Fels. A. O. S., Pawlowski, N. A., Cramer, E. B., Cohn, Z. A. and Scott, W. A. (1982). Human alveolar macrophages produce leukotriene B4. *Proc. Natl. Acad. Sci.*, USA, **79**, 7866–70.

Filley, W. V., Holley, K. E., Kephart, G. M. and Gleigh, G. J. (1982). Identification by immunofluorescence of eosinophil granule major basic protein in lung tissue of patients with bronchial asthma. *Lancet*, **1**, 11–16.

Finnerty, J. P. and Holgate, S. T. (1990). Evidence for the roles of histamine and prostaglandins as mediators in exercise-induced asthma: the inhibitory effect of terfenadine and flurbiprofen alone and in combination. *Eur. Respir. J.*, **3**, 540–7.

Flint, K. C., Leung, K. B. P., Hudspith, B. N., Brostoff, J., Pearce, F. L. and Johnson, N. M. (1985a). Bronchoalveolar mast cells in extrinsic asthma: a mechanism for the initiation of antigen specific bronchoconstriction. *Br. Med. J.*, **291**, 923–63.

Flint, K. C., Leung, K. B. P., Pearce, F. L., Hudspith, B. N., Brostoff, J. and Johnson, N. M. (1985b). Human mast cells recovered by bronchoalveolar lavage: their morphology, histamine release and effects of sodium cromoglygate, *Clin. Sci.*, **68**, 427–32.

Folkerts, G. (1991). *Virus-induced Airway Hyperresponsiveness*. Thesis. Utrecht, The Netherlands.

Folkerts, G., Henricks, P. A. J., Slootweg, P. J. and Nijkamp, F. P. (1988). Endotoxin-induced inflammation and injury of the guinea pig respiratory airways cause bronchial hyporeactivity. *Am. Rev. Respir. Dis.*, **137**, 1441–8.

Folkerts, G., Engels, F. and Nijkamp, F. P. (1989). Endotoxin-induced hyperreactivity of the guinea pig isolated trachea coincides with decreased prostaglandin E2 production by the epithelial layer. *Br. J. Pharmacol.*, **96**, 388–94.

Fournier, M., Lebargy, F., Roy Ladurie, F. le, Lenormand, E. and Pariente, R. (1989). Intraepithelial T-lymphocyte subsets in the airways of normal subjects and of patients with chronic bronchitis. *Am. Rev. Respir. Dis.*, **140**, 737–47.

Franklin, W. (1974). Treatment of severe asthma. *N. Engl. J. Med.*, **290**, 1469–72.

Frigas, E., Loegering, D. A. and Gleigh, G. J. (1980). Cytotoxic effects of the guinea pig eosinophil major basic protein on tracheal epithelium. *Lab. Invest.*, **42**, 35–43.

Frigas, E., Loegering, D. A., Solley, G. O., Farrow, G. M. and Gleigh, G. J. (1981). Elevated levels of eosinophil granule major basic protein in the sputum of patients with bronchial asthma. *Mayo Clin. Proc.*, **56**, 345–53.

Galli, S. J. (1990). New insights into 'The riddle of the mast cells': microenvironmental regulation of mast cell development and phenotypic heterogeneity. *Lab. Invest.*, **62**, 5–33.

Galli, S. J. and Askenase, P. W. (1986). Cutaneous basophil hypersensitivity. In Abramoff, P., Phillips, S. M. and Escobar, M. R. (eds.), *The Reticuloendothelial System: A Comprehensive Treatise*, Vol. IX, Plenum, New York, 321–52.

Galli, S. J., Dvorak, A. M. and Dvorak, H. F. (1984). Basophils and mast cells: morphologic insights into their biology, secretory patterns and function. *Prog. Allergy*, **34**, 1–32.

Gittlen, S. D., MacDonald, S. M., Bleecker, E. R., Liu, M. C., Kagey-Sobotka, A. and Lichtenstein, L. M. (1988). An IgE dependent histamine releasing factor (HRF) in human bronchoalveolar lavage (BAL) fluid. *Fed. Proc.*, **2**, 1232 (Abstract).

Gleigh, G. J., Frigas, E., Loegering, D. A., Wassom, D. L. and Steinmuller, D. (1979). Cytotoxic properties of the eosinophil major basic protein. *J. Immunol.*, **123**, 2925–7.

Goetzl, E. J., Wasserman, S. I. and Austen, K. F. (1975). Eosinophil polymorphonuclear function in immediate hypersensitivity. *Arch. Pathol.*, **99**, 1–4.

Goldie, R. G., Fernandes, L. B., Farmer, S. G. and Hay, D. W. P. (1990). Airway epithelium-derived inhibitory factor. *Trends Pharmacol. Sci.*, **11**, 67–9.

Gordon, J. R., Burd, P. R. and Galli, S. (1990). Mast cells as a source of multifunctional cytokines. *Immunol. Today*, **11(12)**, 458–64.

Hastie, A. T., Loegering, D. A., Gleigh, G. J. and Kueppers, F. (1987). The effect of purified human eosinophil major basic protein on mammalian ciliary activity. *Am. Rev. Respir. Dis.*, **135**, 848–853.

Henricks, P. A. J., Engels, F., Linde, H. J. van der and Nijkamp, F. P. (1991). 13-Hydroxy-linoleic acid induces airway hyperreactivity to histamine in guinea pigs. *Eur. J. Pharmacol.*, **197**, 233–4.

Herscowitz, H. B. (1985). In defence of the lung: paradoxical role of the pulmonary alveolar macrophage. *Ann. Allergy*, **55**, 639–49.

Hmamguchi, Y., Kanakura, Y., Fujita, J., Takeda, S., Nakano, T., Turui, S., Honjo, T. and Kitamura, Y. (1986). Interleukin 4 as an essential factor for *in vitro* clonal growth of murine connective tissue-type mast cells. *J. Exp. Med.*, **165**, 268–73.

Hogg, J. C. and Eggleston, P. A. (1984). Is asthma an epithelial disease? *Am. Rev. Respir. Dis.*, **129**, 207–8.

Holtzman, M. J., Aisaa, H., Nadel, J. A. and Goetzel, E. J. (1983a). Selective generation of leukotriene B4 by tracheal epithelial cells from dogs. *Biochem. Biophys. Res. Commun.*, **114**, 1071–6.

Holtzman, M. J., Fabbri, L. M., O'Byrne, P. M., Gold B. D., Aizawa, H., Walters, E. H., Alpert, S. E. and Nadel, J. A. (1983b). Importance of airway inflammation for hyperresponsiveness induced by ozone. *Am. Rev. Respir. Dis.*, **127**, 686–90.

Horn, B. R., Robin, E. D., Theodore, J. and Van Kessel, A. (1975). Total eosinophil counts in the management of bronchial asthma. *N. Engl. J. Med.*, **292**, 1152–5.

Hseih, K.-H. (1985). Altered interleukin-2 (IL-2) production and responsiveness after hyposensitization to house dust. *J. Allergy Clin. Immunol.*, **76**, 188–94.

Hubscher, T. (1975). Role of the eosinophil in the allergic reaction. I.EDI – an eosinophil-derived inhibitor of histamine release. *J. Immunol.*, **114**, 1379–8.

Hulbert, W. M., McLean, T. and Hogg, J. C. (1985). The effect of acute airway inflammation on bronchial reactivity in guinea pigs. *Am. Rev. Respir. Dis.*, **132**, 7–11.

Hunter, J. A., Finkbeiner, W. E., Nadel, J. A., Goetzl, E. J. and Holtzman, M. J. (1985). Predominant generation of 15-lipoxygenase metabolites of arachidonic acid by epithelial cells from human trachea. *Proc. Natl. Acad. Sci. USA*, **82**, 4633–7.

Irani, A. A., Schechter, N. M., Craig, S. S., Debois, G. and Schwartz, L. B. (1986). Two human mast cell subsets with distinct neural protease compositions. *Proc. Natl. Acad. Sci. USA*, **83**, 4464–6.

Jacques, L., Couture, R., Drapeau, G. and Regoli, D. (1989). Capillary permeability induced by intravenous neurokinins receptor characterization and mechanism of action. *Naunyn Schmiedebergs Arch. Pharmacol.*, **340**, 170–9.

Jarrett, E. E. E. (1984). Mucosal mast cells *in vivo* and *in vitro*. *Immunol. Today*, **5**, 115–18.

Joseph, M., Capron, A., Ameisen, J. C., Capron, M., Vorng, H., Pancre, V.,

Kusnierz, S. P. and Auriault (1986). The receptor for IgE or blood platelets. *Eur. J. Immunol.*, **16**, 306–12.

Kalsner, S. and Richards, R. (1984). Coronary arteries of cardiac patients are hyperreactive and contain stores of amines. A mechanism of coronary spasm. *Science*, **223**, 1435–7.

Katsumata, U., Miura, M., Ichinose, M., Kimura, K., Takahashi, T., Inoue, H. and Takishima, T. (1990). Oxygen radicals produce airway constriction and hyperresponsiveness in anesthetized cats. *Am. Rev. Respir. Dis.*, **141**, 1158–61.

Kirby, J. G., Hargreave, F. E., Gleich, G. J. and O'Byrne, P. M. (1987). Bronchoalveolar cell profiles of asthmatic and nonasthmatic subjects. *Am. Rev. Respir. Dis.*, **136**, 379–83.

Laitinen, L. A., Heino, M., Laitinen, A., Kava, T. and Haahtela, T. (1985). Damage of the airway epithelium and bronchial reactivity in patients with asthma. *Am. Rev. Respir. Dis.*, **131**, 599–606.

Lawson, I. C., Bunting, S., Holzgrefe, H. and Fitzpatrick, F. (1986). Leukotriene B4 contracts guinea pig tracheal strips *in vitro*. *J. Pharmacol. Exp. Ther.*, **227**, 888–92.

Lee, T. C., Lenitran, D. J., Malone, B., Roddy, L. L. and Wasserman, S. I. (1984). Increased biosynthesis of platelet-activating factor in activated human eosinophils. *J. Biol. Chem.*, **259**, 5526–30.

Lett-Brown, M. A., Alam, R. and Grant, J. A. (1989). Regulation of basophil and mast cell activation by cytokines. In Sorg, C. (ed.), *Cytokines Regulating the Allergic Response*, Vol. 2, Karger, Basel, 90–9.

Lin. C.-Y., Kuo, Y.-C., Liu W.-T. and Lin, C.-C. (1988). Immunomodulation of influenza virus infection in the precipitating asthma attacks. *Chest*, **93**, 1234–8.

Lopez, A. F., Williamson, J., Gamble, J. R., Begley, C. G., Harlan, J. M., Klebanoff, S. J., Waltersdorph, A., Wong, G., Clark, S. C. and Vadas, M. A. (1986). Recombinant human granulocyte–macrophage colony-stimulating factor stimulates *in vitro* mature human neutrophil and eosinophil function, surface receptor expression, and survival, *J. Clin. Invest.*, **78**, 1220–8.

Lopez, A. F., Sanderson, C. J., Gamble, J. R., Campbell, H. D., Young, I. G. and Vadas, M. A. (1988). Recombinant human interleukin-5 is a selective activator of human eosinophil function. *J. Exp. Med.*, **167**, 219–24.

Lowell, F. C. (1967). Clinical aspects of eosinophilia in atopic disease. *J. Am. Med. Assoc.*, **202**, 875–8.

MacDermot, J., Kelsey, C. R., Waddell, K. A., Richmond, R., Knight, R. K., Cole, P. J., Dollery, C. T., Landon, D. N. and Blair, I. A. (1984). Synthesis of leukotriene B4 and prostanoids by human alveolar macrophages: analysis by gas chromatography/mass spectrometry. *Prostaglandins*, **27**, 163–77.

Macklam, P. T., Protor, D. F. and Hogg, J. C. (1970). The stability of peripheral airways. *Respir. Physiol.*, **8**, 191–203.

Mannaioni, P. F. and Masini, E. (1988). The release of histamine by free radicals. *Free Rad. Biol. Med.*, **5**, 177–97.

Marin, M. G., Davis, B. and Nadel, J. A. (1977). Effect of histamine on electrical and ion transport properties of tracheal epithelium. *Am. J. Physiol.*, **42**, 735–8.

Martinet, Y., Rom, W. N., Grotendorst, G. R., Martin, G. R. and Crystal, R. G. (1987). Exaggerated spontaneous release of platelet-derived growth factor by alveolar macrophages from patients with idiopathic pulmonary fibrosis. *N. Engl. J. Med.*, **317**, 202–9.

McDonald, D. M. (1987). Neurogenic inflammation in the respiratory tract: actions of sensory nerve mediators on blood vessels and epithelium of the airway mucosa. *Am. Rev. Respir. Dis.*, **136**, S65–S72.

Metcalf, D., Begley, C. G., Johnson, G. R., Nicola, N. A., Vadas, M. A., Lopez,

A. F., Williamson, D. J., Wong, G. G., Clark, S. C. and Wang, E. A. (1986). Biologic properties *in vitro* of a recombinant human granulocute-macrophage colony-stimulating factor. *Blood*, **67**, 37–45.

Michell, E. B., Platt-Mills, T. A. E., Peraira, R. S., Malkovska, V. and Webster, A. D. (1983). Basophil and eosinophil dificiency in a patient with hypogammaglobulinemia associated with thymoma. In Wedgwood, R. J., Rosen, F. S. and Paul, N. W. (eds.), *Primary Immunodeficiency Diseases – Birth Defects*, Original Article Series, Vol. 19, 3rd edn., Alan R. Liss, New York. 331–54.

Miller, L., Blank, U., Metzger, H. and Kinet, J.-P. (1989). Expression of high-affinity binding of human immunoglobulin E by transfected cells. *Science*, **244**, 334–7.

Mitchell, H. W., Willet, K. E. and Sparrow, M. (1989). Perfused bronchial segments and bronchial strip: narrowing vs. isometric force by mediators. *J. Appl. Physiol.*, **66**, 2704–9.

Miyajima, A., Miyatake, S., Schreurs, J., De Vries, J., Arai, N., Yokota, T. and Arai, K.-I. (1988). Coordinate regulation of immune and inflammatory responses by T cell-derived lymphokines. *FASEB J.*, **2**, 2462–3.

Munakata, M., Huang, I., Mitzner, W. and Menkes, H. (1989). Protective role of the epithelium in the guinea pig airway. *J. Appl. Physiol.*, **66**, 1547–52.

Murlas, C. G. and Roum, J. H. (1985a). Bronchial hyperreactivity occurs in steroid-treated guinea pigs depleted of leukocytes by cyclophosphamide. *J. Appl. Physiol.*, **58**, 1630–7.

Murlas, C. G. and Roum, J. H. (1985b). Sequence of pathologic changes in the airway mucosa of guinea pigs during ozone-induced bronchial hyperreactivity. *Am. Rev. Respir. Dis.*, **131**, 314–20.

Nadel, J. A. (1988). Cell to cell communication. Some epithelial metabolic factors affecting airway smooth muscle. *Am. Rev. Respir. Dis.*, **138**, S22–S23.

Naline, E., Devillier, P., Drapeau, G., Toty, L., Bakdach, H., Regoli, D. and Advenier, C. (1989). Characterization of neurokinin effects and receptor selectivity in human isolated bronchi. *Am. Rev. Respir. Dis.*, **140**, 679–86.

Nathan, C. F. (1987). Secretory products of alveolar macrophages. *J. Clin. Invest.*, **79**, 319–29.

Nijkamp, F. P. and Folkerts, G. (1986). Reversal of arachidonic acid-induced tracheal relaxation into contraction after epithelium removal. *Eur. J. Pharmacol.*, **131**, 315–16.

Nijkamp, F. P. and Henricks, P. A. J. (1988). Free radicals in pulmonary disease. In Barnes, P. J., Rodger, I. W. and Thomson, N. C. (eds.), *Asthma: Basic Mechanisms and Clinical Management*, Academic Press, London. 315–33.

O'Byrne, P. M., Walters, E. H., Gold, B. D., Aizawa, H. A., Fabbri, L. M., Alpert, S. E., Nadel, J. A. and Holtzman, M. J. (1984). Neutrophil depletion inhibits airway hyperresponsiveness induced by ozone exposure. *Am. Rev. Respir. Dis.*, **130**, 214–19.

O'Byrne, P. M., Laikauf, G. D., Aizawa, H. A., Bethel, R. A., Ueki, I. F., Holtzman, M. J. and Nadel, J. A. (1985). Leukotriene B4 induces airway hyperresponsiveness in dogs. *J. Appl. Physiol.*, **59**, 1941–6.

Ohnishi, M., Ruhno, J., Bienenstock, J., Doloich, J. and Denburg, J. A. (1989). Hematopoietic growth factor production by cultured cells of human nasal polyp epithelial scrapings: kinetics, ceil source, and relationship to clinical status. *J. Allergy Clin. Immunol.*, **83**, 1091–100.

Oosthuizen, M. J., Engels, F., Esch, B. van, Henricks, P. A. J. and Nijkamp, F. P. (1990). Production of arachidonic acid matabolites by guinea pig tracheal epithelial cells. *Inflammation*, **14**, 401–7.

O'Sullivan, M. R., MacLachlan, N. J., Fleischer, L. N., Olson, N. C. and Brown,

T. T. (1988). Modulation of arachidonic acid metabolism by bovine alveolar macrophages exposed to interferons. *J. Leukocyte Biol.*, **44**, 116.

Parish, W. E. and Luckhurst, E. (1982). T-lymphocyte substance controlling eosinophilia, *Clin. Allergy*, **12**, 475–88.

Pearce, F. L., Flint, K. C., Leung, K. B. P., Hudspith, B. N., Seager, K., Hammond, M. D., Brostoff, J., Geraint-James, D. and Johnson, N. McI. (1987). Some studies on human pulmonary mast cells obtained by bronchoalveolar lavage and by enzymatic dissociation of whole lung tissue. *Int. Allergy Appl. Immunol.*, **82**, 507–12.

Persson, C. G. A. (1987). Leakage of macromolecules from the tracheabronchial microcirculation. *Am. Rev. Respir. Dis.*, **135**, S71–S75.

Peters, S. P., Schulman, E. S., Schleimer, R. P., MacGlashan, J. D. W., Newball, H. H. and Lichtenstein, L. M. (1982). Dispersed human lung mast cells: pharmacologic aspects and comparison with human lung tissue fragments. *Am. Rev. Respir. Dis.*, **126**, 1034–9.

Peters, S. P., Ramesha, C., Naclerio, R. and Lichtenstein, L. M. (1986). Identification of PAF molecular species present in allergic secretions. *Fed. Proc.*, **45**, 1530–4.

Postma, D. S., Koeter, G. H. and Sluiter, H. J. (1989). Pathophysiology of airway hyperresponsiveness. In Weiss, S. T. and Sparrow, D. (eds.), *Airway Responsiveness and Atopy in the Development of Chronic Lung Disease*, Raven Press, New York, 21–71.

Proud, D., Liekrerski, E. S. and Bailey, G. S. (1988). Identification of human lung mast cell kininogenase as tryptase and the relevance of tryptase kininogenase activity. *Biochem. Pharmacol.*, **78**, 1473–80.

Rankin, J. A. (1989). The contribution of alveolar macrophages to hyperreactive airway disease. *J. Allergy Clin. Immunol.*, **83**, 722–9.

Raphael, G. D. and Metcalfe, D. D. (1986). Mediators of airway inflammation. *Eur. J. Respir. Dis.*, **69 (Suppl. 147)**, 44–56.

Renzi, P. M., Sapienza, S., Du, T., Wang, N. S. and Martin, J. M. (1991). Lymphokine-induced airway hyperresponsiveness in the rat. *Am. Rev. Respir. Dis.*, **143**, 375–9.

Rhoden, K. J. and Barnes, P. J. (1989). Effect of hydrogen peroxide on guinea pig tracheal smooth muscle *in vitro*: role of cyclo-ocygenase and airway epithelium. *Br. J. Pharmacol.*, **98**, 325–30.

Salvato, G. (1968). Some histological changes in chronic bronchitis and asthma. *Thorax*, **23**, 168–72.

Schleimer, R. P., MacGlashan, D. W., Peters, S. P., Pinckard, R. N., Adkinson, J. N. F. and Lichtenstein, L. M. (1986). Characterization of inflammatory mediator release from purified lung mast cells. *Am. Rev. Respir. Dis.*, **133**, 614–17.

Schwartz, L. B. (1989). Heterogeneity of mast cells in humans. In Galli, S. J. and Austen, K. F. (eds.), *Mast Cell and Basophil Differentiation and Function in Health and Disease*, Raven Press, New York, 93–116.

Schwartz, L. B., Kawahara, M. S., Hugi, T. E., Vik, D. T., Fearon, D. T. and Austen, K. F. (1983). Generation of C3a anaphylatoxin from human C3 by mast cell tryptase. *J. Immunol.*, **130**, 1891–5.

Sekizawa, K., Caughey, G. H., Lazarus, S. C., Gold, W. M. and Nadel, J. A. (1989). Mast cell tryptase causes airway smooth muscle hyperresponsiveness in dogs. *J. Clin. Invest.*, **83**, 175–9.

Seltzer, J., Bigby, B. G. and Stulbarg, M. (1986). O3-induced change in bronchial reactivity to methacholine and airway inflammation in humans. *J. Appl. Physiol.*, **60**, 1321–61.

Shaw, R. J., Walsh, G. M., Cromwell, O., Moqbel, R., Spry, C. J. F. and Kay, A. B. (1985). Activated eosinophils generate SRS-A leukotrienes following IgG-dependent stimulation. *Nature (London)*, **316**, 150–2.

Shore, S. A., Kariya, S. T., Anderson, K., Skornik, W., Feldman, H. A., Pennington, J., Godleski, J. and Drazen, J. M. (1987). Sulfur-dioxide-induced bronchitis in dogs: effects on airway responsiveness to inhaled and intravenously administered methacholine. *Am. Rev. Respir. Dis.*, **135**, 840–7.

Sibille, Y. and Reynolds, H. Y. (1990). Macrophages and polymorphonuclear neutrophils in lung defense and injury. *Am. Rev. Respir. Dis.*, **141**, 471–501.

Slifman, N. R., Adolphson, C. R. and Gleigh, G. J. (1988). Eosinophils: biochemical and cellular aspects. In Middleton, J. E., Reed, C. E., Ellis, E. F., Adkinson, J. N. F. and Yunginger, J. W. (eds.), *Allergy, Principles and Practice*, CV Mosby, St. Louis, 179–95.

Soter, N. A., Lewis, R. A., Corey, E. J. and Auten, K. F. (1983). Local effects of synthetic leukotrienes (LTC4, LTD4, LTE4, and LTB4) in human skin. *J. Invest. Dermatol.*, **80**, 115–19.

Sparrow, M. P. and Mitchell, H. W. (1991). Modulation by the epithelium of the extent of bronchial narrowing produced by substances perfused through the lumen. *Br. J. Pharmacol.*, **103**, 1160–4.

Tanno, Y., Shindoh, Y. and Takishima, T. (1990). Effects of interleukin-3, interleukin-4, and fibroblasts on cultures of human lung mast cells in bronchoalveolar lavage fluids. *Cell Struct. Func.*, **15**, 137–42.

Thompson, J. E., Scypinski, L. A., Gordon, T. and Sheppard, D. (1986). Hydroxyurea inhibits airway hyperresponsiveness in guinea pigs by a granulocyte-independent mechanism. *Am. Rev. Respir. Dis.*, **134**, 1213–18.

Togias, A. G., Proud, D., Lichtenstein, L. M., Adams, G. K. (III), Norman, P. S., Kagey-Sobotka, A. and Naclerio, R. M. (1988a). The osmolarity of nasal secretions increases when inflammatory mediators are released in response to inhalation of cold, dry air, *Am. Rev. Respir. Dis.*, **137**, 625–9.

Togias, A. G., Proud, D., Lichtenstein, L. M., Kagey-Sobotka, A., and Adams, G. K. (1988b). The osmolarity of nasal secretions increases during the response to inhalation of cold air. *Am. Rev. Respir. Dis.*, **137**, 625–9.

Tomioka, M., Ida, S., Shindoh, Y., Ishihara, T. and Takishima, T. (1984). Mast cells in bronchoalveolar lumen of patients with bronchial asthma. *Am. Rev. Respir. Dis.*, **129**, 1000–5.

Valone, F. H. and Epstein, L. B. (1988). Biphasic platelet-activating factor synthesis by human monocytes stimulated with IL-1-β, tumor necrosis factor, or INF-γ. *J. Immunol.*, **141**, 3945–50.

Vanhoutte, P. M. (1989). Epithelium-derived relaxing factor(s) and bronchial reactivity. *J. Allergy Clin. Immunol.*, **83**, 855–61.

Wanner, A. (1977). Clinical aspects of mucociliary transport. *Am. Rev. Respir. Dis.*, **116**, 73–125.

Wardlaw, A. J., Dunnette, S., Gleich, G. J., Collins, J. V. and Kay, A. B. (1988a). Eosinophils and mast cells in bronchoalveolar lavage fluid in subjects with mild asthma. Relation to bronchial hyperreactivity. *Am. Rev. Respir. Dis.*, **137**, 62–9.

Wardlaw, A. J., Kurihara, K., Moqbel, R., Walsh, G. M., and Kay, A. B. (1988b). Eosinophils in allergic and non-allergic asthma. In Kay, A. B. (ed.), *Clinical Immunology and Allergy: the Allergic Basis of Asthma*, Balliere Tindall, London, 15–36.

Wasserman, S. I., Goetzl, E. J. and Austen, K. F. (1975). Inactivation of slow reacting substance of anaphylaxis by human eosinophil arylsufatase, *J. Immunol.*, **114**, 645–9.

Weiss, E. B. and Bellino, J. R. (1986). Leukotriene-associated toxic oxygen metabolites induce airway hyperreactivity. *Chest*, **89**, 709–16.

White, M. V., Slater, J. E., and Kaliner, M. A. (1987). Histamine and asthma. *Am. Rev. Respir. Dis.*, **135**, 1165–76.

Wilson, J. W., Schrader, J. W. and Pain, M. C. F. (1986). In *Proceedings of the XXXth Congress of the International Union of Physiological Sciences, Vancouver, British Columbia*, 123a (abstract).

Yang, Y. C., Ciarletta, A. B., Temple, P. A., Chung, M. P., Kovacic, S., Witek-Giannotti, J. S., Leary, A. C., Kriz, R., Donahue, R. E., Wong, G. G. *et al.* (1986). Human IL-3 (multi-CSF): identification by expression cloning of a novel hematopoietic growth factor related to murine IL-3. *Cell*, **47**, 3–10.

Zeiger, R. S. and Colten, H. R. (1977). Histaminase release from human eosinophils. *J. Immunol.*, **118**, 540–3.

20

Synergism Between PAF-Acether and IL-5: Relevance for Eosinophil Attraction and Activation

E. Coëffier, D. Joseph and B. B. Vargaftig

20.1 Introduction

An increased number of eosinophils in blood and bronchoalveolar lavage fluid (BAL) is frequently observed in patients with bronchial asthma (DeMonchy et al., 1985), as initially recognized by Hüber and Koessler (1922), but neither the mechanisms of eosinophil recruitment into tissues undergoing allergic reactions nor their pathophysiological role have been completely elucidated (Frigas and Gleich, 1986; Venge, 1990). PAF-acether (1-0-hexadecyl-2-acetyl-sn-glycero-3-phosphorylcholine) and leukotriene (LT) B$_4$ are two recognized inflammatory mediators which share the ability to induce eosinophil chemo-attraction in vitro (Czarnetzki and Mertensmeier, 1985; Wardlaw et al., 1986; Coëffier et al., 1991a) and in vivo (Coyle et al., 1988; Sanjar et al., 1990; Lellouch-Tubiana et al., 1988; Arnoux et al., 1988; Silbaugh et al., 1987).

T lymphocytes may be important in asthma as anticipated from studies where T cell depletion reduced eosinophilia. Three well-characterized factors, interleukin-3 (IL-3) (Lopez et al., 1987), granulocyte–macrophage colony-stimulating factor (GM-CSF) (Metcalf et al., 1986) and interleukin-5 (IL-5) (Sanderson et al., 1985; Yokota et al., 1987) are known to stimulate eosinophilopoiesis in vitro. While IL-3 and GM-CSF are not specific for eosinophils, IL-5, a 115 amino acid protein, recombinant IL-5 are potent and selective stimuli for eosinophil colony formation, growth and differentiation (reviewed in Banchereau, 1990). IL-5 also induces the migration of murine (Yamaguchi et al., 1988; Secor et al., 1990), human (Wang et al., 1989) and guinea pig eosinophils and causes normodense eosinophils to become hypodense (Owen et al., 1989). Recent studies demonstrated that IL-5 accounts for eosinophilopoiesis in helminth-infected mice (Coffman et al., 1990; Sher et al., 1990) and patients (Limaye et al., 1990) and the hypothesis can be raised that IL-5 may account for the recruitment and/or activation of eosinophils in allergic diseases, including bronchial asthma.

The potential role of PAF-acether and of IL-5 as an eosinophil prolifer-ating, activating and/or recruiting mediator in asthma led us to study the effects of recombinant human IL-5 (rhIL-5), PAF-acether and LTB_4, alone or combined, on isolated guinea-pig eosinophils.

20.2 Materials and Methods

Materials and Buffers

Lipid-free bovine serum albumin (BSA), calcium ionophore A23187, formyl-L-methionyl-L-leucyl-L-phenylalanine (FMLP), polymyxin B sul-phate, N-2-hydroxyethylpiperazine-N'-2-ethanesulphonic acid (HEPES), cytochrome c, superoxide dismutase, creatine phosphate, creatine phos-phokinase and metrizamide were from Sigma Chemical Co. (St. Louis, MO). Synthetic PAF-acether (1-0-hexadecyl-2-acetyl-sn-glycero-3-phosphorylcholine) was from Bachem (Budendorf, Switzerland). Aspirin lysine salt (Aspegic[R]) was from Laboratoires Synthélabo (Paris, France). Recombinant human interleukin-5 (rhIL-5) was from Mony's (Beverly Hills, CA, USA). Ovalbumin was from Miles (Naperville, IL, USA). Synthetic lyophilized leukotriene B_4 (LTB_4) was from Amersham (Amer-sham, UK). Lipopolysaccharide (LPS) W E. coli 055:B5 was from Gibco (Paisley, UK). Fura 2 AM was from Calbiochem (La Jolla, USA). BN 52021 and WEB 2086 were supplied respectively by IHB-IPSEN (Le Plessis Robinson, France) and Boehringer Ingelheim (Ingelheim, FRG).

Buffers were L-glumatine-free RPMI 1640, containing 2 g/l sodium bicar-bonate from Eurobio (Paris, France) and Ca^{2+} and Mg^{2+}-free Hank's balanced salt buffer (HBSS) from Gibco (Paisley, UK).

The 48-well microtaxis chambers and the cellulose nitrate filters (3 μm pore size) were purchased from Neuro Probe, Inc. (Cabin John, MD, USA).

Purification of Guinea-pig Eosinophils

Eosinophils were isolated from peritoneal exudates of polymyxin B sulphate-treated guinea-pigs and purified on a discontinuous metrizamide gradient as already described (Coëffier *et al.*, 1991b).

Eosinophil Migration

Eosinophil migration was evaluated on a micro-Boyden chamber using micropore filters with a 3 μm pore size as previously described (Coëffier *et al.*, 1991b). The results are quantitated by counting in fields the number of cells which have migrated to 40 μm through the filter using an optical grid at 400× magnification and are expressed as the number of migrating eosinophils (mean ± SEM) in the presence of the agonist or of the solvent alone.

Superoxide Anion Generation

Superoxide anion production by resting and stimulated eosinophils was determined as the superoxide dismutase (30 μg/ml) inhibitable reduction of cytochrome c as previously described (Coëffier *et al.*, 1991b).

Measurement of $[Ca^{2+}]_i$

$[Ca^{2+}]_i$ was measured as previously described (Coëffier *et al.*, 1991b) after incubation of normodense eosinophils with fura 2 AM.

20.3 Results

Two populations of eosinophils were separated upon the discontinuous metrizamide gradient, one of low density (between 20% and 22% of metrizamide; purity, 63 ± 3%, $n = 27$) and another of normal density (between 22% and 24% of metrizamide), their purity ranging between 71% and 98% (87 ± 1%, mean ± SEM, $n = 36$), Macrophages were the only identified contaminant. We investigate the responses to chemotactic stimuli of both normal and low density eosinophil populations.

Human recombinant IL-5 markedly stimulated chemotaxis of nor-modense eosinophils, as compared with PAF-acether and LTB$_4$. The chemotactic activity of rhIL-5 was dose-dependent and significant between

50 and 1000 ng/ml. In the same conditions, recombinant murine IL-5 was inactive. In contrast, guinea-pig eosinophils did not migrate in the presence of LPS, a potential contaminant. It is noteworthy that, in contrast to its efficacy on normodense eosinophils, rhIL-5 was very poorly effective on hypodense eosinophils. Nevertheless, the baseline migration of the two populations of eosinophils was similar (6 ± 2 and 8 ± 2 migrating eosinophils without stimuli for normodense and hypodense eosinophils respectively). Then normodense eosinophils are used for all further experiments.

To study priming, guinea-pig normodense eosinophils were preincubated for 5 min with rhIL-5 at 50, 100 and 500 ng/ml or buffer and then introduced into the upper compartment of the Boyden chamber and stimulated with PAF-acether at 1, 10 and 100 nM and LTB_4 1 and 10 nM. Under those conditions, eosinophil migration by PAF-acether was significantly enhanced. This priming was dose dependent for rhIL-5. The spontaneous migration of eosinophils is also stimulated by rhIL-5. By contrast, rhIL-5 failed to enhance migration induced by LTB_4 (Fig. 20.1). Finally, FMLP, used up to 1 μM, failed to induce eosinophil chemotaxis alone or associated to rhIL-5. Recombinant human tumor necrosis factor α (TNFα) also failed to prime PAF-acether-induced migration.

We would like to know whether the effect of priming with IL-5 removed by washing. In four experiments, normodense eosinophils were exposed to 100 ng/ml rhIL-5 for 5 min, washed or not, and placed in the wells for PAF-acether-induced migration. Without washing, priming effect with IL-5 was observed. Removal of rhIL-5 suppressed priming of PAF-acether, even though the direct stimulation of rhIL-5 and PAF-acether persisted (Fig. 20.2). Since priming could only be demonstrated under conditions of co-incubation of rhIL-5 and PAF-acether, and this led to total duration of migration of 2 hours, no time-dependent study could be performed for duration of incubation of eosinophils with rhIL-5. The effect of rhIL-5 was observed after only a few minutes of incubation with eosinophils, suggesting that protein biosynthesis is not required.

Interference of BN 52021 and WEB 2086 with the migration of guinea-pig normodense eosinophils induced by PAF-acether and rhIL-5 was studied (Coëffier et al., 1991b). Eosinophil migration by PAF-acether was significantly reduced when the normodense cells were preincubated with the two PAF-acether antagonists. BN 52021 and WEB 2086 also inhibited, but less efficiently, eosinophil migration induced by rhIL-5. Inhibition was also concentration dependent but rose to a plateau around 60%. Both are claimed to be specific for PAF-acether and indeed they suppress different effects of PAF-acether on eosinophils, including the enhanced locomotion. In vivo, BN 52021 and WEB 2086 decreased eosinophil accumulation in the broncho-alveolar lavage fluid and lungs.

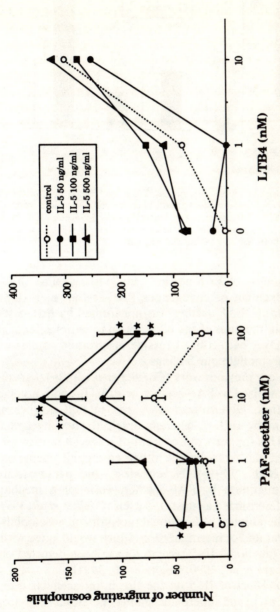

Fig. 20.1 Priming by rhIL-5 of PAF-acether-induced migration of guinea-pig normodense eosinophils. The normodense eosinophils were pre-incubated for 5 min at 37 °C under stirring with buffer (0) or rhIL-5 at 50, 100 and 500 ng/ml. They were then stimulated by buffer, PAF-acether 1 nM, 10 nM and 100 nM or LTB_4 1 and 10 nM. Results are expressed as the number of eosinophils migrating (mean ± SEM of four to seven experiments). * $P < 0.05$; ** $P < 0.01$; *** $P < 0.001$, t test on the results from paired samples between control and agonist (mean ± SEM of three to six experiments).

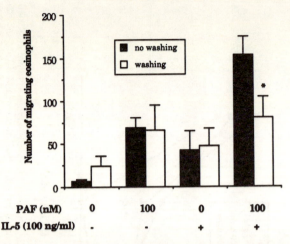

Fig. 20.2   Normodense eosinophils were pre-incubated for 5 min at 37 °C under stirring with buffer or rhIL-5 at 100 ng/ml and washed or not. Then the cell suspensions were added to the upper compartments of the Boyden chamber, buffer (0) and PAF-acether 100 nM. Results are expressed as in Fig. 20.1 (mean ± SEM of four experiments). * $P < 0.05$, t test on the results from paired samples between no washing and washing.

Partial effectiveness of PAF-acether antagonists against rhIL-5 might indicate an involvement of endogenous PAF-acether in rhIL-5-induced chemo-attraction, but PAF-acether was not formed by rhIL-5-stimulated eosinophils, within the limit of the bioassay on rabbit platelet aggregation after Bligh and Dyer extraction. Cross-desensitization studies were thus performed, to substantiate our findings.

We knew from our previous work (Coëffier *et al.*, 1991a) that eosinophils can be auto-desensitized to PAF-acether or to LTB_4, with no evidence of cross-desensitization. Desensitization by and to PAF-acether markedly reduced migration by rhIL-5, whereas desensitization by and to LTB_4 failed to do so. This supports our concept of a special interaction of IL-5 and PAF-acether, unshared by the other eosinophil chemo-attractant, LTB_4 (Coëffier *et al.*, 1991b). Nevertheless, and paradoxically, when primed for the migration by PAF-acether, eosinophils incubated with rhIL-5 were not desensitized against IL-5 itself (Coëffier *et al.*, 1991b). This indicates either the absence of functional receptors on eosinophils or their very rapid turnover and/or internalization, which would agree with the fact that specific and functional IL-5 receptors have been detected on human eosinophils (Chihara *et al.*, 1990; Migita *et al.*, 1991).

We studied the effect of IL-5 on the rise in intracellular free calcium concentration ($[Ca^{2+}]_i$) and superoxide anion generation. PAF-acether and LTB_4 stimulated a rapid and transient rise in intracellular free calcium concentration in normodense eosinophils above baseline. rhIL-5 alone failed to induce elevation of intracellular free calcium concentration. The

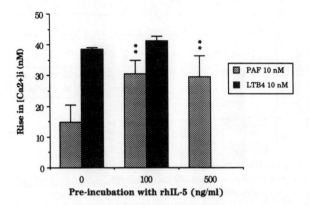

Fig. 20.3   For measuring $[Ca^{2+}]i$, normodense eosinophils (1×10^7/ml; purity, $90 \pm 1\%$ of eosinophils, $n = 3$) were incubated for 30 min at 37 °C with 2.5 μM fura-2-AM, washed three times and resuspended to a final concentration of 3×10^6 cells/ml before addition of PAF-acether, LTB_4 or rhIL-5 alone or associated, and fluorescence was measured. Data represent the mean $\pm$ SEM. ** $P < 0.01$, t test on the results from paired samples between agonist alone and agonist + rhIL-5.

preincubation of normodense eosinophils with rhIL-5 induced a significant increase in the rise in intracellular free calcium concentration induced by 10 nM PAF-acether (Fig. 20.3). By contrast, preincubation of guinea-pig normodense eosinophils with rhIL-5 failed to prime the intracellular free calcium concentration rise induced by LTB_4 10 nM. The dose of rhIL-5 required to prime for PAF-acether-induced rise in $[Ca^{2+}]_i$ was 100 ng/ml.

Superoxide anion generation by normodense eosinophils was only observed at concentrations of PAF-acether and LTB_4 above 10 nM. rhIL-5 alone failed to induce elevation of superoxide anion generation from basal values. The preincubation of normodense eosinophils with rhIL-5 induced a significant increase in superoxide anion generation induced by 10 nM PAF-acether (Fig. 20.4). By contrast, preincubation of guinea-pig normodense eosinophils with rhIL-5 failed to prime the superoxide anion generation induced by LTB_4 10 nM. The dose required to prime for PAF-acether-induced superoxide anion generation was 500 ng/ml.

20.4 Discussion

We showed that rhIL-5 induces the chemo-attraction of guinea-pig eosinophils at concentrations between 50 and 1000 ng/ml, under conditions where PAF-acether and LTB_4, but neither LPS, a potential contaminant, nor recombinant murine IL-5 or rhTNFα, were effective. It is noteworthy that, in contrast to its efficacy on normodense eosinophils, rhIL-5 was very

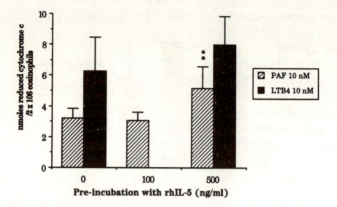

Fig. 20.4 For superoxide anion generation, 80 μM cytochrome c were added to 500 μl of normodense eosinophils (4 × 10⁶/ml, purity, 87 ± 1, n = 3 to 9). Reaction was started by adding PAF-acether, LTB$_4$ or rhIL-5 alone or associated, reduction of cytochrome c was monitored at 550 nm at 37 °C. Data represent the mean ± SEM. ** $P<0.01$, t test on the results from paired samples between agonist alone and agonist + rhIL-5.

poorly active on hypodense eosinophils, as also reported for LTB$_4$ and PAF-acether (Coëffier *et al.*, 1991a).

Alone, rhIL-5 failed to induce a significant elevation of [Ca^{2+}]$_i$ and superoxide anion generation. Under similar conditions, PAF-acether was effective on the former at 1–1000 nM, and on the latter at concentrations at least ten-fold higher. LTB$_4$ induced the elevation of [Ca^{2+}]$_i$ at 1–10 nM and also required higher concentrations for superoxide generation.

One important finding reported here is that rhIL-5 primes for migration, [Ca^{2+}]$_i$ and superoxide generation by PAF-acether but not by LTB$_4$. Less rhIL-5 was required for priming for chemo-attraction by PAF-acether than for priming [Ca^{2+}]$_i$, the generation of superoxide ions requiring larger amounts of rhIL-5.

A selective interaction between rhIL-5 and PAF-acether, also unshared with LTB$_4$, was noted with respect to desensitization and drug antagonism. Thus, IL-5 induces the migration and/or activation of eosinophils from mice, guinea-pig and humans.

Recently, Bischoff *et al.* (1990) demonstrated that rhIL-5 also primes for an enhanced histamine release and generation of LTC$_4$ from human basophils in response to C5a but, as in our case, could not reach a conclusion with respect to the mechanism. Thus, IL-5 primes both eosinophils and basophils, which indeed share many functional and structural similarities, including a postulated common basophil–eosinophil progenitor (Denburg *et al.*, 1985).

Other cytokines enhance the responses of eosinophils, such as rhGM-CSF, rhIL-3 and rhTNFα with respect to eosinophil cytotoxicity (Silberstein *et al.*, 1986; Rothenberg *et al.*, 1988; Silberstein and David, 1986) and calcium ionophore-induced generation of LTC_4 (Silberstein *et al.*, 1986; Rothenberg *et al.*, 1988; Roubin *et al.*, 1987). In our hands, rhTNFα was completely inactive, with respect both to direct activation and to priming of eosinophils by PAF-acether or LTB_4.

T lymphocytes may be important in asthma (Gerblich *et al.*, 1984; Corrigan *et al.*, 1988; Corrigan and Kay, 1990) as anticipated from studies where T cell depletion reduced eosinophilia (Basten and Beeson, 1970). The induction of eosinophil migration *in vitro* by biosynthetic rhIL-5 in a dose-dependent manner and the potentiation of PAF-acether-induced migration, rise in $[Ca^{2+}]_i$ and superoxide generation provide a mechanism by which T lymphocytes might regulate the activation of eosinophils *in vivo*.

The interaction between PAF-acether and rhIL-5, which is clearly selective for rhIL-5 and PAF-acether, since LTB_4 was excluded, probably does not involve new protein synthesis, in view of the short delays required for priming and for desensitization. In addition, the fact that priming was removed by washing rhIL-5 from the cells suggests that no hit-and-run phenomenon is involved and that rhIL-5 must be present continuously to enhance the eosinophil responsiveness to PAF-acether. Likely explanations for synergism, which are being investigated, include an enhanced expression of PAF-acether receptors and particularly an enhanced phospholipase C activity, with consequent augmentation of leukotriene production.

Whatever the mechanisms of the selective interactions between PAF-acether and rhIL-5, and in view of the potential relevance of both mediators in pathology, it is clear that agents capable of inhibiting the effects or the synthesis of IL-5 may be useful in diseases characterized by eosinophil infiltration, including asthma.

References

Arnoux, B., Denjean, A., Page, C. P., Nolibe, D., Morley, J. and Benveniste, J. (1988). Accumulation of platelets and eosinophils in baboon lung after PAF-acether challenge. Inhibition by ketotifen. *Am. Rev. Respir. Dis.*, **137**, 855–60.

Banchereau, J. (1990). Interleukine-5. *Med. Sci.*, **6**, 954–7.

Basten, A. and Beeson, P. B. (1970). Mechanism of eosinophilia. II. Role of the lymphocyte. *J. Exp. Med.*, **131**, 1288–305.

Bischoff, S. C., Brunner, T., Deweck, A. L. and Dahinden, C. A. (1990). Interleukin-5 modifies histamine release and leukotriene generation by human basophils in response to diverse agonists. *J. Exp. Med.*, **172**, 1577–82.

Chihara, J., Plumas, J., Gruart, V., Tavernier, J., Prin, L., Capron, A. and Capron, M. (1990). Characterization of a receptor for interleukin-5 on human eosinophils: variable expression and induction by granulocyte/macrophage colony-stimulating factor. *J. Exp. Med.*, **172**, 1347–51.

Coëffier, E., Joseph, D. and Vargaftig, B. B. (1991a). LTB$_4$, a potent chemotactic factor for purified guinea-pig eosinophils: interference of PAF-acether antagonists. *Int. J. Immunopharmacol.*, **13**, 273–80.

Coëffier, E., Joseph, D. and Vargaftig, B. B. (1991b). Activation by human recombinant IL-5 of guinea-pig eosinophils. Selective priming to PAF-acether and interference of its antagonists. *J. Immunol.*, **147**, 2595.

Coffman, R. L., Seymour, B. W. P., Hudak, S., Jackson, J. and Rennick, D. (1990). Antibody to interleukin-5 inhibits helminth-induced eosinophilia in mice. *Science*, **245**, 308–10.

Corrigan, C. J., Hartnell, A. and Kay, A. B. (1988). T-lymphocyte activation in acute severe asthma. *Lancet*, **i**, 1129–32.

Corrigan, C. J. and Kay, A. B. (1990). T-lymphocytes and their products in chronic asthma. In Bierman, C. W. and Lee, T. H. (eds.), *Immunology and Allergy Clinics of North America*, Saunders, Philadelphia, **10**(2), 319.

Coyle, A. J., Urwin, S. C., Page, C. P., Touvay, C., Villain, B. and Braquet, P. (1988). The effect of the selective PAF antagonist BN 52021 on PAF- and antigen-induced bronchial hyper-reactivity and eosinophils accumulation. *Eur. J. Pharmacol.*, **148**, 51–8.

Czarnetzki, B. M. and Mertensmeier, R. (1985). *In vitro* and *in vivo* chemotaxis of guinea-pig leukocytes toward leukotriene B$_4$ and its ω-oxidation products. *Prostaglandins*, **30**, 5–10.

DeMonchy, J. G. R., Kauffman, H. K., Venge, P., Koeter, G. H., Jansen, H. M., Sluiter, H. J. and DeVries, K. (1985). Bronchoalveolar eosinophilia during allergen-induced late asthmatic reactions. *Am. J. Respir. Dis.*, **131**, 373–6.

Denburg, J. A., Telyzin, S., Messner, H., Jamal, B. L. N., Ackerman, S. J., Gleich, G. J. and Bienenstock, J. (1985). Heterogeneity of human peripheral blood eosinophil-type colonies: evidence for a common basophil-eosinophil progenitor. *Blood*, **66**, 312–18.

Frigas, E. and Gleich, G. J. (1986). The eosinophil and the pathophysiology of asthma. *J. Allergy Clin. Immunol.*, **77**, 527–37.

Gerblich, A. A., Campbell, A. E. and Schuyler, M. R. (1984). Changes in T-lymphocyte subpopulations after antigenic bronchial provocation in asthmatics. *N. Engl. J. Med.*, **310**, 1349–52.

Huber, H. L. and Koessler, K. K. (1922). The pathology of bronchial asthma. *Arch. Intern. Med.*, **30**, 689–760.

Lellouch-Tubiana, A., Lefort, J., Simon, M. T., Pfister, A. and Vargaftig, B. B. (1988). Eosinophil recruitment into guinea pig lungs after PAF-acether and allergen administration. *Am. Rev. Respir. Dis.*, **137**, 948–54.

Limaye, A. P., Abrams, J. S., Silver, J. E., Ottesen, E. A. and Nutman, T. B. (1990). Regulation of parasite-induced eosinophilia — selectively increased interleukin-5 production in helminth-infected patients. *J. Exp. Med.*, **172**, 399–402.

Lopez, A. F., To, L. B., Yang, Y.-C., Gamble, J. R., Shannon, M. F., Burns, G. F., Dyson, P. G., Juttner, C. A., Clark, S. and Vadas, M. A. (1987). Stimulation of proliferation, differentiation, and function of human cells by primate interleukin-3. *Proc. Natl. Acad. Sci. USA*, **84**, 2761–5.

Metcalf, D., Begley, C. G., Johnson, G. R., Nicola, N. A., Vadas, M. A., Lopez, A. F., Williamson, D. J., Wong, G. G., Clark, S. C. and Wang, E. A. (1986). Biologic properties *in vitro* of a recombinant human granulocyte–macrophage colony-stimulating factor. *Blood*, **67**, 37–45.

Migita, M., Yamaguchi, N., Mita, S., Higuchi, S., Hitoschi, Y., Yoshida, Y., Tomonaga, M., Matsuda, I., Tominaga, A. and Takatsu, K. (1991). Characterization of the human IL-5 receptors on eosinophils. *Cell. Immunol.*, **133**, 484–97.

Owen, W. F., Rothenberg, M. E., Petersen, J., Weller, P. F., Silberstein, D., Sheffer, A. L., Stevens, R. L., Soberman, R. J. and Austen, K. F. (1989). Interleukin-5 and phenotypically altered eosinophils in the blood of patients with the idiopathic hypereosinophilic syndrome. *J. Exp. Med.*, **170**, 343–8.

Rothenberg, M. E., Owen, W. F., Silberstein, D. S., Woods, J., Soberman, R. J., Austen, K. F. and Stevens, R. L. (1988). Human eosinophils have prolonged survival, enhanced functional properties, and become hypodense when exposed to human interleukin-3. *J. Clin. Invest.*, **81**, 1986–92.

Roubin, R., Elsas, P. P., Fiers, W. and Dessein, A. J. (1987). Recombinant human tumour necrosis factor (rhTNF) enhances leukotriene biosynthesis in neutrophils and eosinophils stimulated with the Ca^{2+} ionophore A23187. *Clin. Exp. Immunol.*, **70**, 484–90.

Sanderson, C. J., Warren, D. J. and Strath, M. (1985). Identification of a lymphokine that stimulates eosinophil differentiation *in vitro*. Its relationship to interleukin-3, and functional properties of eosinophils produced in cultures. *J. Exp. Med.*, **162**, 60–74.

Sanjar, S., Aoki, S., Boubekeur, K., Chapman, I. D., Smith, D., Kings, M. A. and Morley, J. (1990). Eosinophil accumulation in pulmonary airways of guinea-pigs induced by exposure to an aerosol of platelet-activating factor: effect of antiasthma drugs. *Br. J. Pharmacol.*, **99**, 267–72.

Secor, W. E., Stewart, S. J. and Colley, D. G. (1990). Eosinophils and immune mechanisms. VI. The synergistic combination of granulocyte–macrophage colony-stimulating factor and IL-5 accounts for eosinophil-stimulation promoter activity in *Schistosoma mansoni*-infected mice. *J. Immunol.*, **144**, 1484–9.

Sher, A., Coffman, R. L., Hieny, S., Scott, P. and Cheever, A. W. (1990). Interleukin-5 is required for the blood and tissue eosinophilia but not granuloma formation induced by infection with *Schistosoma mansoni*. *Proc. Natl. Acad. Sci. USA*, **87**, 61–5.

Silbaugh, S. A., Stengel, P. W., Williams, G. D., Herron, D. K., Gallagher, P. and Baker, S. R. (1987). Airway sensitization and lung granulocyte infiltration in the guinea-pig. *Am. Rev. Respir. Dis.*, **136**, 930–4.

Silberstein, D. S. and David, J. R. (1986). Tumor necrosis factor enhances eosinophil toxicity to *Schistosoma mansoni* larvae. *Proc. Natl. Acad. Sci. USA*, **83**, 1055–9.

Silberstein, D. S., Owen, W. F., Gasson, J. C., DiPersio, J. F., Golde, D. W., Bina, J. C., Soberman, R., Austen, K. F. and David, J. R. (1986). Enhancement of human eosinophil cytotoxicity and leukotriene synthesis by biosynthetic (recombinant) granulocyte–macrophage colony-stimulating factor. *J. Immunol.*, **137**, 3290–4.

Venge, P. (1990). The human eosinophil in inflammation. *Agents Actions*, **29**, 122–6.

Wang, J. M., Rambaldi, A., Biondi, A., Chen, Z. G., Sanderson, C. J. and Mantovani, A. (1989). Recombinant human interleukin-5 is a selective eosinophil chemoattractant. *Eur. J. Immunol.*, **19**, 701–5.

Wardlaw, A. J., Moqbel, R., Cromwell, O. and Kay, A. B. (1986). Plateletactivating factor. A potent chemotactic and chemokinetic factor for human eosinophils. *J. Clin. Invest.*, **78**, 1701–6.

Yamaguchi, Y., Hayashi, Y., Sugama, Y., Miura, Y., Kasahara, T., Kitamura, S., Torisu, M., Mita, S., Tominaga, A., Takatsu, K. and Suda, T. (1988). Highly purified murine interleukin-5 (IL-5) stimulates eosinophil function and prolongs *in vitro* survival. IL-5 is an eosinophil chemotactic factor. *J. Exp. Med.*, **167**, 1737–42.

Yokota, T., Coffman, R. L., Hagiwara, H., Rennick, D. M., Takebe, Y., Yokota, K.,

Gemmell, L., Shrader, B., Yang, G., Meyerson, P., Luh, J., Hoy, P., Pène, J., Brière, F., Spits, H., Banchereau, J., De Vries, J., Lee, F. D., Arai, N. and Arai, K.-I. (1987). Isolation and characterization of lymphokine cDNA clones encoding mouse and human IgA-enhancing factor and eosinophil colony-stimulating factor activities: relationship to interleukin-5. *Proc. Natl. Acad. Sci. USA*, **84** 7388–92.

21

Contribution of Histopathology to the Understanding of Asthma

M. Fournier

21.1 Introduction

The clinical definition of asthma includes a spontaneous and drug-induced reversibility of diffuse airway obstruction, and an increased responsiveness of the airways to a wide variety of stimuli. On the basis of histological studies, the airways of asthmatic patients are also known to display inflammatory changes of the mucosal layer. However, to what extent this airway inflammation accounts for or can help in predicting and treating the clinical manifestations of that disease remains a central question.

Indeed, scores of mucosal damage calculated upon examination of bronchial samples of asthmatics have proven to correlate well with the response of the airways to pharmacological stimuli.

In addition, the efficacy of glucocorticoids in controlling the clinical symptoms of asthma provides a strong argument for a link between mucosal inflammation and airway obstruction.

However, the broad spectrum of the clinical forms of asthma, the variability of the responses to treatment, and the clinical evidence that atopic and late onset asthma may differ in many ways suggest that this link between airway inflammation and airflow limitation is complex. The purpose of this paper is to help in delineating the contribution of histopathology to the understanding of the disease.

21.2 Identification of Pathological Changes in the Airways of Asthmatic Patients

Since the first descriptions of pathological changes in the airways of asthmatic patients, a hundred years ago, two methods have been followed to document the structural abnormalities of the airways: examination of lung specimens obtained post mortem from patients that have died of status asthmaticus and, more recently, histological studies of bronchial biopsies obtained through bronchoscopic procedures.

Pathology in Status Asthmaticus

Upon opening of the pleural cavities, the lungs appear overinflated and fail to collapse. The airways are filled with mucous plugs and areas of atelectasis are frequently observed (André-Bougarau *et al.*, 1972). In a minority of patients, saccular bronchiectasis is present. The dominant microscopic feature is the mucous plugging which usually spreads along the bronchial tree and may occlude completely the airway lumen. However, quasinormal peripheral airways may coexist with adjacent occluded bronchioles. Apart from containing remnants of eosinophils and proteinaceous exudates, the mucous plugs are often attached to the surrounding epithelium. This epithelium is either in place or disrupted from the basement membrane whose increased thickness is another prominent histological feature.

Increased numbers of goblet cells and focal zones of squamous metaplasia are usually observed along the epithelial layer. The eosinophilic infiltration of all the airway layers at any level of the bronchial tree has been noted by all observers, although its importance may vary from one case to another. The thickening of the subepithelial layers and of the submucosa results from the presence of oedema, an increased amount of muscle, and perhaps to a lesser extent from an hypertrophy of the gland mass. Of interest is the observation that bronchial smooth muscle is not only hypertrophic but also disarranged, with formation of whirls.

A unique opportunity of autopsic studies, however, is the possibility of documenting histologic changes of the peripheral airways and accompanying vessels. Saeta *et al.* (1991) performed recently a quantitative analysis of the bronchioles and adjacent arteries in the lungs of six asthmatic patients who died suddenly during an asthma attack. They observed an inflammatory process in the wall of the pulmonary arteries adjacent to occluded and inflamed bronchioles. An important finding from their study is that both peripheral airways and arteries are infiltrated with eosinophils and mononuclear cells; another finding is that pulmonary arteries do not display the common features of chronic hypoxy, i.e. an increased medial and intimal thickness.

Other quantitative analyses during autopsies are clearly needed to document further the vascular involvement in various forms of asthma. These studies could also help in delineating the effect of previous treatment with steroids on the eosinophilic infiltration of bronchovascular structures.

Pathology in Other Forms of Asthma

Fibre optic bronchoscopy with bronchoalveolar lavage and endobronchial biopsy has proven safe in asthmatic subjects, except in those with very responsive airways (Djukanovic *et al.*, 1991).

However, even with a careful premedication, local reactions may be observed following immediately the introduction of the fibroscope into the central airways: an oedema may develop rapidly, along with the flooding of fluids and secretions in the airway lumen. These reactions can be blocked with topical or instillated adrenergic agents; they represent a direct example of the hypersensitivity of the airways in asthma. However, for evident reasons, histological changes occurring in the airways during an attack of asthma are unknown. All histological studies (Beasley *et al.*, 1989; Bousquet *et al.*, 1990; Dunnil, 1960; Heino *et al.*, 1990; Jeffery *et al.*, 1989; Laitinen *et al.*, 1985; Naylor, 1962), indeed, have been performed through examination of bronchial biopsies obtained from asthmatic patients with normal spirometry or with a mild obstructive ventilatory pattern. Traditionally, for ethical reasons, the biopsies are taken only in the central airways; therefore, the knowledge of the pathological changes occurring in peripheral airways is mainly provided through indirect ways, i.e. examination of bronchoalveolar lavage products and cells. Another problem linked to sampling bronchial specimens through fibroscopy is the artifactual damage of the epithelium (Soderberg *et al.*, 1990); this limitation is of importance since the epithelial layer regulates muscular tone, interferes with local T-cell function, and is also a target of the inflammatory process in asthma.

Nevertheless, it seems that in asthma there is no significant difference in the cell populations and their state of activation in mucosal samples obtained from different sites. The detailed analysis of the pathological changes (listed in Table 21.1) observed in other forms than status asthmaticus does not provide supplementary specific information. The most striking observation is that the bronchial mucosa displays histological abnormalities even in the mildest forms of asthma. Another point is that damage to the epithelium is not uniform along the bronchial tree: areas of normal epithelium are usually observed adjacent to areas shedding cells and, in some places, areas in which only basal cells seem to be present.

Extensive work through cooperative studies is now needed to elaborate a pathological classification of the asthmatic syndrome, as suggested by Holgate. Indeed a considerable amount of histological data are required to

Table 21.1   Histological changes in the airways of asthmatic patients

Lumen
  Epithelial clumps (Creola bodies)
  Remnants of eosinophils (Charcot Leyden crystals)
  Mucous casts (Curshman's spirals), proteinaceous exudate
Epithelium
  Intra- and intercellular oedema
  Goblet cell hyperplasia
  Leukocyte infiltration
  Epithelial disruption
  Squamous cell metaplasia
Thickening of the basement membrane
Subepithelial layer
  Vascular congestion–neovascularization
  Modification of intercellular spaces through
      exudation of fluid,
      excess deposition of interstitial matrix, or
      infiltration with eosinophils, lymphocytes
Smooth muscle
  Hypertrophy–hyperplasia
Hypertrophy of submucosal glands

Table 21.2   Structural changes of the airways in connection with repair processes

Basal–goblet cell hyperplasia
Squamous cell metaplasia
Subbasement membrane collagen deposition
Neovascularization
Myofibroblast differentiation–proliferation

provide a pathological basis for the various clinical forms of that disease and to help in delineating both the response to treatment and the prognosis. In addition, this work could enhance understanding of repair processes at the mucosal level (Table 21.2).

21.3 Histology as a Tool for Specific Investigations

Drug Side-effects

Repeated applications of glucocorticoids to the skin are known to induce local atrophy and this caused important concern when these drugs were commonly used for long-term inhalation treatment of severe asthmatics. Several studies (Fournier *et al.*, 1990; Gerber *et al.*, 1985; Laursen *et al.*, 1988; Lundgren *et al.*, 1988) addressed this point through histological examination of bronchial samples before and after treatment with inhaled steroids. The duration of treatment varied from 3 months (in a double-blind, steroid vs placebo study (Fournier *et al.*, 1990)) to 10 years. Although bronchial mucosal atrophy is still difficult to define, no specific histological lesion was found to develop upon steroid inhalation. In addition, colonization of the intrathoracic airways with bacteria or fungi was found to be very uncommon (Fournier *et al.*, 1990).

Pharmacology, Pathophysiology, Bronchial Provocation

In the studies cited above, the effect of long-term steroid inhalation on mucosal damage was also investigated.

The investigators quantitated some of the histological lesions either directly (cumulative length of denuded epithelium, total volume or number of migrating cells in the mucosal–submucosal layer, thickness of the basement membrane) or indirectly (number of epithelial cells recovered by bronchoalveolar lavage). On average, a better control of the disease, on a clinical and/or spirometric basis, was associated with a regression of some histological lesions, such as an increase in the number of ciliated cells, or a decrease in the infiltration of the lamina propria with mononuclear cells; this latter observation seemed to occur rapidly upon steroid treatment since a 1 week administration of 0.5 mg/kg of prednisone per day resulted in a significant decrease in the concentration of mononuclear cells in patients with chronic asthma (Gerber *et al.*, 1985). However, the ability of steroids to decrease the collagen deposition beneath the basement membrane remains to be proven. In other words, there is no clear relationship between a better control of the disease and specific changes of the bronchial mucosa upon steroid treatment.

In fact, the normalization of the lung function and the disappearance of clinical symptoms with corticosteroids may coexist with an abnormal and persistant airway reactivity. Indeed, airway hyperreactivity has been shown to correlate with some of the mucosal histological lesions, particularly epithelial loss, and its consequence, mucosal hyperpermeability. The combined use of antigenic bronchial provocation along with histological examination of the bronchial mucosa showed a rapid increase in the cellularity of the lamina propria, although no single population showed a statistically significant disproportionate increase (Beasley *et al.*, 1989); interestingly, these authors observed that this influx of migrating cells was not associated with changes in the extent of mast cell degranulation or in the heterogeneity of the eosinophil granule matrix and core.

21.4 Histology-derived Techniques

Upon adequate preparation, ultrastructural studies (Andrè-Bougaran *et al.*, 1972; Jeffery *et al.*, 1989; Kantelip *et al.*, 1984; Laitinen *et al.*, 1985) can be conducted on airway specimens. Although time consuming, these studies has proven useful in identifying the increased thickness of the reticular lamina of the epithelial basement membrane, in the observation of cilia morphology and intraepithelial nerve fibres, in the characterization of changes in cell ultrastructure (mast cell and eosinophil granules, lymphocytes), and in the identification of platelets in the extravascular spaces. This problem of the identification of migrating cells – particularly the lymphocytes – within the bronchial tissue is now more easily addressed through immunohistological work.

However, an obvious limitation for the combined use of multiple monoclonal antibodies is the small number of cryostat sections that can be obtained from each biopsy. T-lymphocytes, recognized as cells binding anti-CD3 (T-cells) antibodies, are known to populate both the epithelial layer and the lamina propria of the central airways of normal subjects (Fournier *et al.*, 1989); in contrast, B-cells are far less numerous and concentrate deeper in the mucosa and in the submucosa, together with plasma cells. Among T-cells, CD8+ cells (suppressor–cytoxic T-cells) predominate over CD4+ cells (helper T-cells) in the epithelium while CD4+ cells seem more numerous in the lamina propria. Although few studies have been conducted in asthmatic patients (Azzawi *et al.*, 1990; Foresi *et al.*, 1990; Hamid *et al.*, 1991; Paggiaro *et al.*, 1990; Poulter *et al.*, 1990), it seems, at least in those with stable atopic asthma, that the bronchial mucosa contains increased numbers of T-lymphocytes of both subsets, as compared with normal subjects and non-asthmatic patients. Furthermore, a greater proportion of these mucosal T-cells presents surface activation markers, such as HLA-DR and/or interleukin-2 receptor (CD25) (Azzawi *et al.*, 1990; Foresi *et al.*, 1990).

Activated T-cells are suspected to play a central role in eosinophil production and function through the release of soluble mediators (Clutterbuck *et al.*, 1988; Lopez *et al.*, 1988); the co-infiltration of the bronchial mucosa with activated T-lymphocytes and activated eosinophils (Heino *et al.*, 1990), that is the binding of EG2 antibodies which recognize the secreted form of the eosinophilic cationic protein, provides strong support for such a T-lymphocyte–eosinophil interaction in asthma (Azzawi *et al.*, 1990). Indeed, Hamid *et al.* (1991) succeeded in demonstrating that mucosal biopsies from asthmatics contained cells that expressed mRNA for IL-5, an interleukin which promotes the terminal differentiation of the eosinophil precursor, and which enhances the effector capacity of mature eosinophils. These investigators found also a correlation between IL-5 mRNA expression, and the number of CD25+ and EG2+ cells and total eosinophil count. In fact, this study demonstrates that *in situ* hybridization work is feasible on mucosal biopsies, and provides direct evidence for the cellular localization of IL-5 mRNA in bronchial asthma. This combined use of immunohistochemical and *in situ* hybridization techniques is probably the best approach to study immunoregulation for asthma (Djukanovic *et al.*, 1990), particularly the local production of other cytokines, such as the granulocyte macrophage colony stimulating factor (GM-CSF).

Finally, the suspected role of a loss of vasointestinal peptide (VIP) and/or an increase in substance P immunoreactive nerve fibres in the airway hyperreactivity of asthmatics has also been addressed through immunohistochemical work. Indeed, in two successive studies (Ollerenshaw *et al.*, 1989, 1991), the same group reported the absence of VIP and an increase in both the number and the length of substance P immunoreactive nerve fibres in the lungs of asthmatics, suggesting that neuropeptides may be involved in the pathophysiology of asthma.

References

André-Bougaran, J., Pariente, R., Legrand, M., Cayrol, E. and Brouet, G. (1972). Aspect ultrastructural de l'état de mal asthmatique. *Nouv. Presse Méd.*, **1**, 2457–62.

Azzawi, M., Bradley, B., Jeffery, P. K., Frew, A. J., Wardlaw, A. J., Knowles, G., Assouli, B., Collins, J. V., Durham, S. and Kay, A. B. (1990). Identification of activated T-lymphocytes and eosinophils in bronchial biopsies in stable atopic asthma. *Am. Rev. Respir. Dis.*, **142**, 1407–13.

Beasley, R., Roche, W. R., Roberts, J. A. and Holgate, S. T. (1989). Cellular events in the bronchi in mild asthma and after bronchial provocation. *Am. Rev. Respir. Dis.*, **139**, 806–17.

Bousquet, J., Chanez, P., Lacoste, J. Y., Barneon, G., Ghavanian, N., Enander, I., Venge, P., Ahlstedt, S., Simony-Lafontaine, J., Godard, P. and Michel, F. B. (1990). Eosinophilic inflammation in asthma. *N. Engl. J. Med.*, **323**, 1033–9.

Clutterbuck, E. J., Hirst, E. M. A. and Sanderson, C. J. (1989). Human interleukin-5 (IL-5) regulates the production of eosinophils in human bone marrow cultures: comparison and interaction with IL-1, IL-3, IL-6 and GM-CSF. *Blood*, **73**, 1504–12.

Djukanovic, R., Roche, W. R., Wilson, J. W., Beasley, C. E. W., Twentyman, O. P., Howarth, P. H. and Holgate, S. T. (1990). Mucosal inflammation in asthma. *Am. Rev. Respir. Dis.*, **142**, 434–57.

Djukanovic, R., Wilson, J. W., Lai, C. K. W., Holgate, S. T. and Howarth, P. H. (1991). The safety aspects of fiberoptic bronchoscopy, bronchoalveolar lavage and endobronchial biopsy in asthma. *Am. Rev. Respir. Dis.*, **143**, 772–7.

Dunnil, M. S. (1960). The pathology of asthma, with special reference to changes in the bronchial mucosa. *J. Clin. Pathol.*, **13**, 27–33.

Foresi, A., Bertorelli, G., Pesci, A., Chetta, A. and Olivieri, D. (1990). Inflammatory markers in bronchoalveolar lavage and in bronchial biopsy in asthma during remission. *Chest*, **98**, 528–35.

Fournier, M., Lebargy, F., Leroy-Ladurie, F., Lenormand, E. and Pariente, R. (1989). Intraepithelial T-lymphocyte subsets in the airways of normal subjects and of patients with chronic bronchitis. *Am. Rev. Respir. Dis.*, **140**, 737–42.

Fournier, M., Renon, D., Leroy-Ladurie, F., Pappo, M. and Pariente, R. (1990). Tolérance bronchique à l'inhalation de béclométasone. Etude histologique et microbiologique chez l'asthmatique. *Presse Med.*, **19**, 1441–4.

Gerber, F., Fournier, M. and Pariente, R. (1985). Effets des glucocorticoïdes dans l'asthme à dyspnée continue: étude histologique et immunohistologique de la muqueuse. *Rev. Mal. Respir.*, **2**, 313–17.

Hamid, Q., Azzawi, M., Ving, S., Moqbel, R., Wardlaw, A. J., Corrigan, C. J., Bradley, B., Durham, S. R., Collins, J. V., Jeffery, P. K., Quint, D. J. and Kay, A. B. (1991). Expression of mRNA for interleukin-5 in mucosal bronchial biopsies from asthma. *J. Clin. Invest.*, **87**, 1541–6.

Heino, M., Juntunen-Backman, K., Leijala, M., Rapola, J. and Laitinen, L. A. (1990). Bronchial epithelial inflammation in children with chronic cough after early lower respiratory tract illness. *Am. Rev. Respir. Dis.*, **141**, 428–32.

Jeffery, P. K., Wardlaw, A. J., Nelson, F., Collins, J. Y. and Kay, A. B. (1989). Bronchial biopsies in asthma. An ultrastructural, quantitative study and correlation with hyperreactivity. *Am. Rev. Respir. Dis.*, **140**, 1745–53.

Kantelip, B., Delage, J., Molina, C. and Fonck, Y. (1984). Etude ultrastructurale de biopsies bronchiques obtenues au cours d'une fibroscopie effectuée en période d'accalmie intercrise chez des asthmatiques adultes. *Ann. Pathol.*, **4**, 97–104.

Laitinen, L. A., Heino, M., Laitinen, A., Kava, T. and Haahtela, A. (1985). Damage of the airway epithelium and bronchial hyperreactivity in patients with asthma. *Am. Rev. Respir. Dis.*, **131**, 599–606.

Laursen, L. C., Taudorf, E., Borgeskov, S., Kobayashi, T., Jensen, M. and Weeke, B. (1988). Fiberoptic bronchoscopy and bronchial mucosal biopsies in asthmatics undergoing long term high-dose budesonide aerosol treatment. *Allergy*, **43**, 284–8.

Lopez, A. F., Sanderson, C. J., Gamble, J. R., Campbell, H. R., Young, I. G. and Vadas, M. A. (1988). Recombinant human interleukin-5 is a selective activator of human eosinophil function. *J. Exp. Med.*, **167**, 219–24.

Lundgren, R., Soderberg, M., Morstedt, P. and Stenling, R. (1988). Morphological studies of bronchial mucosal biopsies from asthmatics before and after ten years of treatment with inhaled steroids. *Eur. Respir. J.*, **1**, 883–9.

Naylor, B. (1962). The shedding of the mucosa of the bronchial tree in asthma. *Thorax*, **17**, 69–72.

Ollerenshaw, S., Jarvis, D., Woolcock, A., Sullivan, C. and Scheibner, T. (1989). Absence of immunoreactive vasoactive intestinal polypeptide in tissue from the lungs of patients with asthma. *N. Engl. J. Med.*, **320**, 1244–8.

Ollerenshaw, S. L., Jarvis, D., Sullivan, C. E. and Woolcock, A. J. (1991). Substance P immunoreactive nerves in airways from asthmatics and no asthmatics. *Eur. Respir. J.*, **4**, 673–82.

Paggiaro, P. L., Bacci, E., Paoletti, P., Bernard, P., Dente, F., Marchetti, G., Talini, D., Menconi, G. F. and Giuntini, C. (1990). Bronchoalveolar lavage and morphology of the airways after cessation of exposure in asthmatic subjects sensitized to toluene diisocyanate. *Chest*, **98**, 536–42.

Poulter, L. W., Power, C. and Burke, C. (1990). The relationship between bronchial immunopathology and hyperresponsiveness in asthma. *Eur. Respir. J.*, **3**, 792–9.

Saetta, M., Distefano, A., Rosina, C., Thiene, G. and Fabbri, L. (1991). Quantitative structural analysis of peripheral airways and arteries in sudden fatal asthma. *Am. Rev. Respir. Dis.*, **143**, 138–43.

Soderberg, M., Hellstrom, S., Sandstrom, T., Lundgren, R. and Bergh, A. (1990). Structural characterization of bronchial mucosal biopsies from healthy volunteers: a light and electron microscopical study. *Eur. Respir. J.*, **3**, 261–6.

22

Immunopathology of Chronic Bronchial Inflammation: Contribution of Animal Models

J. R. Lapa e Silva, D. Guerreiro, N. C. Munro, L. W. Poulter and P. J. Cole

22.1 Introduction

It is widely accepted that chronic bronchial inflammation is one of the main features of the asthmatic syndrome. The study of mechanisms leading to chronic bronchial inflammation of various aetiologies, as well as the dissection of the components of this inflammation, might have implications for the understanding of asthma. We have used bronchiectasis as a model of chronic bronchial disease and looked into the immunopathogenesis of the condition.

Bronchiectasis is a chronic bronchopulmonary disease characterized by irreversible dilatation of one or more bronchi, usually associated with chronic purulent sputum production. The affected bronchi are the seat of persistent inflammation, which may lead to scarring and shrinkage of the lung and ultimately, in some cases, to cor pulmonale and death. Cole (1989) described that 83% of patients with the disease have wheezing and airflow obstruction, some of them reversible upon therapy. The prevalence of bronchial hyperreactivity in those patients is also significantly higher than in controls (Pang *et al.*, 1989).

Since the days of Laennec, bronchiectasis has been defined mainly on morphological grounds, and the pathological finding of irreversible dilatation of a bronchus provides the ultimate diagnosis of the condition. Whitwell (1952) regarded bronchiectasis as a destructive inflammatory process. His main contribution to the understanding of the pathogenesis of bronchiectasis was the proposal of a new subgroup – follicular bronchiectasis. He also noted that the lymphoid tissue, although prominent, was only part of an extensive mural inflammation and has implied that this inflammation played an important role on the pathogenesis of the condition. However, despite the fact that the disease has been known for almost 200 years, its pathogenesis remains obscure.

In 1984 a new hypothesis for the pathogenesis of the disease was proposed by Cole. Over a period of five years, he observed more than 300 patients complaining of daily production of infected sputum. Many of these patients proved to have bronchiectasis and the clinical data originating from this group were intriguing: the patients were relatively young, slightly more frequently women, mainly never or ex-smokers and often had associated sinusitis and purulent posterior nasal discharge. He observed that these patients, rather than presenting a syndrome of classical immunity deficiency, were mounting an appropriate immune response to normally absent intrabronchial microorganisms, or even an overresponse, as suggested by the appearance of auto-antibodies in some or association with autoimmune diseases. A considerable number of patients presented a progressive form of the disease that led to scarring and shrinkage of the lung, and finally to cor pulmonale and death (Cole, 1984). He then proposed a 'vicious circle' hypothesis, by which the lesions seen in bronchiectasis are the result of a sequence of host-mediated biological events stimulated by the avirulent colonizing microbes which, although intended to protect the lung's integrity against insults, in fact damage the lung and impair its defence mechanisms. Thus, increasing colonization by microorganisms in turn elicits more, and chronic, host-mediated inflammation – and hence a 'vicious circle' with resulting progressive lung damage.

We have studied this host-mediated inflammatory reaction with respect to its immunologic components. The question as to whether local cellular immune responses in the bronchial wall might contribute to the inflammation associated with bronchiectasis was addressed by comparing samples of bronchial mucosa from bronchiectasis patients with those from controls by immunohistochemical methods (Lapa e Silva *et al.*, 1989a, 1990a; Lapa e Silva, 1991). Intense infiltration of mononuclear cells was seen in bronchi from all bronchiectasis samples and was organized into follicles in half of them. The major component of the infiltrates was the T-lymphocyte but increments of monocyte–macrophages were also seen. B-lymphocytes were only present in samples displaying follicles. In the majority of samples the predominant T cell subset was the CD8+. The T cells co-expressed activation markers and CD45RO antigens. These findings suggest that in bronchiectasis a bronchial cellular immune reaction forms part of the inflammatory response.

Advances in understanding of the pathogenesis of bronchiectasis clearly indicate the need for a new animal model of experimental bronchiectasis incorporating the information from the literature (Tannenberg and Pinner, 1942; Cheng, 1954; Ventura and Domaradzki, 1967; Cash *et al.*, 1979) with concepts of pathogenesis of the disease developed in the past decade, particularly the 'vicious circle' hypothesis. This requires restriction of the bronchial lumen to induce defective mucociliary clearance, chronic infection by a pathogen known to be important in human disease, and should result in histopathological changes similar to those seen in the human disease. Guerreiro has achieved this model (Guerreiro *et al.*, 1990), which was used to investigate different aspects of the immunopathogenesis of bronchiectasis (Lapa e Silva *et al.*, 1989b, 1990b; Lapa e Silva, 1991).

22.2 Methods

Animals and Surgical Technique

Bronchiectasis was induced in specific pathogen-free Wistar rats (Charles Rivers Ltd., Margate, UK). Young rats, 6–8 weeks old, were operated on using the technique devised by Guerreiro. In brief, 160 g animals were anaesthetized with an intramuscular injection of 20 µl of Hypnorm (Janssen Pharmaceutical Ltd., Marlow, UK), intubated with a 4FG cannula (Portex Ltd., Hythe, UK) under direct vision and connected to a small animal ventilator (Harvard Apparatus Ltd., Edenbridge, UK). The rats were ventilated with 0.05% halothane (ICI Pharmaceuticals, Cheshire, UK) in 100% oxygen. A right thoracotomy was performed through the 5th intercostal space. The apical lobe bronchus was partially ligated with 7/0 prolene (Ethicon Ltd, UK) together with a needle from an insulin-injecting microsyringe (Terumo Europe N.V., Leuven, Belgium), ligating the bronchus to an internal diameter of 0.45 mm, corresponding to the external diameter of the needle. A volume of 20 µl of bacterial suspension was then injected into the ligated bronchus, the lungs were inflated with a 5 ml syringe, and the chest wall was closed.

Bacteria

Pseudomonas aeruginosa (P455) was isolated from a bronchiectasis patient. Frozen organisms were cultured in Oxoid Nutrient Broth no. 2, centrifuged, and the cell pellet washed twice and finally resuspended in phosphate-buffered saline (PBS). Viable counts were undertaken and the suspension was adjusted by nephelometry (Evans Electrosellenium Ltd., Halstead, UK) to contain 1×10^8 viable colony-forming units per ml.

Experimental Design

Five groups of animals were studied: test group, partial apical lobe bronchus ligation followed by distal intrabronchial injection of live *P. aeruginosa* (Pa + LIG); control group I, animals received intrabronchial injection of the same number of live bacteria without bronchial ligation (Pa + NOLIG); control group II, partial ligation of the apical lobe bronchus followed by intrabronchial injection of 20 μl of sterile PBS (PBS + LIG); control group III, sham operation (S), achieved by thoracotomy without bronchopulmonary manipulation; normal controls (N), to allow comparisons between the littermates.

The development of experimental bronchiectasis was studied exploring the histopathology and immunopathology of the experimental condition, involving a total of 135 rats. Five animals of each group were killed at the following time points:

Groups	Time since surgery (weeks)							Total
	2	4	8	12	16	20	24	
Pa + LIG	5*	5	5	5	5	5	5	35
Pa + NOLIG	5	5	5	5	ND	ND	5	25
PBS + LIG	5	5	5	ND	ND	ND	ND	15
SHAM	5	5	ND	5	ND	ND	5	20
NORMAL	5	5	5	5	5	5	5	35
TOTAL	25	25	20	20	10	10	20	130

*, number of animals used; ND, not done.

One additional set of five normal controls were killed at time zero to establish baseline parameters.

Also, markers of cell activation were employed to investigate whether the development of pathology described in the previous expriment resulted in changes in cellular phenotype denoting activation.

Techniques

Animals were killed with an overdose of 0.5 ml of Hypnorm (Janssen Pharmaceutical Ltd., Marlow, UK) and exsanguinated by cardiac puncture. Lung lavage was performed by instilling six aliquots of 5 ml sterile

PBS through a 4FG cannula (Portex Ltd., Hythe, UK) inserted into the trachea. The contents of the thorax were excised 'en bloc'. The apical lobe of the right lung was dissected, a small cannula was inserted into the bronchus and the lobe was inflated gently with 1 ml of Histocon (Polysciences, Inc., Warrington, USA). The lung was then mounted on cork, covered with OCT compound (Miles Laboratories Inc., Illinois, USA) and snap frozen in isopentane cooled by liquid nitrogen. Serial sections were used to evaluate co-expression of different antigens by a given cell type. Conventional histology stains were performed.

The lung lavage liquid was placed onto *P. aeruginosa* Isolation Agar (Oxoid, Basingstoke, UK) and 7% Blood Agar (Oxoid) plate for aerobic culture growth. The number of colonies present on the Blood Agar were counted. Colonies on Isolation Agar which were Gram-negative bacilli were subcultured for oxidase tests to confirm the presence of *P. aeruginosa*. Tissue samples were also cultured.

Indirect immunoperoxidase was the main method used for the immunohistochemical studies of immunocompetent cells present in the rat lung (Janossy and Amlot, 1987). The following panel of monoclonal antibodies was employed: MRC OX-52 (Serotec, Oxford, UK) recognizes all rat T-lymphocytes (Robinson *et al.*, 1986); MRC OX-19 (Serotec, Oxford, UK) recognizes a determinant expressed on all rat thymocytes and peripheral T cells (Dallman *et al.*, 1984); MRC OX-19 and MRC OX-52 were used together to enhance the staining (Holt and Schon-Hegrad, 1987); MRC OX-8 (Serotec, Oxford, UK) reacts against membrane glycoproteins present on rat CD8 positive cytotoxic–suppressor T cells (Barclay, 1981; Dallman *et al.*, 1982); W3/25 (Sera-Lab, Crawley, UK) recognizes a determinant present in CD4 positive helper–inducer T cells and in many macrophages and dendritic cells (Mason *et al.*, 1983); ED1 (kindly supplied by Dr C. Dijkstra) recognizes all rat macrophages and dendritic cells (Dijkstra *et al.*, 1985); MRC OX-6 (Serotec, Oxford, UK) identifies a monomorphic determinant of the rat Ia antigen, present on B-lymphocytes, some macrophages, activated T cells and certain epithelial cells (Barclay and Mayrhofer, 1981); MRC OX-39 (Serotec, Oxford, UK) recognizes expression of the activation marker interleukin-2 receptor on the T cells (Patterson *et al.*, 1987); MRC OX-12 recognizes a determinant on rat kappa light chain (Hunt and Fowler, 1981). The sections from each group of animals stained with the same antibody were randomized and evaluated in a 'blind' manner. Three compartments of the lung were assessed: bronchial epithelium; bronchus-associated lymphoid tissue (BALT); peribronchial lamina propria. The number of positive cells were counted on each compartment, using the Solitaire Plus Image Analysis System (Seescan Imaging PLC, Cambridge, UK) and the results expressed by the number of positive cells per unit area (10 000 μm^2).

The quantitation of the major histocompatibility complex class II Ia antigen was achieved by using the MRC OX-6 monoclonal antibody and optical densitometry was performed by using the same morphometric system. The relative expression of Ia staining was determined in each compartment and the results expressed as the mean $\pm$ SD of arbitrary units obtained in the readings.

Statistical analysis was performed using Student's t-test for unpaired data. The results were considered significant when $p = < 0.05$.

22.3 Results

The development of histopathological and immunopathological changes in rats was studied in the test group and compared with the different controls. Bronchial dilatation was consistently observed in 29/35 animals of the Pa + LIG group (3/5 rats at week 2, 4/5 at week 4, 5/5 at weeks 8 and 12, 4/5 at weeks 16, 20, and 24). The apical lobes from two rats at 20 and 24 weeks were totally replaced by fibrous tissue, making it impossible to distinguish the presence of bronchial dilatation. This ranged from isolated distal dilatation and distortion of the bronchioli, to saccular dilatation compromising proximal and distal bronchi. More dilatation and lung destruction were observed at progressive time points. None of the 95 animals from the control groups developed any kind of bronchial dilatation.

Some form of damage to the bronchial epithelium affected all rats of the Pa + LIG group at all time points. Exfoliation, ulceration, goblet cell hyperplasia, and metaplasia were noted. Mucosal foldings, similar to that seen in different forms of human bronchiectasis, were also present in some specimens. Epithelial damage was seen at week 2 in 5/5 rats of the Pa + NOLIG group, in 2/5 rats of the PBS + LIG group, and in 2/5 of the S group but no animals from either of these groups exhibited such damage from 4 weeks onwards, apart from mild goblet cell hyperplasia in a few specimens.

Bronchial wall infiltration by both acute and chronic inflammatory cells was the most consistent histological finding, present in all animals of the Pa + LIG group at all time points. Peribronchial fibrosis was present in the Pa + LIG group in 2/5 animals at week 2, 4/5 at week 4, and in all animals at later time points. None of the 95 animals of the control groups developed fibrosis.

There was no significant difference in the number and distribution of lymphoid follicles between the groups at any time point but an expansion of the bronchus-associated lymphoid tissue (BALT) was seen in the rats of the Pa + LIG group. From 2 weeks onwards a number of lymphoid aggregates situated deeper in the lung parenchyma and apparently not associated with a bronchus began to appear *de novo* in the Pa + LIG group. If BALT and follicular structures were considered together, statistical significance was reached when compared with the number of lymphoid aggregates seen in normals. Hilar and intrapulmonary lymph nodes, some of them much enlarged, also appeared in this group. The other groups failed to show these changes.

The involvement of immunocompetent cells in the development of the histopathological changes in the animals undergoing the experimental procedures was examined in each of the lung compartments analysed. The *p* values presented here compare test or experimental control groups with normal controls by Student's *t*-test.

Significant intraepithelial infiltration of T-lymphocytes in the Pa + LIG group was first noticed at week 2 when compared with the N group, mainly as a result of an increase of CD4 positive cells ($p \leqslant 0.01$). Subsequently, this increase in the number of intraepithelial T cells was mainly due to an increment in the number of CD8 positive cells ($p < 0.003$ at week 4, $p = 0.0001$ at week 8, $p < 0.0001$ at week 20). Equivalent numbers of both subsets were seen at 24 weeks. No such increments were seen in the other experimental groups when compared with group N. A significant increase in ED1 positive macrophages was noted in the Pa + LIG group when compared with group N at weeks 2 ($p < 0.03$), 8 ($p < 0.005$), and 24 ($p = 0.02$) but no statistical significance was reached at the other time points. In the Pa + NOLIG group an increment in the number of intraepithelial macrophage-like cells was noted only at week 2 ($p < 0.01$) and none was seen in the PBS + LIG or S groups.

No OX-12 positive cells were ever seen infiltrating the bronchial epithelium of test or control groups of rats.

With regard to immunocompetent cell proliferation in the BALT, a highly significant ($p < 0.0001$) increase in the number of T cells infiltrating the BALT of animals of the Pa + LIG group was first noticed at week 2, when compared with group N. This increase was almost entirely due at this stage to increased numbers of CD4 positive helper T cells ($p = 0.001$). Similar results were obtained when the Pa + LIG group was compared with the Pa + NOLIG ($p < 0.0001$ for T cells, $p < 0.003$ for CD4 positive cells), PBS + LIG ($p < 0.0001$ for T cells, $P < 0.01$ for CD4 positive cells), and S groups ($p < 0.0004$ for T cells, $p = 0.003$ for CD4 positive cells). In none of the control animals in these three groups was such an increase in the cell numbers seen at any time point. Subsequently, T cell numbers decreased but remained statistically different from N at all time points. An inversion of the CD4/CD8 ratios was seen at weeks 8 and 16, and at the other time points there were similar numbers of both subsets or slight predominance of CD4 positive cells.

The macrophage-like cell population in the BALT of animals from the Pa + LIG group did not demonstrate the same dramatic increase as that seen in the T cell population, when compared with group N, but was significantly increased at weeks 2 ($p \leq 0.01$) and 12 ($p < 0.02$).

Cells of the B-lymphocyte lineage, as determined by the monoclonal antibody OX-12, showed a significant increase in the Pa + LIG group from week 4 onwards compared with the normal controls but no differences were seen between the experimental control groups and the normal animals at any time point.

For peribronchial infiltration, a different pattern of infiltration to that in previously described compartments was noted in the bronchial lamina propria. A less marked but highly significant increase in the numbers of T cells present in the Pa + LIG group was seen at all time points, steadily increasing up to 8 weeks, declining at 16 weeks, then increasing again in a bi-phasic mode (Fig. 22.1). In some animals, mainly at week 8, this infiltration was so massive as to form a continuous sheath. This T cell increment was initially due to both subsets, with a slight predominance of CD4 positive cells at the first time point but from 8 weeks onwards a predominance of CD8 positive cells over the CD4 positive cells or equivalent numbers of both phenotypes were noted.

A significant increase in the macrophage population was also present in the Pa + LIG group compared with controls at all time points. In the Pa + NOLIG, PBS + LIG, and S groups, a small but significant increase in the T cell and macrophage populations was seen at week 2 but the numbers of positive cells were not different from group N after 4 weeks.

Significant increase in numbers of B-lymphocytes were noted at all time points when the Pa + LIG group was compared with normal controls but no differences were seen between the experimental control groups and the normal animals at any time point.

Significantly higher proportions of T cells expressing OX-39 in animals of the Pa + LIG compared with the other three groups included in this study were seen in all compartments examined, principally in the lamina propria ($p < 0.0001$). The number of OX-39 positive cells in rats from the Pa + LIG group was higher at the initial time points as compared with later points. Ia antigen was expressed by bronchial epithelial cells and by many mononuclear cells infiltrating the lung compartments of the Pa + LIG group but not by cells in the control groups. This Ia expression was quantitated in the different compartments of the lung (Fig. 22.2). Highly significant differences were seen in the Ia readings obtained in the Pa + LIG group when compared with the other three groups, particularly in the epithelium ($p < 0.0001$ vs N; $p = 0.0001$ vs Pa + NOLIG; $p = 0.0003$ vs S) but also in the lamina propria ($p < 0.0001$ vs N; $p < 0.01$ vs Pa + NOLIG; $p < 0.03$ vs S). In the BALT the differences were less remarkable ($p = 0.006$ vs N; $p < 0.01$ vs Pa + NOLIG). No differences could be established between the readings from the Pa + NOLIG and S groups when compared with group N.

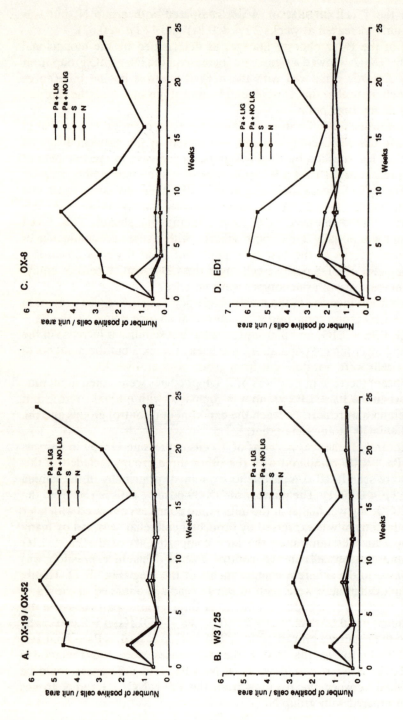

Fig. 22.1 Changes in the composition and frequency of immunocompetent cells infiltrating the peribronchial areas of animals with experimental bronchiectasis compared with controls. The graphs show changes in frequency of immunocompetent cells in the lamina propria of test and control groups of rats. PBS + LIG and S groups are represented together. Standard deviations are omitted for clarity. See text for specificity of monoclonal antibodies.

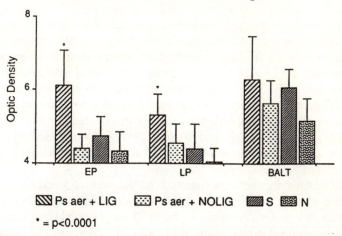

Fig. 22.2 Expression of MHC class II antigens in lung compartments of test and control groups of rats. The bar graph shows the results of optical densitometry of lung compartments of test and control groups of rats. The results are expressed in arbitrary units.

22.4 Discussion

Chronic bronchial inflammation is now regarded as a pivotal mechanism involved in bronchial hyperreactivity and asthma. Recent publications have dissected the basic components of this inflammatory reaction, as it became clear that non-specific as well as immune specific mechanisms take part in the reaction. The presence of T-lymphocytes exhibiting phenotypic characteristics of activated cells either in the circulation of patients with severe asthma (Corrigan *et al.*, 1988) or in bronchial biopsies of stable atopic asthmatics (Azzawi *et al.*, 1990), mainly of the CD4+ subset, suggested that cell-mediated immune mechanisms have also a role to play in the pathogenesis of the condition.

As far as bronchiectasis is concerned, Guerreiro's model described here closely mirrors human bronchiectasis, both histopathologically and immunopathologically. Introduction of *P. aeruginosa* into a rat bronchus after its partial ligation produced a reliable model of bronchiectasis and chronic bronchial inflammation in which to study the pathogenesis of both conditions. Such experiments confirm that the combination of partial bronchial ligation and intrabronchial presence of viable *P. aeruginosa* are necessary for the emergence of bronchiectasis. The mere presence of the bacterium in a previously normal bronchus or the impairment of the mucociliary clearance without infection did not result in the emergence of the bronchial dilatation or chronic inflammation. Similar requirements were found by others (Tannenberg and Pinner, 1942; Cheng, 1954; Ventura and Domaradzki, 1967). Damaging insults to the human bronchial tree especially in genetically predisposed individuals (or those with underlying disease) may compromise the first line bronchial defence mechanism of mucociliary clearance and predispose the individual to microbial colonization of the bronchial tree. The host inflammatory response fails to eliminate these microbial colonists and becomes chronic, damaging adjacent lung tissue in the process. This chronic inflammation and tissue damage further reduce mucociliary clearance (Cole and Wilson, 1989), allowing increased microbial colonization. The end result of such a chronic inflammatory process is bronchiectasis and progressive lung damage.

Bronchiectasis in the experimental model was characterized by the infiltration of large numbers of T cells, increased MHC class II expression, emergence of follicles and other findings. The development of this cellular immune response during evolution of bronchiectasis and the demonstration that it was at its height at the time when the rats developed histologically apparent bronchiectasis raise the possibility that this reaction might be causal. In established bronchiectasis, the continuing presence of large numbers of T-lymphocytes and macrophages in all lung compartments suggests an ongoing acquired immune response. The time studies used to compare development of the inflammatory lesions disclosed that during the development of bronchiectasis an early expansion of the T-lymphocyte population took place in the BALT, with an almost fourfold increase in the numbers of T cells as compared with the age-matched normal controls, together with the development of T cell follicles in the lung parenchyma. The major T cell subset both in the BALT and in the newly formed lymphoid aggregates during the first weeks of the inflammatory process was the CD4 positive helper subset. This situation was then superseded by a gradual increase in the numbers of CD8 positive cytotoxic–suppressor cells. Such changes would be compatible with recruitment of lymphocytes from the circulation in response to antigens in the bronchial lumen. As the majority of these cells are CD4 positive helper cells, it could be postulated that this is similar to a type IV hypersensitivity reaction. Potentially, the BALT acts as the draining lymphoid organ and the deeper follicles represent the outcome of perivascular accumulations of recruited T cells. This situation is reminiscent of the Mantoux reaction in man (Poulter et al., 1982), particularly as a minor but significant population of non-lymphoid macrophage cells is present in the locality possibly acting as antigen presenting cells (Unanue and Allen, 1987).

Also in the epithelium and peribronchial area, an early and highly significant accumulation of T-lymphocytes was apparent, and at the onset of the process a small predominance of CD4 positive over CD8 positive T cells was also observed. From week 8 onwards a predominance of CD8 positive cells, or an equilibrium between the two major subsets, was present in the bronchiectatic animals. Whether this predominance of the CD8 positive subset was an attempt to control the cell-mediated immune response, or whether it represented the emergence of a cytotoxic population itself involved in the tissue damaging events, are questions yet to be answered.

The time-dependent study showed clearly that severe inflammatory changes preceded the development of bronchiectasis. The presence of a small but statistically significant population of OX-39 (interleukin-2 receptor) positive T cells in the lamina propria, BALT, and other lymphoid aggregates in rats with experimental bronchiectasis suggested that these T cells were activated. The increased expression of class II MHC antigens by the epithelium and mononuclear cells infiltrating the peribronchial areas was further evidence of cellular activation. In the human condition, T-lymphocytes also exhibit signs of cell activation and immunological commitment, with increased expression of HLA-DR and CD45RO antigens (Lapa e Silva, 1991). These data strongly suggest that T-lymphocytes are very important for the development of experimental bronchiectasis. This immune response may cause at least part of the tissue damage seen in the experimental condition described here.

The use of animal models of bronchial hyperreactivity could shed new light on the immunopathogenesis of asthma and related disorders. Frew et al. (1990) have used a model of late-phase asthmatic reaction in the guinea pig to investigate the kinetics of T-lymphocyte and eosinophil accumulation but employed a limited number of monoclonal antibodies. The technology used to investigate the immunopathology of experimental bronchiectasis could now be applied to well-established models of bronchial hyperreactivity (Pretolani et al., 1988), in order to dissect basic immunopathogenetic mechanisms involved in asthma.

Acknowledgements

We are indebted to Dr Philippa Roberts for preparing some animals, to Mr H. Todd for the bacteriological studies, and to Ms Aida Condez for technical help. JRLS was partially supported by the Brazilian Research Council and by the Federal University of Rio de Janeiro. The work at the RFHSM was partially supported by a grant from the British Lung Foundation to LWP.

References

Azzawi, M., Bradley, B., Jeffery, P. K., Frew, A. J., Wardlaw, A. J., Knowles, G., Assoufi, B., Collins, J. V., Durham, S. and Kay, A. B. (1990). Identification of activated T-lymphocytes and eosinophils in bronchial biopsies in stable atopic asthma. *Am. Rev. Respir. Dis.*, **142**, 1407–13.

Barclay, A. N. (1981). The localization of populations of lymphocytes defined by monoclonal antibodies in rat lymphoid tissues. *Immunology*, **42**, 593–600.

Barclay, A. N. and Mayhofer, G. (1981). Bone marrow origin of Ia-positive cells in the medulla of rat thymus. *J. Exp. Med.*, **153**, 1666–71.

Cash, H. A., Woods, D. E., McCollough, B., Johanson, W. G., Jr, and Bass, J. A. (1979). A rat model of chronic respiratory infection with *Pseudomonas aeruginosa*. *Am. Rev. Respir. Dis.*, **119**, 453–9.

Cheng, K. K. (1954). The experimental production of bronchiectasis in rats. *J. Pathol. Bacter.*, **67**, 89–98.

Cole, P. J. (1984). In Davies, R. J. (ed.), *Strategies for the Management of Chronic Bronchial Sepsis*, Medicine Publishing Foundation, Oxford, 1–20.

Cole, P. J. (1989). In Reeves, D. and Geddes, A. (eds.), *Recent Advances in Infection 3*, Churchill Livingstone, Edinburgh, 141–51.

Cole, P. J. (1990). In Brewis, R. A. L., Gibson, G. J. and Geddes, D. M. (eds.), *Respiratory Medicine*, Bailliere Tyndall, London, 726–59.

Cole, P. and Wilson, R. (1989). Host–microbial interrelationships in respiratory infection. *Chest*, **95** (Suppl.), 217S–221S.

Corrigan, C. I., Hartnell, A. and Kay, A. B. (1988). T-lymphocyte activation in acute severe asthma. *Lancet*, **i**, 1129–31.

Dallman, M. J., Mason, D. W. and Webb, M. (1982). The roles of host and donor cells in the rejection of skin allografts by T cell-deprived rats injected with syngeneic T cells. *Eur. J. Immunol.*, **12**, 511–18.

Dallman, M. J., Thomas, M. L. and Green, J. R. (1984). MRC OX-19: a monoclonal antibody that labels rat T-lymphocytes and augments *in vitro* proliferative responses. *Eur. J. Immunol.*, **14**, 260–7.

Dijkstra, C. D., Dopp, E. A., Joling, P. and Kraal, G. (1985). The heterogeneity of mononuclear phagocytes in lymphoid organs: distinct macrophage subpopulations in the rat recognized by monoclonal antibodies ED1, ED2, and ED3. *Immunology*, **54**, 589–99.

Frew, A. J., Moqbel, R., Azzawi, M., Hartnell, A., Barkans, J., Jeffery, P. K., Kay, A. B., Scheper, R. J., Varley, J., Church, M. K. and Holgate, S. T. (1990). T-lymphocytes and eosinophils in allergen-induced late-phase asthmatic reactions in the guinea pig. *Am. Rev. Respir. Dis.*, **141**, 407–13.

Guerreiro, D., Heard, B., Rohde, J., Todd, H., Sheppard, M. and Cole, P. J. (1990). Quantitation of experimental bronchiectasis. *Eur. Respir. J.*, **3**, 296s.

Holt, P. G. and Schon-Hegrad, M. A. (1987). Localization of T cells, macrophages and dendritic cells in rat respiratory tract tissue: implications for immune function studies. *Immunology*, **62**, 349–56.

Hunt, S. V. and Fowler, M. H. (1981). A repopulation assay for B and T-lymphocytes stem cells employing radiation quimeras. *Cell Tissue Kinet.*, **14**, 445–64.

Janossy, G. and Amlot, P. (1987). In Klaus, G. G. B. (ed.), *Lymphocytes. A Practical Approach*, IRL Press, Oxford, 67–108.

Lapa e Silva, J. R. (1991). Acquired immune responses in the lung: their relevance to bronchiectasis. *Ph.D. Thesis*, University of London, London, 1–278.

Lapa e Silva, J. R., Jones, J. A. H., Cole, P. J. and Poulter, L. W. (1989a). The immunological component of the cellular inflammatory infiltrate in bronchiectasis. *Thorax*, **44**, 668–73.

Lapa e Silva, J. R., Guerreiro, D., Noble, B., Poulter, L. W. and Cole, P. J. (1989b). Immunopathology of experimental bronchiectasis. *Am. J. Respir. Cell Mol. Biol.*, **1**, 297–304.

Lapa e Silva, J. R., Poulter, L. W. and Cole, P. J. (1990a). In Challacombe, S. J., Stokes, C. R. and MacDonald, T. T. (eds.), *Advances in Mucosal Immunology*, Kluwer, Dordrecht, 636–7.

Lapa e Silva, J. R., Guerreiro, D., Munro, N. C., Noble, B., Cole, P. J. and Poulter, L. W. (1990b). In Challacombe, S. J., Stokes, C. R. and MacDonald, T. T. (eds.), *Advances in Mucosal Immunology*, Kluwer, Dordrecht, 821–4.

Mason, D. W., Arthur, R. P., Dallman, M. J., Green, J. R., Spickett, G. P. and Thomas, M. L. (1983). Functions of rat T-lymphocyte subsets isolated by means of monoclonal antibodies. *Immunol. Rev.*, **74**, 57–82.

Pang, J., Chan, H. S. and Sung, J. Y. (1989). Prevalence of asthma, atopy, and bronchial hyperreactivity in bronchiectasis: a controlled study. *Thorax*, **44**, 948–51.

Patterson, D. J., Jefferies, W. A., Green, J. R., Brandon, M. R., Corthesy, P., Puklavec, M. and Williams, M. R. (1987). Antigens of activated rat T-lymphocytes including a molecule of 50 000 M detected only on CD4 positive T blasts. *Mol. Immunol.*, **24**, 1281–90.

Poulter, L. W., Seymour, G. J., Duke, O., Janossy, G. and Panayi, G. (1982). Immunohistological analysis of delayed-type hypersensitivity in man. *Cell. Immunol.*, **74**, 358–69.

Pretolani, M., Lefort, J. and Vargaftig, B. B. (1988). Active immunization induces lung hyperresponsiveness in the guinea pig: pharmacological modulation and triggering role of the booster injection. *Am. Rev. Respir. Dis.*, **138**, 1572–8.

Robinson, A. P., Puklavec, M. and Mason, D. W. (1986). MRC OX-52: a rat T-cell antigen. *Immunology*, **57**, 527–31.

Tannanberg, J. and Pinner, M. (1942). Atelectasis and bronchiectasis. An experimental study concerning their relationship. *J. Thor. Surg.*, **11**, 571–616.

Unanue, E. R. and Allen, P. M. (1987). The basis for the immunoregulatory role of macrophages and other dendritic cells. *Science*, **236**, 551–7.

Ventura, J. and Domaradzki, M. (1967). Pathogenesis of experimental bronchiectasis in laboratory rats. *Arch. Pathol.*, **83**, 80–5.

Whitwell, F. (1952). A study of the pathology and pathogenesis of bronchiectasis. *Thorax*, **7**, 213–99.

Poster Abstracts

TOXOCARA CANIS: THE INFLAMMATORY RESPONSE IN THE LUNGS OF EXPERIMENTALLY INFECTED MICE IS CHARACTERIZED BY EOSINOPHILS AND TRACHEAL HYPOREACTIVITY

J. BUIJS[1] and F. P. NIJKAMP[2]. 1. Nat. Inst. Public Health and Env. Hyg. BILTHOVEN. 2. Fac. Pharmacy, University of UTRECHT, The Netherlands.

Toxocara spp the large round worms for which dogs and cats are the definitive hosts may infect other mammals including man. The tissue migrating phase of this parasite causes 'Visceral Larva Migrans' (VLM) in the latter hosts. The inflammatory response of the lungs of mice was investigated in a longitudinal study. BALB/c mice infected orally with 1000 *Toxocara* ova induced multifocal inflammatory reactions which persisted for $\geq$ 3 months. Perivascular- and partial peribronchiolar cuffs were observed consisting of mixed cellular infiltrates in which eosinophils were prominent. Bronchoalveolar lavages (BAL) were performed and the collected cells analyzed. The number of cells in the BAL fluid increased 5–7 fold (day 7–28 post-infection (p.i.)). The population consisted of eosinophils (ca 60%), lymphocytes (ca 30%) and macrophages (ca 10%). About 30% of the lymphocytes reacted with anti-Thy-$1,2^+$ and anti-L$_3$T$_4^+$ MoAbs. $\leq$ 1% of the lymphocytes were Lyt-2 positive. The effect of the persisting inflammatory reaction on tracheal reactivity was investigated by performing carbachol cumulative dose-response curves at various days p.i.. The trachea showed a hyporeactive response from day 7 p.i. which persisted until 3 months p.i. It was concluded that a primary *Toxocara* infection in mice causes persistent inflammation in the lungs which is accompanied by a hyporeactive response of the trachea to the cholinergic agonist carbachol.

INDUCTION OF AIRWAY HYPERREACTIVITY BY SUBSTANCE-P (SP) IN THE GUINEA PIG

R. EISENBURGER, I. SCHEMAINDA and K. SEIBEL,
Dept. of Pharmacology, Klinge Pharma GmbH, Weihenstephanerstr. 28, 8000 MUNICH 80, F. R. Germany

Different animal models of airway hyperreactivity enable us to investigate the possible mechanism involved in the pathogenesis of this phenomenon and allow us to develop novel therapeutic agents which may be of benefit in asthma. With regard to this aim, some pharmacological facets of a new model of airway hyperreactivity induced by infusion of substance P (SP), were compared with hyperreactivity induced by platelet activating factor (PAF) in anaesthetized guinea pigs.

After intravenous infusion of 40 µg/kg SP or 600 ng/kg of PAF, over a period of 60 minutes, a 5–10 fold increase in bronchial reactivity to 3 µg/kg i.v. methacholine is induced.

Our experiments have shown that:
- the genesis of SP-hyperreactivity, as well as that induced by PAF, takes place in spite of bilateral cervical vagotomy
- mepyramine is without effect in SP- or PAF-induced hyperreactivity
- atropine does not inhibit the increase in bronchial reactivity in both models
- FR 111099, a specific PAF-antagonist, does not inhibit the SP-induced hyperreactivity in contrast to that induced by PAF-infusion
- prednisolone is effective in the SP- as well as in the PAF-induced hyperreactivity
- the development of SP-induced hyperreactivity in contrast to that induced by PAF is not associated with a pulmonary recruitment and concomitant decrease of platelets in the blood circulation

From these data we conclude that:
- in the genesis of airway hyperreactivity a vagal-reflex-mediated contribution is improbable. In addition, in both models of hyperreactivity we can exclude any involvement of cholinergic receptor mechanism
- both models are independent of histamine-release
- in the SP-induced hyperreactivity, as well as in the PAF-induced hyperreactivity, inflammatory cells seem to be involved as the corticosteroids are effective in these airway-hyperreactivity models
- induction of SP-hyperreactivity does not seem to be platelet-dependent in contrast to PAF-hyperreactivity

EFFECTS OF TYPE IV PHOSPHODIESTERASE (PDE) INHIBITORS ON SEPHADEX-INDUCED EOSINOPHILIA AND HYPERRESPONSIVENESS.

J. R. S. ARCH, S. M. LAYCOCK, H. SMITH and B. A. SPICER, Smith-Kline Beecham Pharmaceuticals, Yew Tree Bottom Road, Epsom, KT18 5XQ, UK

Injection of rats with Sephadex particles (0.5 mg i.v. of G200) on days 0, 2 and 5 elicits a selective increase in blood and lung eosinophil numbers, associated with hypersensitivity of the resistance to artificial respiration produced by i.v. 5-hydroxytryptamine (5-HT) and hyperreactivity of lung parenchymal strips to 5-HT. Dexamethasone and isoprenaline, given prior to each dose of Sephadex, reduced these effects, but aminophylline (100 mg/kg, p.o.) inhibited significantly only the blood eosinophilia (Spicer *et al.*, 1990, Cook, 1990). The more potent and type IV-selective PDE inhibitors denbufylline (D) and rolipram (R) (IC_{50} values approx. 1μM) have now been evaluated in this model. They were given 30 min before each dose of Sephadex and measurements were made on days 7 or 8.

D (6.25 and 25 mg/kg, p.o.) and R (10 mg/kg, p.o.) significantly reduced blood eosinophilia to 66 ± 12 (D, 6.25), 48 ± 6 (D, 25) and $46 \pm 4\%$ (R) of Sephadex control values (cf. 14% in saline-treated controls). D (25) also significantly reduced the area under the 5-HT concentration response curve (1.4×10^{-9} to 1.2×10^{-4} M) *in vitro* to $30 \pm 4\%$ of Sephadex control values (cf. 27% in saline-treated controls) and increased the ED_{30} (95% confidence intervals) value to 5-HT *in vivo* from 15.6 (12.9–18.9) to 20.7 (17.8–23.8) μg/kg, i.v. (cf. 26.6 (22.7–31.5) in saline-treated controls). ($n \geq 6$ in all cases.) R reduced the response to 5-HT *in vitro* (55% of controls) but was not evaluated *in vivo*.

Since eosinophilia and airways hyperresponsiveness are features of asthma, these results indicate that type IV PDE inhibitors have potential in the treatment of the disease.

- Cook, R. M. (1990). Eosinophil accumulation in rats injected with Sephadex particicules. *Clin. Expt. All.*, **20**, 511–17.
- Spicer, B. A., Baker, R. C., Hatt, P. A., Laycock, S. M. and Smith, H. (1990). The effects of drugs on Sephadex-induced eosinophilia and lung hyperresponsiveness in the rat. *Br. J. Pharmacol.*, **101**, 891–898.

COMPARISON OF TWO RAT MODELS WITH INFLAMMATION-RELATED BRONCHIAL HYPERREACTIVITY

O. H. Wilhelms, J. Koehnke, P. Kroschel, Ch. Lemmermann, M. Linssen, L. Lipponer, W. Seilnacht, Medical Research, Boehringer Mannheim GmbH

Spontaneous inhalation of: ovalbumin antigen aerosol (OVA) or i.-v. administration of sephadex particles (S i.v.) are both suitable for an induction of bronchial inflammation (BI) in actively immunized rats. This B.I. is accompanied by bronchial hyperreactivity 24 h after challenge.

Sprague Dawley rats were actively immunized against ovalbumin on day 0, and challenged on day 14–16 either by OVA or S. i.v. (2 mg) 24 h before performing bronchoalveolar lavage (BAL) or measurement of the degree of bronchial hyperreactivity in separate groups ($n = 8$–12) of anaesthetized rats with the Konzett-Roessler-air overflow method. BAL fluid (BALF) was analyzed for an increase of the 'total' (L_T) and 'small-sized leukocyte' number (L_{ss}), protein and several proteinases, and of lumino-amplified chemiluminescence of BALF leukocytes after stimulation with opsonized zymosan.

Both challenges OVA and S.i.v. induced a significant and apparently equipotent bronchial inflammation, as all the above mentioned BALF parameters were significantly and approximately equally increased compared to saline controls.

Bronchial hyperreactivity following OVA challenge, however, was restricted to 5-HT-aerosol, whereas S. i.v.-challenge induced an unspecific bronchial hyperreactivity which was detected for OVA, 5-HT- and ACh-aerosol.

Differential leukocyte counts showed additional differences in the mechanism of B.I. in both models: eosinophils were significantly increased only following pretreatment with S. i.v., but not 24 h after OVA challenge.

Differences in the inhibitory profiles of dexamethasone and cyclosporine A on bronchial hyperreactivity and on BAL parameters underline further that both rat models for bronchial hyperreactivity differ in their mechanisms.

BRONCHIAL INFLAMMATION AFTER AEROSOL INDUCED ANAPHYLACTIC REACTION IN BROWN NORWAY RATS

J. P. TARAYRE, M. ALIAGA, M. BARBARA, N. MALFETES, S. VIEU, J. TISNE-VERSAILLES – Centre de Recherche Pierre Fabre, 81106 Castres, France

In comparison to normal animals or to animals sensitized but exposed to NaCl aerosol, Brown Norway rats, actively sensitized (10 mg/kg, ovalbumin i.m.; killed Bordetella pertussis i.p.) and exposed to a 10%-ovalbumin aerosol 12–14 days after sensitization, showed an increase in the number of neutrophils and eosinophils in bronchoalveolar lavage (BAL) fluid 24 h after the challenge. In passively sensitized Brown Norway rats exposed to ovalbumin aerosol no inflammation appeared in BAL fluid 24 h after the anaphylactic reaction. Various drugs were administered twice after the anaphylactic reaction at +5 min. and +5 h, and have been experimented on the 24-h inflammation obtained in actively sensitized rats.

Dexamethasone acetate (6.25 mg/kg × 2 i.p.) and theophylline (50 mg/kg × 2 i.p.) decreased the number of eosinophils and neutrophils. Ketotifen fumarate (12.5 mg/kg × 2 i.p.), cetirizine dihydrochloride (12.5 mg/kg × 2 i.p.), salbutamol (2 mg/kg × 2 i.p.), disodium cromoglycate (50 mg/kg × 2 i.p.) reduced the number of eosinophils. Tioxamast decreased the number of eosinophils at 12.5 mg/kg × 2 (i.p. and p.o.). At higher doses (50 mg/kg × 2 i.p.; 150 mg/kg × 2 p.o.), it reduced the number of eosinophils and neutrophils. Indomethacin (5 mg/kg × 2 i.p.), mepyramine maleate (12.5 mg/kg × 2 i.p.) and atropine sulfate (1 mg/kg × 2 i.p.) were inactive. Hence 24-h inflammation after an aerosol induced anaphylactic reaction in actively sensitized Brown Norway rats appears a good model to study an IgE-mediated bronchial inflammation.

INFLUENCE OF THE ROUTE OF ADMINISTRATION IN THE INDUCTION OF BRONCHIAL HYPERREACTIVITY AFTER A PASSIVE ANAPHYLACTIC SHOCK IN THE GUINEA PIG

J. P. TARAYRE, M. ALIAGA, N. MALFETES, M. BARBARA, S. VIEU, J. TISNE-VERSAILLES – Centre de Recherche Pierre Fabre, 81106 Castres, France

The possible generation of bronchial hyperreactivity to histamine or carbamylcholine after a passive anaphylactic shock in guinea pigs has been studied according to the respective administration route of the mediator and of the antigen. After an anaphylactic shock induced by aerosol challenge in conscious guinea pigs, we obtain a hyperreactivity to histamine and carbamylcholine inhalation respectively 1–3 h and 1–2 h after the shock. When the anaphylactic shock is caused in conscious guinea pigs by an intravenous (i.v.) injection of antigen, we could not obtain a bronchial hyperreactivity to histamine inhalation. After an anaphylactic shock by i.v. injection of antigen in anaesthetized and ventilated guinea pigs, the i.v. administration of histamine induces a maximum hyperreactivity 10 minutes after the shock, which decreases 20 minutes after it. Besides, when after an anaphylactic shock induced by aerosol challenge in conscious guinea pigs we investigate one hour later the hyperreactivity to the i.v. injection of histamine in the same anaesthetized and ventilated animal, we do not obtain a hyperreactivity. In conclusion, under the experimental conditions used, we could obtain a bronchial hyperreactivity to the systemic administration of a mediator after a passive anaphylactic shock only if mediator and antigen (to induce the shock) were administered by the same route.

ACTIVE SENSITIZATION OF GUINEA PIGS WITH A BOOSTER INJECTION OF ANTIGEN INDUCES A MODIFICATION OF THE SENSITIVITY OF THE PAF-INDUCED BRONCHOCONSTRICTION AND OF THE RECRUITMENT OF EOSINOPHILS INDUCED BY AN INSTILLATION OF PAF

S. DESQUAND, J. LEFORT AND B. B. VARGAFTIG, Unité de Pharmacologie Cellulaire, Unité Associée Institut Pasteur-INSERM n° 285, 75015, Paris, France

Lungs isolated from actively sensitized guinea pigs with a booster injection of antigen exhibit a bronchopulmonary hyper-responsiveness to various agonists *in vitro* and particularly to platelet activating factor (PAF), which is partially accounted for by an increased metabolism of arachidonic acid through the lipoxygenase pathway (Pretolani *et al.*, 1988 and 1989). This led us to compare, *in vivo*, bronchoconstriction induced by the intratracheal (i.t.) instillation of 1 µg of PAF to naive and to actively sensitized and boosted guinea pigs. The PAF-induced bronchoconstriction in both groups of animals were reduced by the injection of the H1 antagonist mepyramine (500 µg/kg., i.v.) and blocked by the administration of the PAF antagonist BN 52021 (1 mg, i.t.) ($p < 0.05$). By contrast, the cyclooxygenase inhibitor aspirin (50 mg/kg; i.v.), which blocked PAF-induced bronchoconstriction in non-sensitized guinea pigs, became inactive when they were actively sensitized with a booster injection of antigen. We also investigated whether the modifications of the sensitivity of PAF-induced bronchoconstriction to aspirin induced by immunisation with a booster injection involve the content of the inflammatory cells of the bronchoalveolar lavage (BAL) or their behaviour. No differences in the macrophage, eosinophil, lymphocyte and neutrophil contents of the BAL of both naive and boosted guinea pigs pretreated with mepyramine and aspirin were noted 10 min after the instillation of PAF as compared to the contents observed in animals receiving the solvent of PAF. By contrast, 60 min later, the number of eosinophils was increased in normal as well as in boosted guinea pigs. Under those conditions, it was also noted that the number of eosinophils was statistically higher in BAL of boosted guinea pigs as compared to those of naive animals ($p < 0.05$). Thus, active sensitization with a booster injection of antigen operates as a trigger for pulmonary inflammation, modifying the recruitment of inflammatory cells into the airways when guinea pigs are instilled with PAF and making bronchoconstriction less dependent on cyclooxygenase derivatives.

- Pretolani, M., Lefort, J. and Vargaftig, B. B. (1988). Active immunization induces lung hyper-responsiveness in the guinea pig – Pharmacologic modulation and triggering role of the booster injection. *Am. Rev. Respir. Dis.*, **138**, 1572–8.
- Pretolani, M., Lefort, J., Dumarez, C. and Vargaftig, B. B. (1989). Role of lipoxygenase metabolites for the hyper-responsiveness to platelet activating factor of lung from actively sensitized guinea pig. *J. Pharmacol. Exp. Ther.*, **248**, 353–9.

SALMETEROL INHIBITS NEUTROPHIL ACCUMULATION IN RAT LUNG

A. T. Nials, C. J. Whelan and *C. J. Vardey*, Department of Peripheral Pharmacology, Glaxo Group Research Ltd., Ware, Herts SG12 0DP, UK

Salmeterol is a long-acting β_2-adrenoceptor agonist which has been developed for the treatment of asthma. We have shown previously that in addition to its long-lasting bronchodilator effects, salmeterol has anti-inflammatory properties in guinea pig lung, inhibiting both plasma protein extravasation (Whelan and Johnson, 1990), and the accumulation of granulocytes induced by lipopolysaccharide (LPS) or platelet activating factor (Whelan and Johnson, 1991). In this study, we have investigated whether salmeterol also exhibits anti-inflammatory activity in rat lung, a species in which β-agonists are weak bronchodilators. We have compared the effects of salmeterol with those of the short-acting β_2-adrenoceptor agonist, salbutamol.

Male Wistar rats ($\sim$300 g) were exposed to aerosols of β_2-agonists (0.01–30 mM) or vehicle for 2 min (Whelan and Johnson, 1990). After 30 min, the animals were challenged with aerosolized lipopolysaccharides (LPS) (100 μg.ml^{-1}) for 10 min. Four hours later, the rats were killed (pentobarbitone, i.p.) and the lungs lavaged twice with 5 ml phosphate-buffered saline containing heparin, 10 u.ml^{-1}. Total and differential leucocyte counts were performed on aliquots of the bronchoalveolar lavage fluid (BALF). From these data, neutrophils.ml^{-1} BALF were calculated.

In vehicle-treated rats, LPS increased the neutrophil content of BALF from 1.1 ($\pm$0.7) to 250.9 ($\pm$36.4) $\times$ 10^3 neutrophils.ml^{-1} (mean $\pm$ SEM, n = 14), 4 h after challenge. However, salmeterol pretreatment caused a dose-related decrease in LPS-induced neutrophil accumulation with 38.3% $\pm$ 8.1 and 63.0% $\pm$ 6.4 (n = 4) inhibition at 0.1 and 1 mM nebuliser concentrations, respectively. In contrast, salbutamol aerosols (0.1–30 mM) had no significant effect on neutrophil accumulation. Propranolol (5 mg.kg^{-1}, s.c.), administered 30 min before exposure to aerosolized salmeterol (1 mM), abolished the inhibition of neutrophil accumulation.

Thus salmeterol, but not salbutamol, inhibits LPS-induced neutrophilia in rat lung, and these effects appear to be mediated through its ability to cause prolonged activation of β-adrenoceptors. These findings provide further evidence for anti-inflammatory effects of salmeterol.

• Whelan, C. J. and Johnson, M. (1990). The antiinflammatory effects of inhaled salmeterol and salbutamol in guinea pig lung. *Br. J. Pharmacol.*, **101**, 598P.
• Whelan, C. J. and Johnson, M. (1991). Salmeterol inhibits granulocytes accumulation in guinea pig lung. *Br. J. Pharmacol.*, **102**, 176P.

IN VIVO MODELS OF EOSINOPHILIA

D. FATTAH, J. WRIGHT, K. PAGE & B. CHAMPION, Immuno-regulation Group, Biochemistry Department, Glaxo Group Research Ltd., Greenford, Middlesex, UB6 OHE, UK

Eosinophilia is a hallmark of allergic and parasitic diseases, and these cells play an important role in the associated tissue damage, particularly in asthma. We are investigating the role of interleukin-5 (IL-5) in the differentiation and activation of eosinophils *in vivo*. BALB/c mice infected with the parasite *Mesocestoides corti* developed an eosinophilic response that was completely blocked by the IL-5-specific monoclonal antibody, TRFK5, even when administered after onset of the eosinophilia. Administration of recombinant human IL-5 also induced a similar blockable eosinophil response. Serum levels of IgA, IgG1 and IgM, but not IgG2a or IgE, were elevated following IL-5 administration (up to 20-fold for IgG1). Somewhat surprisingly, infection of either *M.corti* or IL-5 into T-cell deficient mice (athymic BALB/c or C.B-17 *scid*) also induced an eosinophilic response which was inhibited by TRFK5. Studies are underway to identify the cellular source of IL-5 in these T-cell deficient mice.

GLUCOCORTICOID STABILIZATION OF EOSINOPHILS: AN *IN VITRO* MODEL

C. E. Lawrence and F. B. De Brito.
Rhône-Poulenc Rorer Ltd., Dagenham Research Centre,
Rainham Road South, Dagenham, Essex, RM10 7XS, UK

Few models have been reported that are able to demonstrate an effect of glucocorticoids on eosinophil activity *in vitro* raising the suggestion that the cells may be affected indirectly *in vivo*. In experiments involving hypereosinophilic bone marrow cultures, we observed a marked cellular accumulation of eosinophil peroxidase when dexamethasone was present. The possibility, that eosinophil degranulation was occurring in these cultures and that glucocorticoids could inhibit this, prompted us to study the phenomenon further.

Femoral bone marrow from mice infected two weeks previously with *Mesocestoides corti*, was prepared as a single cell suspension in RPMI 1640 tissue culture media supplemented with foetal calf serum, glutamine, sodium bicarbonate, HEPES buffer, sodium pyruvate and antibiotics. The cells (10^5–10^6/ 100 μL) were plated into a 96-well microtitre plate containing steroid (10^{-8} M–10^{-5} M) or vehicle (0.01% dimethylsulphoxide) and incubated at 37°C/5% CO_2 for up to seven days. Plates were then centrifuged, supernates discarded, and cell pellets assayed for eosinophil peroxidase (EPO) as described by Strath *et al.*, (1985).

Increased cell associated EPO in bone marrow cultures was only observed when the glucocorticoids dexamethasone, prednisolone or hydrocortisone were present. Progesterone was without such effect. The increase in cell-EPO was related to the concentration of cells and glucocorticoid present in the cultures and depended on the duration of incubation of cultures. The earliest detectable rise in enzyme was day 4. Peak levels of enzyme were reached on days 6–7. Cytosmear preparations of these later cultures showed very few but mainly eosinophilic cells. Maximal EPO levels were observed at 10^{-7} M with all three glucocorticoids. Enzyme accumulation was not observed in glucocorticoid treated cultures of bone marrow cells derived from normal (i.e. non-hypereosinophilic) mice.

It would thus appear that EPO accumulation in bone marrow cells occurs only when eosinophils and glucocorticoids are present and that several days are required for the effect to manifest. The effect is highly reproducible and simple to perform and should facilitate mechanistic studies in a potential model of eosinophil function.

- Strath, M., Warren, D. J., and Sanderson, C. J. (1985). Detection of eosinophils using an eosinophil peroxydase assay. Its use as an assay for eosinophil differentiation factors. *J. Immunol. Methods*, **83**, 209–15.

EXPRESSION OF HLA-DR AND ICAM 1 ON BRONCHIAL EPITHELIAL CELLS OF ASTHMATIC PATIENTS

A. M. VIGNOLA, A. M. CAMPBELL, A. RIVIER, P. CHANEZ, A. M. PINEL*, B. FREISS*, L. DUSSOURD D'HINTERLAND*, J. BOUSQUET, F. B. MICHEL, P. GODARD, Hôpital Aiguelongue, 34059 Montpellier Cedex and *Pierre Fabre, 31520 Ramonville-St Agne, Toulouse, France

BACKGROUND: Interactions between different cell types play an important role in the pathogenesis of asthma. Recent evidence has suggested that bronchial epithelial cells may be capable of the presentation of antigen to T-Lymphocytes, thus up-regulating the inflammatory response.

METHODS: Epithelial cells obtained by bronchial brushing from 6 normal subjects and 6 asthmatics were examined using a confocal fluorescence scanning laser microscope system. Epithelial cells were identified by their typical morphology and HLA-DR and ICAM-1 molecules were revealed by immunofluorescence.

RESULTS: Immunofluorescence results have shown that epithelial cells obtained from asthmatic subjects express increased levels of HLA-DR and ICAM than those from normals. These two markers appear to be localized directly below the apical membrane and thus may play an important role in cellular interactions between bronchial epithelial cells and cells present in the airway lumen.

CONCLUSIONS: These findings suggest that epithelial cells may be involved in antigen presentation and that this involvement may be increased in asthma.

SENSORY NEUROPEPTIDE INVOLVEMENT IN THE MECHANISM OF ACTION OF LEVODROPROPIZINE IN EXPERIMENTAL INDUCED COUGH

A. LAVEZZO, G. MELILLO, G. CLAVENNA and C. OMINI, Research and Development Laboratories, Dompé Farmaceutici S.p.a., MILAN, Italy

Levodropropizine (LDP) is a well known antitussive drug which does not interact with opioid receptors. In order to further characterize the peripheral site and the mechanism of action of LDP, we investigated its activity in different models of experimentally induced cough. In particular the involvement of sensory neuropeptides on the mechanism of action of LDP was evaluated. The peripheral site of action of LDP was confirmed by injecting the drug intracerebroventricularly (icv). In these experiments, LDP (40 µg/50 µl, icv) did not prevent electrically induced coughing. On the other hand, codeine (5 µg/ 50µl, icv) markedly prevented coughing. A difference in the potency ratio of LDP and codeine was demonstrated in capsaicin induced cough. In fact, after oral administration codeine was about 2–3 times more potent than LDP. In addition, after aerosol administration the two compounds were equipotent suggesting a peripheral site of action for LDP.

The involvement of sensory neuropeptides in the mechanism of action of LDP is suggested by the results obtained in capsaicin desensitized guinea pigs. In a model of vagal induced cough the activity of LDP is markedly reduced by the depletion of sensory neuropeptides by capsaicin, whereas the effect of codeine is not affected by capsaicin pretreatment. A further support for the involvement of sensory neuropeptides in LDP activity comes from the results obtained after repeated administration of capsaicin. In these experiments, LDP seems to prevent the release of sensory neuropeptides due to capsaicin. In particular, the capsaicin capacity to induce cough is decreasing with time due probably to depletion of sensory neuropeptides. LDP seems to prevent the tachyphylaxis induced by capsaicin.

MODIFICATION BY CGRP OF AIRWAY CONTRACTILE RESPONSES IN NORMAL AND SENSITIZED GUINEA PIGS.

A. CADIEUX and C. LANOUE, Department of Pharmacology, Faculty of Medicine, University of Sherbrooke, Sherbrooke (Quebec), Canada J1H 5N4

Calcitonin gene-related peptide (CGRP) has been studied in relation to non-vascular smooth muscle tone control in mammalian respiratory tract. We previously reported that bronchoconstriction can be blocked by CGRP in rat, guinea pig and man and that spasmogens against which the inhibitory effect of the peptide is exerted are amongst mediators encountered in bronchial asthma. In the present work, the inhibitory action of CGRP on agonist-induced bronchoconstriction was assessed in airways obtained from actively sensitized guinea pigs to ovalbumin. Sensitization was performed by injecting 100 mg i.p. and 100 mg s.c. on day 1 and a further 10 mg i.p. on day 8. Animals were killed 2 weeks later. All experiments were carried out *in vitro* and lung parenchymal strips were used as target tissues.

Our results showed that CGRP blocked in a concentration-related manner contractions induced by substance P (SP) 5×10^{-8} M, 5-hydroxytryptamine (5-HT) 5×10^{-7} M and histamine 10^{-8} M, on parenchymal strips from untreated animals. Addition of thiorphan 10^{-6} M increased response to SP but did not influence serotoninergic and histaminergic receptor responses, neither did it alter the inhibitory effect of CGRP (10^{-6} M). In both cases (in presence or in absence of thiorphan), maximal decreases in contractions evoked by SP, 5-HT and histamine following the administration of CGRP amounted to 65, 47 and 20% respectively. In airways from actively sensitized guinea pigs, the ability of CGRP to block SP-induced response was decreased by 60% while that elicited by 5-HT was reduced by more than 85%. Pre-incubation of the tissues with thiorphan, phosphoramidon, captopril or bestatin (all 10^{-6} M) did not prevent the loss of CGRP biological activity. However we observed that the effect of CGRP on 5-HT-evoked contraction was more susceptible to treatment with peptidases blocking agents than it was on SP-induced response.

We conclude that the protecting effect offered by CGRP on airway smooth muscle tension can be strongly influenced in hyperreactive airway disorders.

(Supported by the Fonds de la Recherche en Santé du Québec).

ANTI-INFLAMMATORY EFFECTS OF CORTICOTROPIN-RELEASING FACTOR (CRF) ON THE UPPER AND LOWER RESPIRATORY TRACT OF RATS

E. T. WEI and S. M. SERDA, School of Public Health, University of California, Berkeley, CA 94720, USA

Various investigators, notably Persson (1988) and Barnes (1986), have suggested that microvascular leakage and neurogenic mechanisms in the upper respiratory tract account for some of the inflammatory changes of asthma. We call attention to CRF and other peptides of the CRF superfamily, such as urotensin and sauvagine, which inhibit microvascular leakage and neurogenic inflammation in animal models. Topical application of CRF onto hamster cheek pouch mucosa attenuates histamine and bradykinin induced vascular leakage. In the rat, CRF prevents protein extravasation in the trachea after antidromic stimulation of the vagus, after subcutaneous injection of substance P, or after exposure to formaldehyde vapors. Surprisingly, CRF also inhibits edema formation in the lower respiratory tract: a subcutaneous dose higher than 6 µg/kg administered to anesthetized rats 1 hr before intravenous epinephrine, 90 nmol/kg, decreases both pulmonary edema and mortality. The anti-inflammatory effects of CRF were not due to secondary release of adrenal steroids. The therapeutic potential of CRF in asthma remains to be investigated.

- Barnes, P. J. (1986). Asthma as an axon reflex. Lancet, Feb. 1, 242–244
- Persson, C. G. A. (1988). Plasma exudation and asthma. *Lung*, **166**, 1–23

REDUCED CORTISOL RESERVE IN ASTHMATIC SUBJECTS

H REDIER[1], *M HAMMOND*[2], N BRESSOT[1], A CRASTES DE PAULET[3], B DESCOMPS[3] & Ph GODARD
[1]CLINIQUE DES MALADIES RESPIRATOIRES 34059 Montpellier, [2]BAYER UK, Stoke Poges, Bucks, SL2 4LY, UK, [3]INSERM U58, Montpellier 34090, France.

Subgroups of guinea pigs have been identified that show high allergic responsiveness associated with an increased rate of urinary cortisol excretion (Francis and Hammond 1991). Eicosanoid mediator-release was also enhanced in this group, an effect similar to that observed in the *ex vivo* release of leukotriene B4 from alveolar macrophages of asthmatic subjects (Damon *et al.*, 1989).

Groups of therapy withdrawn asthmatic subjects showing immediate (I, n = 6) or dual (D, n = 5) bronchial reactions were compared with normal subjects (n = 10) with respect to their basal cortisol metabolism and also following stimulation by Synacthen or allergen. Determinations were also made of cortisol plasma-binding and auto-antibodies to lipocortin (Goulding *et al.*, 1989).

Measurement	Normal Subjects ($\pm$ ISD)	Asthmatic Subjects ($\pm$ ISD)
Total Cortisol Excretion (Basal) (nmoles/24h)	121.89 ± 21.0	89.2 ± 40.2*
Time to 50% Total Daily Cortisol Excretion	10 to 16.00h	00 to 12.00h
17-OH Prog (Salivary) Mean pmol/L	101.6 ± 36.8	84.2 ± 70.1
SYNACTHEN Test % Increase t + 60 min	81.2 ± 31.7	83.9 ± 33.9
Plasma-Binding % Free (*Cort. Saliv.*) – Basal	2.96 ± 0.087	3.95 ± 1.09*
(Cort. Plasma) – t + 60 min	6.3 ± 1.87	8.07 ± 2.07*
Transcortin ug/ml	38.8 ± 6.8	35.7 ± 6.2^{d}
Lipocortin Autoantibodies Median IgG (IQR)	20 (18–31)	43 (24–54)[+]

[+]$P < 0.05$ (Mann Witney 'U') *$P < 0.05$ (t-test) [d] differential effect I vs D

Allergen challenge induced much smaller increases in plasma cortisol than those seen following challenge with Synacthen, particularly in those patients producing a dual reaction. From these results, there is a strong indication of deficiencies in asthmatics in respect of cortisol secretion, precursor availability, plasma binding and lipocortin auto-antibodies which could in combination produce suppression of cortisol protective activity.

[2] Present address Bayer UK, Newbury, Berks, RG13 1JA

- Damon, M., Chavis, C., Daures, J. P., Crastes de Paulet, A., Michel, F. B. and Godard, P. (1989). Increased generation of the arachidonic metabolites LTB4 and 5-HETE by human alveolar macrophages in patients with asthma: effect in vitro of nedocromil sodium. *Eur. Respir. J.*, **2**, 202–209
- Francis, H. and Hammond, M. (1991). *Clin. Exp. Allergy*, in press
- Goulding, N. J., Podgorsky, M. R., Hall, N. D., Flower, R. J., Browning, J. L., Pepinsky, R. B. and Maddison, P. J. (1989). Autoantibodies to recombinant lipocortin-1 in rhumatoid arthritis and systemic lupus erythematosus. *Ann. Rheum. Dis.*, **48**, 843–850

EFFECT OF THE Ca^{2+}-ACTIVATED K$^+$-CHANNEL ANTAGONISTS, CHARYBDOTOXIN (ChTX) AND IBERIOTOXIN (IbTX) ON ISOLATED AIRWAY SMOOTH MUSCLE

T. R. Jones and L. Charette, Merck Frosst Centre for Therapeutic Research, P. O. Box 1005, Pointe Claire-Dorval, Québec, Canada, H9R 4P8

Airway smooth muscle plasma membranes are rich in K$^+$ channels of various types. ChTX is a potent blocker of high conductance Ca^{2+}-activated K$^+$ channels (P$_{K,Ca}$) in smooth muscle and produces a concentration-dependent contraction of guinea pig trachea (Jones *et al.*, 1991). In the present study, pharmacologic experiments were performed on carbachol-contracted (0.34 μM) guinea pig trachea contracted further with ChTX in order to determine if P$_{K,Ca}$ play a role in the relaxation responses to cAMP dependent and cAMP-independent bronchodilators. Concentration-relaxation curves to salbutamol $\geq$ sodium nitroprusside $>$ isoproterenol $>>$ dibutyryl cAMP = aminophylline were inhibited by ChTX (180 nM). In contrast, ChTX (180 nM) failed to produce a significant inhibition of the relaxation response curves to the ATP-dependent K$^+$-channel agonists, BRL-34915 and pinacidil. IbTX purified from Buthus tamulus scorpion venom is more selective and more potent than ChTX at blocking P$_{K,Ca}$ (Galvez *et al.*, 1990). IbTX produced similar concentration-dependent contractions of GPT but was approximately 3-fold more potent as a functional antagonist of salbutamol and isoproterenol. At 60 nM IbTX completely blocked relaxation to salbutamol but did not inhibit BRL-34915 induced relaxation at 60 or 180 nM. These findings support the hypothesis that P$_{K,Ca}$ may have a physiological role in controlling resting membrane potential in airway smooth muscle. Furthermore, relaxation to certain bronchodilators and in particular, the β$_2$ agonist, salbutamol may be dependent on P$_{K,Ca}$.

• Galvez, A., Gimenez-Gallego, G., Reuben, J. P., Roy-Contancin, L., Feigenbaum, P., Kaczorowski, G. J. and Garcia, M. L. (1990). Purification and characterization of a unique, potent, peptidyl probe for the high conductance calcium-activated potassium channel from venom of the scorpion *Buthus tamulus*.
  J. Biol. Chem. **265:** 11083–11090.
• Jones, T. R., Charette, L., Garcia, M. L. and Kaczorowski, G. J. (1990). Selective inhibition of relaxation of guinea-pig trachea by charybdotoxin, a potent Ca^{++}-activated K$^+$ Channel Inhibitor.
  J. Pharmacol. Exp. Therap. **255:** 697–706

TRACHEAL RELAXANT AND BRONCHODILATOR EFFECTS OF THE NOVEL K$^+$-CHANNEL OPENER HOE 234

H. C. Englert, K. Wirth, D. Gehring, M. Hropot and B. A. Schöl-kens, Hoechst AG, POB 800320, D-6238 Frankfurt/M. 80

HOE 234, (3S,4R)-3-Hydroxy-2,2-dimethyl-4-(2-oxo-1-pyrrolidinyl)-6-phenylsulfonylchroman hemihydrate, was investigated for its smooth muscle relaxant effects in guinea pig airways and compared with lemakalim (BRL 38227), the active enantiomer of cromakalim. In isolated tracheal rings HOE 234 and lemakalim attenuated spontaneous tone or tone induced by histamine, carbachol and prostaglandin E_2 (PGE$_2$). The respective IC$_{50}$-values, µM, were (for lemakalim in parenthesis): 0.013 (0.13); 0.045 (1.2); 0.032 (0.26); 0.016 (0.10). In a wash out experiment following relaxation of spontaneous tone HOE 234 showed a twofold longer duration of action than an equieffective dose of lemakalim.

In anesthetized animals pulmonary resistance (R$_L$) was assessed via whole body plethysmography. HOE 234 and lemakalim given either intravenously (i.v.) or by inhalation showed a dose related inhibition of the histamine (0.5–2 µg/kg i.v. at 5 min intervals) induced increase (200%) of R$_L$. HOE 234 was more potent with ID$_{50}$-values (lemakalim in parenthesis) being 4.1 (14.3) µg/kg after i.v. and 0.85 (5.6) µg/kg after inhalation administration and had an up to twofold longer duration of action. Administration of 30 µg/kg i.v. HOE 234 during continuous bronchoconstriction maintained by infusion of histamine decreased R$_L$ for more than 20 min whereas the effect of 100 µg/kg i.v. lemakalim disappeared within 4 min.

These results show that HOE 234 is effective against the contractile response to asthma mediators in guinea pig airways and compares favourable with lemakalim. Moreover it acts on acute existing bronchospasms and has therefore the potential to act against asthma attacks.

EFFECTS OF THE NOVEL POTASSIUM CHANNEL OPENER HOE 234 ON CHLORIDE SECRETION IN CANINE TRACHEAL EPITHELIUM

M. HROPOT, H. C. ENGLERT, P. HAINZ, E. KLAUS, and B. A. SCHÖLKENS, Hoechst AG, POB 800320, 6230 FRANKFURT am MAIN 80, Germany

Hoe 234, (3S,4R)-3-Hydroxy-2,2-dimethyl-4-(2-oxo-1-pyrrolidinyl)-6-phenylsulfonylchroman hemihydrate, a novel potassium channel opener is effective against contractile response to asthma mediators in guinea pig airways and acts on acute existing bronchospasms. It has been shown that bradykinin (BK), neurokinin A (NKA), and PGE_2 are potent stimulators of luminal chloride secretion in tracheal epithelium probably by increasing production of intracellular cAMP. Moreover, increased epithelial chloride secretion is an early event of the response to specific allergen challenge in the airway mucosa. The aim of this study was to investigate if the BK-, NKA-, or PGE_2-induced chloride secretion can be influenced by the potassium channel opener Hoe 234. For this purpose the membranous portions of the dog trachea were dissected and mounted in the Ussing chamber. These tissues were bathed on both sides by Ringer bicarbonate solution and oxygenated at 32°C. Short-circuit current (ISC), a measure of the luminal chloride secretion, and membrane conductance were measured. Hoe 234 does not induce the epithelial chloride secretion itself, whereas, salbutamol is a potent stimulator of this event when applied to the mucosal side of the tracheal tissue. Preincubation of tracheal tissues with Hoe 234 (10^{-6}-10^{-4} mol/l, applied on mucosal side) dose-dependently decreases the short-circuit current after addition of BK (10^{-6} mol/l), NKA (10^{-7} mol/l) and PGE_2 (10^{-6} mol/l), the IC_{50} values being about 5×10^{-5} mol/l). Hoe 234 is significantly less effective when applied to the serosal side of the tracheal tissue. In conclusion, the novel potassium channel opener Hoe 234 does not induce the luminal chloride secretion, but distinctly decreases BK-, NKA-, and PGE_2-induced chloride secretion in canine tracheal epithelium. The predominant site of action of Hoe 234 is the luminal side of the tracheal tissue, indicating its interference with chloride channels.

PAF-INDUCED HYPERREACTIVITY IN THE GUINEA-PIG IS INHIBITED BY Ro 31-6930 AND SALMETEROL

P. M. PACIOREK, A. M. SPENCE, P. R. GATER and J. F. WATERFALL, Dept. Biology, Roche Products Ltd., Welwyn Garden City, Herts AL7 3AY, UK

It has been reported that potassium channel openers inhibit airway hyperreactivity at non-bronchodilator doses and that this property may be of importance in the resolution of airway hyperreactivity in asthma (Chapman *et al.*, 1990). In the anaesthetized guinea-pig, bronchoconstriction following a submaximal dose of ACh (5–30 µg/kg^{-1}, i.v.) was determined before and after graded infusion of PAF (200ng/kg^{-1} total dose, i.v.). The potassium channel opener Ro 31-6930 (Paciorek *et al.*, 1990) or the long acting β agonist salmeterol were administered as a bolus dose of 1µg kg^{-1}, i.v. plus co-infusion with PAF of a further total of 1µg kg^{-1}, i.v. Following infusion of PAF alone, the response to ACh increased to 206.5 ± 16.5% (pre-infusion = 100%). In animals which received Ro 31-6930 or salmeterol the responses to ACh after PAF infusion were 80.9 ± 19.0 and 130.9 ± 4.4% respectively. At these doses, Ro 31-6930 and salmeterol had no effect on responsiveness to ACh in guinea-pigs which did not receive PAF. It is concluded that Ro 31-6930 and salmeterol prevent airway hyperreactivity at doses which have no bronchodilator activity.

- Chapman, I. D., Kristersson, A., Mazzoni, L., Amsler, B. and Morley, J. (1991). Reversal of induced airway hyperreactivity by potassium channel openers: PCO 400 and cromakalim. *Br. J. Pharmacol.*, **102**, 335P
- Paciorek, P. M., Cowlrick, I. S., Perkins, R. S., Taylor, J. C., Wilkinson, G. F. and Waterfall, J. F. (1990). Evaluation of the bronchodilatator properties of Ro 31-6930, a novel potassium channel opener, in the guinea pig. *Br. J. Pharmacol.*, **100**, 289–294

SYNTHESIS AND IN VITRO STUDY OF THE PREVENTION OF BRONCHOSPASMS OF 8-ARYL OR 8-HETEROARYL THEOPHYLLINES

A. RACHED*, G. BAZIARD-MOUYSSET*, J. BELLAN*, M. PAYARD*, F. KINIFFO** and C. ADVENIER**.
*Faculté de Pharmacie, Département de chimie, 31 Allées J. Guesde, 31000 – TOULOUSE
**Faculté de Médecine Paris-Ouest, Departement de pharmacologie, 15, Rue de l'Ecole de Médecine, 75270 PARIS

We have synthesized eight new theophyllines substituted by aromatics groups or heterocycles which we believe have an antiallergic or a spasmolytic effect.

Tested in vitro in relation to the bronchospasms caused by acetylcholine and histamine, three compounds have proven to be as active as theophylline:

	Histamine-induced bronchoconstriction pD_2 ($-\log EC_{50}$)	Acetylcholine-induced bronchoconstriction pD_2 ($-\log EC_{50}$)
Theophylline	4,10	3,50
Compound I	3,75	–
Compound IV	4,75	4,00
Compound VI	4,40	3,55

The furanic compound was found to be about four times more active than theophylline control.

RESPONSE OF HUMAN ISOLATED BRONCHIAL PREPARATIONS TO ACETYLCHOLINE AND MUSCARINIC ANTAGONISTS: EFFECT OF EPITHELIUM REMOVAL.

M. G. MATERA*, X. NOREL, *I. GORENNE*, M. CAZZOLA*, F. ROSSI* and C. BRINK. *Institute of Pharmacology and Toxicology, 1st Faculty of Medicine and Surgery, University of Naples, Italy and CNRS-URA 1159, Centre Chirurgical Marie-Lannelongue, 133 av. de la Résistance, 92350 Le Plessis-Robinson, France

The aim of this investigation was to evaluate the effects of acetylcholine (ACh) and muscarinic antagonists on intact and epithelium denuded human bronchi. Bronchial rings were set up in 10 ml organ baths containing Tyrode's solution at 37°C and gassed with 5% CO_2 in O_2. Force (contraction and relaxation) was recorded isometrically and expressed in grams (mean $\pm$ SEM) and agonist potency was indicated by pD_2 value ($-\log$ of EC_{50}). Removal of the epithelium did not significantly modify the ACh response (intact, 2.26 $\pm$ 0.3 g and denuded, 2.86 $\pm$ 0.8 g; N = 8, P > 0.1) nor the bronchial sensitivity to ACh (pD_2 values; intact, 4.40 $\pm$ 0.2 and denuded, 4.68 $\pm$ 0.1; N = 8, P > 0.1). Atropine (ATR, non-selective muscarinic antagonist) and parafluorohexahydrosiladyphenidol (pFHHSiD, M_3 selective antagonist) reversed ACh-induced tone. These antagonists shifted to the right the ACh curves. The pK_B values: $-\log$ [concentration of antagonist/(dose ratio -1)] were: intact, 8.23 $\pm$ 0.1 and denuded, 8.49 $\pm$ 0.1 (N = 4, P > 0.1) with ATR; intact, 7.06 $\pm$ 0.4 and denuded, 7.70 $\pm$ 0.3 (N = 3, P > 0.1) for pFHHSiD. These data suggest that muscarinic receptors in the epithelium may not alter the cholinergic contraction in human airways.

CELLULAR MECHANISMS IN THE GENERATION OF SUPEROX-
IDE PRODUCTION FROM GUINEA PIG PERITONEAL MAC-
ROPHAGES

L. J. Wood and N. C. Turner
Dagenham Research Centre, Rhône-Poulenc-Rorer Ltd, Dagenham, Essex
RM10 7XS UK

In this study we have examined the cellular mechanisms involved in
superoxide generation by peritoneal macrophages following stimulation with
a range of soluble or particulate stimuli. Cells were obtained by peritoneal
lavage of horse serum pretreated guinea-pigs and purified by centrifugation
on a discontinuous Percol gradient (55% and 70%). Macrophages (purity >
85%, viability > 95%) were recovered from the surface of the 55% layer,
washed and resuspended in Hanks buffer saline solution (HBSS). 5×10^5
cells were incubated with drugs for 5 minutes at 37°C prior to the addition
to 96 well microtitre plates containing PAF, FMLP $(10^{-9}-10^{-5})$,
PMA$(10^{-12}-10^{-8})$ and OPZ(0.01−1mg/ml) for a further 5 minutes. Superoxide generation was measured by the reduction of p-iodonitrotetrazolium
violet (INTV).

PAF(EC$_{50}$ 7×10^{-9}M), FMLP(EC$_{50}$ 1.5×10^{-8}M), PMA(EC$_{50}$ $2.7 \times$
10^{-10}M) and OPZ elicited dose-related increases in reduction of INTV that
were inhibited by Staurosporine, Mepacrine and Superoxide Dismutase
(SOD) but not Rolipram (see table).

	Increase in O$_2^-$. generation			
	PAF 10^{-6}M	FMLP 10^{-5}M	PMA 10^{-8}M	OPZ 1mg/ml
Control	0.67 ± 0.10	0.61 ± 0.10	0.62 ± 0.11	0.47 ± 0.03
Rolipram (100μM)	0.68 ± 0.04	0.55 ± 0.04	0.78 ± 0.10	0.52 ± 0.07
+PGE$_2$(1μM)				
Staurosporine (0.1μM)	0.50 ± 0.10	0.42 ± 0.10	0.48 ± 0.09	0.50 ± 0.10
Staurosporine(1μM)	0.24 ± 0.04	0.13 ± 0.04	0.19 ± 0.01	0.32 ± 0.06
Mepacrine(100μM)	0.18 ± 0.04	0.14 ± 0.04	0.23 ± 0.04	0.11 ± 0.02
SOD(100μg/ml)	0.18 ± 0.02	0.27 ± 0.02	0.34 ± 0.04	0.28 ± 0.02

We conclude that the protein kinase C pathway may be involved in the
respiratory burst of guinea-pig macrophages not only to PMA but also to
soluble (PAF, FMLP) and phagocytic stimuli (OPZ). The lack of effect of
Rolipram with a stimulus to adenylate cyclase suggests however that either
protein kinase A is not involved in the regulation of superoxide generation by
these cells or that the cells do not have the Type IV phosphodiesterase
isoenzyme. The potent action of Mepacrine suggests that protein kinase C
stimulation of superoxide generation may involve a phospholipase A$_2$/C
mediated step.

• PAF: platelet activating factor
• FMLP: formyl-methionine-leucine-phenylalanine
• PMA: phorbol myristate acetate
• OPZ: opsonized zymosan

RESPONSE TO ANTI-IgE IN HUMAN PULMONARY AR-TERIES: REGULATION BY ENDOTHELIUM

J. L. ORTIZ, C. LABAT, X. NOREL, *I. GORENNE*, J. VERLEY and C. BRINK, CNRS-URA D1159, Centre Chirurgical Marie Lannelongue, 133 Av. de la Résistance, 92350 Le Plessis-Robinson, France

Human pulmonary arteries from 8 patients who had undergone surgery for lung carcinoma were cut as rings, and set up in organ baths containing Tyrode's solution gassed with 5% CO_2 in O_2. The relaxant effects are shown as percent of contractions (mean ± SEM). Following a contraction with noradrenaline (10 μM: 1.37 ± 0.10 grams), the tissues relaxed when challenged with anti-(human-IgE) (a-IgE; 1/1000; 31 ± 5%) and histamine (0.1 μM; 67 ± 10%). These relaxations were dependent on the presence of an intact endothelium. Atropine (1 μM), FPL 55712 (10 μM) or the nitric-oxide-inhibitor, L-N^{G}nitroarginine (L-NOARG; 300 μM) did not alter the a-IgE response. This a-IgE relaxation was significantly inhibited by either chlorpheniramine (1 μM: 12 ± 4%) or indomethacin (1.7 μM: 13 ± 3%). Furthermore, a combination of indomethacin and L-NOARG (30 μM) completely blocked the action of a-IgE (2 ± 2%). These results demonstrate that a-IgE can induce a relaxation in isolated vessels and suggest that this effect is mediated by histamine stimulation of endothelial cells via products of the cyclooxygenase and nitric-oxide-pathways.

INFLUENCE OF HUMAN SERUM ALBUMIN ON STIMULATED cAMP PRODUCTION IN HUMAN PERIPHERAL BLOOD MONO-NUCLEAR CELLS.

M. J. E. FISCHER, A. J. M. VAN OOSTERHOUT* AND F. P. NIJKAMP*. Dept. of Pharmaceutical Chemistry and Dept. of Pharmacology*, Faculty of Pharmacy, University of Utrecht, P. O. Box 80.082, 3508 TB Utrecht, The Netherlands

Albumin has been shown to interfere with cellular processes. An influence on growth modulation, steroid production and receptor interference through structural changes in biological membranes has been demonstrated. Activities of albumin are often presumed to originate from substances bound to albumin. In the present study we investigated the effect of albumin on receptor-stimulated cAMP production in human peripheral blood mononuclear cells (PBMC). In our experiments with a variety of cAMP receptor stimuli, serum albumin was added. PBMC were isolated from buffy coats. Incubations were performed with 5×10^6 cells/ml in RPMI-1640 in the presence or absence of albumin and the cells were subsequently stimulated with receptor agonists coupled to adenylate cyclase. Accumulated cAMP was measured in a competitive protein binding assay. Control experiments revealed no binding of agonists to albumin and no interference with the assay. The buffer capacity of the medium however was insufficient to maintain stable pH. This had large effects on cAMP production. After improvement the pH was checked during experiments. Albumin, at concentrations above 0.1% dose dependently inhibited both basal and agonist stimulated cAMP levels in PBMC. The inhibitory effect of albumin was present with different receptor stimuli like isoprenaline, histamine, forskolin and prostaglandin E_2. A reduction of 30–60% (cell batch dependent) with 0.5% albumin was found in relation to experiments without albumin. Incubation time had no influence on the reduction. A washing step after a 20 hour incubation did not reverse the albumin-induced cAMP inhibition. Specific structural interactions are not likely as high ratios of fatty acid bound to albumin did not affect isoprenaline stimulated cAMP production, although this changed the 3D structure of albumin. Albumin of bovine origin is more effective and chicken albumin is less. At this moment no explanation for this behavior can be provided.

It seems that albumin binds to or influences receptors inside the membrane of the PBMC and in that way partially blocks the binding of agonists. This process most likely is not receptor specific and as the active part of the forskolin stimulated adenylate cyclase buried deep inside the membrane is affected, changes in the fluidity of the membrane may be involved. Also an allosteric interaction with the outer membrane part of the adenylate cyclase cannot be excluded.

OXYGEN SPECIES RELEASED BY BLOOD MONOCYTES FROM HEALTHY AND ASTHMATIC SUBJECTS.

I. Vachier, M. Damon, Ch Le Doucen, *F. B. Michel, A. Crastes de Paulet, *Ph Godard. INSERM U. 58, 60 rue de Navacelles, *Clinique des Maladies Respiratoires, Montpellier, France.

Knowing that alveolar macrophages are differentiated from blood monocytes and that alveolar macrophages are activated in asthmatic patients, the aim of our study was to determine if blood monocytes present the same activation state as alveolar macrophages from asthmatic patients compared to healthy subjects, studying their ability to release oxygen species and superoxide dismutase activity, with conventional, chemiluminescence and video-imaging assays.

This study was performed on blood monocytes from 24 asthmatic patients and 18 healthy subjects. Lucigenin-chemiluminescence (CL) showed that blood monocytes in suspension released more superoxide anion in asthmatic patients with significant differences from 4 min to 8 min after stimulation ($p < 0.01$). Hydrogen peroxide measured by luminol-dependent CL was higher in asthmatic patients with significant differences from time 4 min ($p < 0.005$). When horse radish peroxidase was added to the reaction mixture responses were higher and significant differences were shown between asthmatic patients and healthy subjects ($p < 0.05$). Video-imaging camera assays were performed with blood monocytes in adherence under the same conditions of CL. Two groups of asthmatic patients were isolated: allergic asthmatic patients (AA) and non-allergic ones (nA). Nonallergic patients had the highest quantity of anion release, but no difference had been seen between healthy subjects and allergic asthmatic patients. When we studied blood monocytes in adherence with conventional ferricytochrome c assays to measure superoxide anions, blood monocytes from asthmatic patients were more activated than those from healthy subjects ($p < 0.01$). Individual kinetics showed a plateau from 30 min except for 3 asthmatic patients in which there was a continuous increase. These 3 asthmatic patients had an asthma attack 12 hours before the prelevement. Superoxide dismutase (SOD)-chemiluminescence assays showed that in blood monocytes from asthmatic patients there were smaller quantities of free SOD in stimulated and non stimulated blood monocytes ($p < 0.01$). In the 3 asthmatic patients who were near crisis no SOD was detected. These data show that blood monocytes from asthmatic patients were more activated than those from healthy subjects suggesting that in asthma, these cells could be primed in vivo.

Index

307